HEMATOLOGY:
Principles and Procedures

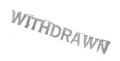

HEMATOLOGY:
Principles and Procedures

Barbara A. Brown B.A., M.T. (ASCP), M.S.

Supervisor, Department of Hematology
Tufts New England Medical Center Hospital
Boston, Massachusetts

FOURTH EDITION

Lea & Febiger   *Philadelphia*   *1984*

Lea & Febiger
600 Washington Square
Phildelphia, PA 19106
U.S.A.

First Edition, 1973
  Reprinted, 1974
Second Edition, 1976
  Reprinted, 1977, 1978, 1979
Third Edition, 1980
  Reprinted, 1981, 1982
Fourth Edition, 1984

Library of Congress Cataloging in Publication Data

Brown, Barbara A.
  Hematology: principles and procedures.

  Bibliography: p.
  Includes index.
  1. Blood—Examination. 2. Hematology. I. Title.
[DNLM: 1. Hematologic diseases—Diagnosis—Laboratory
manuals. WH 25 B877h]
RB45.B76 1984   616.1′5   83-24849
ISBN 0-8121-0927-9

PRINTED IN THE UNITED STATES OF AMERICA

Print Number: 4   3   2   1

Preface

Again, I am very grateful to have had the opportunity to write a fourth edition of this book. As with the previous editions, the purpose of the book remains the same: to give the new student a basic knowledge of hematology. It may also be used by the medical technologist who has been away from the field to review the basic principles of hematology and to become up to date in the areas of instrumentation and procedures. Laboratory supervisors may find the book helpful in the preparation of their own laboratory procedure manuals.

The subject of each chapter remains the same, although the order of the chapters has been changed slightly as a result of suggestions that I received from people using previous editions. Chapter 1, "Basic Laboratory Techniques," remains with few changes. Chapter 2 is now "Routine Hematology Procedures," which has been updated, as has Chapter 3, "Hematopoiesis." The black and white photographs remain, in an attempt to have the student look more closely at nuclear and cytoplasmic detail rather than depending solely on color for cell identification. Chapter 4 is now "Special Hematology Procedures," to which the non-specific esterase stain, chloroacetate esterase stain, and isopropanol precipitation test have been added. In Chapter 5, "Coagulation," the theory has been updated and procedures for Fletcher factor and antithrombin III have been added. A large number (26) of diseases have been added to Chapter 6. The disorders are not discussed in great detail for two reasons: (1) lack of space; (2) since the purpose of the book is instruction at the bench, I feel it more important to emphasize testing, instrumentation, and troubleshooting. Chapter 7, "Automation," has been updated and expanded in an attempt to keep up with the many new hematology instruments being developed. Again, because of space, only those instruments in relatively widespread use are outlined.

For this new edition, I greatly appreciated the suggestions and material that I received from Bio/Data Corporation (James Eichelberger), Coulter Electronics, Inc. (Steve Otto), Geometric Data Corporation (Paul Rust), Lancer Division of Sherwood Medical Industries, Inc. (Evon Creech), Medical Laboratory Automation, Inc. (John J. Hartnett), Miles Lab-Tek Division (Brent L. Riley), Ortho Diagnostic Systems, Inc. (Collette Murphy), and Warner-Lambert Company (Kathy Smith and Jane G. Lenahan).

My thanks and appreciation to Philip R. Daoust, M.D., and Estelle Stetz, M.D. for their review of part of the manuscript.

I am most appreciative of the efforts of Mary Eldridge for her many hours spent typing the manuscript. My thanks also to Nan W. Brown and Mary R. Donahoe for their help with the manuscript and for their assistance with the tedious job of proofreading.

As in the first three editions, I am again indebted to James J. Bonner for his art work. I also wish to thank the Copy Editing Department of Lea & Febiger for their valuable assistance with the manuscript.

This fourth edition of the book was built on the previous three editions, which were made possible with the help of many other people whom I wish to acknowledge and thank: Beth Conley, Thomas Gould, M.D., Arianne Graddick, Steven Halpern, Bettina Martin, Douglas A. Nelson, M.D., Kathleen Yount, and, last but not least, Theresa Kuszaj who has helped with the proofreading of all four editions.

For this and previous editions of the book, I express my sincere appreciation to the publishing company of Lea & Febiger for their help.

Randolph, MA.   Barbara A. Brown

Contents

5. COAGULATION

6. DISEASES

7. AUTOMATION

1

Basic Laboratory Techniques

Hematology is defined as the study of blood and today is concerned primarily with the study of the formed elements of the blood.

COMPOSITION OF BLOOD

The total blood volume in an adult is about 6 liters, or 7 to 8% of the body weight. Approximately 45% of this amount is composed of the formed elements of the blood: *red blood cells, white blood cells,* and *platelets.* The remaining 55% of the blood is the fluid portion, termed *plasma.* Approximately 90% of the plasma is water. The remaining 10% is composed of proteins (albumin, globulin, and fibrinogen), carbohydrates, vitamins, hormones, enzymes, lipids, and salts.

The blood may be thought of as a transportation system. As it circulates throughout the body, oxygen is transported from the lungs to the tissues, products of digestion are absorbed in the intestine and carried to the various tissues of the body, and substances produced in various organs are transferred to other tissues for use. Cellular elements of the blood may also be transported to fight infection or aid in blood coagulation. At the same time, waste products from the tissues are picked up by the blood to be excreted through the skin, kidneys and lungs.

If coagulation is prevented, the formed elements of the blood can be separated from the liquid portion, or plasma. If blood is allowed to clot, the liquid portion expressed from the clot is termed *serum* and differs from plasma in the loss of fibrinogen, which was utilized to form the fibrin threads of the blood clot.

COLLECTION OF BLOOD

The medical technologist most often comes in contact with a patient during the process of blood collection or of bone marrow aspiration. The patient in a hospital is anxious, fearful, and in ill health. He is anxious about his physical condition; he fears because he does not know what will happen next; and he is physically uncomfortable as a result of his sickness or injury. He is also separated from his known surroundings and family. For these reasons, a person's mental attitude is often at its worst when he is in the hospital as a patient. It is important, therefore, for the medical technologist to show the patient, at all times, the kindness and understanding that could mean so much.

When the technologist is dealing with a child, his approach is doubly important. This may be the first time the child has had a blood test. If it turns out to be a horrendous experience, it will be remembered and feared by the child for many years. Therefore, it is important to gain the child's confidence before proceeding with the blood collection. The child should be told what is going to happen. He should not be told that the puncture will not hurt.

1

In doing this, the child's confidence will be lost because what he or she is told is false.

The techniques used in obtaining blood are not learned overnight. They are an art that must be developed by study, observation, and practice, until the technologist has the necessary skill and self-confidence.

Skill, patience, understanding—these are the qualities of a good phlebotomist.

Microsampling

Microsampling refers to blood collection from the finger, toe, or heel and is frequently used for the following types of patients:

1. *Newborn infants.* The blood is generally obtained from the heel or big toe because these two areas are larger and more accessible than the fingertip. Newborns do not have a large blood supply, and it would be dangerous to remove the volume of blood involved in a venipuncture.
2. *Young children.* If only a small amount of blood is needed, the tip of the third or fourth finger is usually punctured.
3. *Adults.* When a patient has poor veins, or when the veins cannot be used because of intravenous (I.V.) infusions, the tip of the third or fourth finger may be used to obtain blood.

EQUIPMENT

1. Alcohol, 70% (v/v).
2. Dry gauze pads or cotton balls.
3. Sterile blood lancet (Fig. 1)
4. Appropriate pipets, diluting fluids, and tubes for microsampling.

PROCEDURE

1. Rub the puncture site on the appropriate finger or toe vigorously with a gauze pad that has been moistened well with 70% alcohol. (This cleanses the area and increases the circulation.)
2. Wipe the area dry with gauze or cotton. (Gauze is preferable because small pieces of the cotton may stick to the finger and interfere with the collection of blood.)
3. Using the sterile blood lancet, make a deep puncture on the side of the fingertip, midway between the edge and midpoint of the fingertip (Fig. 2). (A deep puncture is no more painful than a superficial one, gives a much better blood flow, and makes it unnecessary to repeat the procedure.)
4. Using dry gauze, wipe away the first drop of blood, making certain the area is completely dry.
5. Apply moderate pressure, approximately 1 cm behind the site of the puncture to obtain a drop of blood.
6. Release this pressure immediately to allow recirculation of the blood.
7. Repeat steps 5 and 6 until enough blood has been collected.
8. Apply a piece of gauze to the puncture site, using slight pressure until the bleeding has stopped.

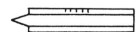

Fig. 1. Blood lancet.

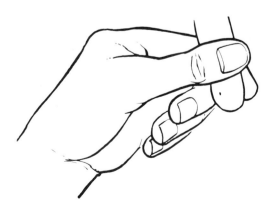

Fig. 2. Site of fingertip puncture.

DISCUSSION

1. The finger should not be squeezed tightly. This causes tissue juice to mix with and dilute the blood.
2. When collecting blood for hematology tests, the finger must be wiped dry after each test. (Platelets clump immediately in the blood at the puncture site.)
3. The preceding procedure may be used for a heel stick, toe stick, and the rare ear lobe puncture.
4. Because of platelet adhesiveness and aggregation at the site of puncture, it is advisable to collect the platelet count and blood smears first (if requested) when samples for a number of tests are to be obtained.
5. The values for the red blood count, hematocrit, hemoglobin, and platelets are lower in capillary blood than in venous blood. Therefore, when possible and if the patient is old enough, the venipuncture is performed.
6. An automatic lancet for microsampling techniques is available. This device, the Autolet (see Fig. 3), is manufactured by Owen Mumford Ltd., Woodstock, Oxfordshire, England, and is available through most hospital laboratory distributors in the United States. The Autolet is a small, portable device that rapidly and automatically makes a standardized, painless incision in the fingertip or heel. The disposable, sterile, Monolet lancet (manufactured by Sherwood Medical, Inc.) is used in the Autolet.

Venipuncture

A venipuncture must be performed with care. The veins of a patient are the main source of blood for testing and the entry point for medications, intravenous solutions, and blood transfusions. Because there are only a limited number of easily accessible veins in a patient, it is important that everything be done to preserve their good condition and availability. Part of this responsibility lies with the medical technologist.

The recommended procedure is to have the patient lie down. If this is not possible, he should sit in a sturdy, comfortable chair with his arm firmly supported on a table or chair arm and easily accessible to the technologist. A patient should never stand or sit on a high stool during any process of blood collection. The technologist must be ready for the occasional patient who faints during this procedure, but this rarely occurs with hospital inpatients who are lying flat in bed.

EQUIPMENT

1. Alcohol, 70% (v/v).
2. Dry gauze pad.
3. Tourniquet.
4. Appropriate test tubes for tests ordered.
5. Vacutainer holder or syringe (Figs. 4 and 5).
6. Band-Aid.
7. Needle (Figs. 4 and 6). The choice of needle depends on the size of the vein. The most commonly used needle is the 20-gauge. The higher

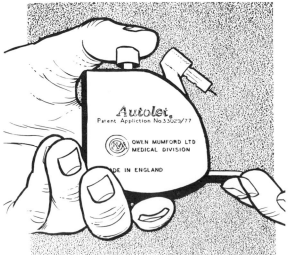

Fig. 3.   Autolet.

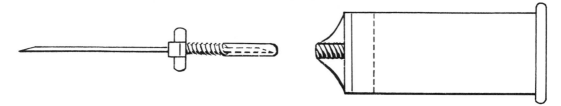

Fig. 4.   Vacutainer holder and multisample needle.

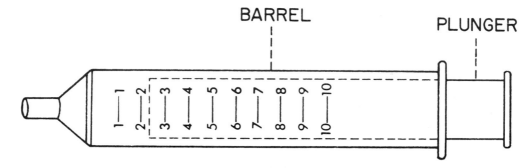

Fig. 5.   Syringe.

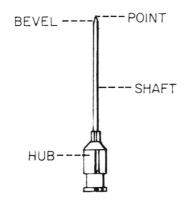

Fig. 6.   Hypodermic needle.

the gauge number, the smaller the diameter, or bore, of the needle. For small veins, a 21- or 22-gauge needle is recommended. The length of needle used is chosen by the individual technologist. The two most widely used needle lengths are 1 inch and 1½ inches. Blood may be obtained from most deep veins with a 1-inch needle.

PROCEDURE

1. *Make certain you have accurately identified the patient.* For inpatients, this may be done by checking the wristband. When collecting blood from an outpatient, ask him his name. A tube of blood mislabeled for type and cross match can end in a patient's death.
2. Prepare equipment (syringe and needle or Vacutainer assembly).
3. Apply the tourniquet several inches above the puncture site, as shown in Figs. 7 and 8, just tightly enough to be uncomfortable to the patient.
4. Ask the patient to make a tight fist. This makes the vein more easily palpable.
5. Select a suitable vein for puncture (Fig. 9). The three main veins of the arm, which are the sites of the majority of venipunctures, are the cephalic, median cephalic, and the median basilic. (It is not necessary to learn the names of these veins. They are named here only as a method of identification for referral.) Generally,

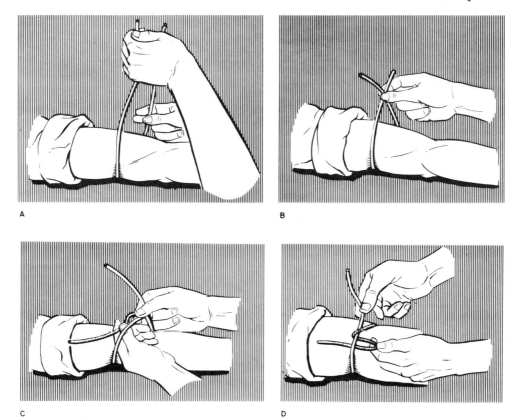

Fig. 7. Method of tourniquet application. A. Stretch the tourniquet to obtain the correct amount of tension. B. Grasp both sides of the tourniquet with the right hand while continuing to maintain the proper tension. C. With the left hand, reach through the loop and grasp the left side of the tourniquet. D. With the left hand, pull the tourniquet halfway through the loop. Release hands carefully.

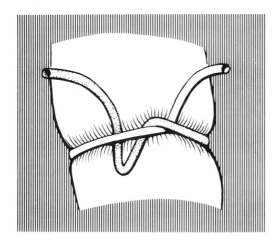

Fig. 8. Front view of tourniquet on arm. To release the tourniquet, carefully pull the end of the tourniquet on the left (shaded end).

the median cephalic is the vein of choice because it is usually well anchored in tissue and does not roll when the vein is punctured. The median basilic vein, at the inner edge of the arm, tends to roll in many patients. The cephalic vein is located on the edge of the outer part of the arm where the outside skin tends to be a little tougher. These points are mentioned only as a precaution. Using the index finger of your left hand, palpate the arm until you have found the best vein. It should feel similar to an elastic tube. (A frequent error made by students and technologists is the failure to find the best vein because of carelessness or haste.)

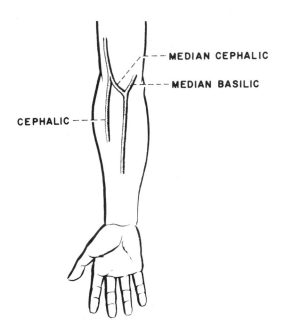

Fig. 9. Major veins of the arm.

6. Cleanse the puncture area with 70% alcohol. Do not touch this area again with your finger or with any other unsterile object.

7. If you are using a syringe, move the plunger up and down in the barrel once or twice to make sure that it does not stick. Expel all air from the syringe before proceeding.

8. Grasp the patient's arm just below the puncture site, pulling the skin tight with your thumb.

9. Hold the syringe, or Vacutainer assembly, with the opposite hand between the thumb and last three fingers. Rest the index finger against the hub of the needle to serve as a guide.

10. The needle should point in the same direction as the vein and be on a line with it at an angle approximately 15° to the arm.

11. The vein should be entered slightly below the area where it can be seen. In this way, there is more tissue available to serve as an anchor for the needle.

12. A prominent vein may be entered quickly with a one-step puncture of the skin and vein. When the veins are deeper or the entry more difficult, a two-step procedure should be followed. First, the skin is punctured, and then, if need be, the left index finger may be used to palpate above the puncture site to confirm the exact location of the vein. The second step is to puncture the vein.

13. If a syringe is used, the blood flows into it when the needle enters the vein. Care should be taken when pulling back on the plunger. Do not pull back with too much force because this may cause the blood to hemolyze; the force may pull the wall of the vein down on top of the bevel of the needle, causing the blood flow to stop; or the needle may inadvertently be pulled out of the vein.

14. If the Vacutainer assembly is being used, as soon as the needle is in the vein, push the tube firmly but carefully in as far as it will go, ensuring that the needle is kept steady.

15. The tourniquet may be loosened as soon as the blood enters the tube or syringe, or it may be left on until the process is complete. It should be noted, however, that if the tourniquet is left on too long, the blood in this area will have an increased concentration of cells (hemoconcentration). The patient may open his fist as soon as the blood begins to flow.

16. Release the tourniquet before the needle is removed from the vein.

17. Apply a clean, dry gauze to the puncture site and quickly withdraw the needle.

18. Have the patient apply gently pressure to the point of puncture for several minutes until the bleeding has stopped and then apply a Band-Aid. The patient may also keep his arm straight, elevating it above the heart.

19. If a syringe is employed, remove the needle before expelling the blood

into the appropriate tubes. This process must be done quickly before the blood begins to clot.

DISCUSSION

1. In the event that you have been unable to puncture the vein immediately, use your free index finger to locate the vein. It may be that the needle has not gone deeply enough, or perhaps it is slightly to the left or right of the vein. Do not attempt to puncture the vein from that location. This is painful to the patient and may cause tissue damage. Withdraw the needle until the point is almost to the surface of the skin and then redirect the needle. This procedure is acceptable if the needle is close to the vein, but care should bc takcn that the patient is not caused too much pain. Sometimes a second venipuncture is necessary.

2. If a patient is receiving intravenous infusions into both arms, it is acceptable to puncture the vein 3 to 4 inches below the site of the I.V. device.

3. A technologist or student should not stick a patient more than three times. If the blood sample has not been obtained after the second attempt, it is usually advisable to call another technologist. By this time, both you and the patient have lost confidence.

4. It is important that pressure be applied to the site of the venipuncture. Failure to follow this procedure leads to a hematoma (bleeding into the tissues).

5. If the area surrounding the puncture site begins to swell while blood is being withdrawn, this usually indicates that the needle has gone through the vein or that the bevel of the needle is halfway out of the vein and blood is leaking into the tissues. The tourniquet should be released and the needle withdrawn immediately, with pressure applied to the site.

6. In some instances, it is almost impossible to locate a vein in the arm. In such a case, the veins of the lower arm, wrist, or hand may be used or, as a last resort, an ankle vein. The student should gain a reasonable amount of skill and confidence before attempting a venipuncture in these areas.

7. When a venipuncture must be carried out on a small child, it may be necessary to release the tourniquet when the blood starts to enter the syringe. Children's veins are small and collapse quickly because blood is removed from the vein faster than it enters it. Therefore, release the tourniquet carefully to improve the blood circulation.

8. When performing a venipuncture in the lower arm, hand, ankle, or on small children, a syringe or small Vacutainer assembly is generally used. When a venipuncture is required for a patient with poor or small veins, it is also advisable to use a syringe or a small Vacutainer. The use of standard-size Vacutainers tends to collapse these veins.

9. When disposing of the used needle, place it in a specially prepared container provided for this purpose. Never throw it directly into the wastebasket.

10. Regardless of the disease the patient has, be careful not to stick yourself with his needle. If this happens, report it to your supervisor as soon as possible on the day of the accident.

11. When using the Vacutainer collection system, the multisample Vacutainer needle should be used if more than one tube of blood is to be collected from the patient. It contains a rubberlike sleeve which covers the shorter shaft of the needle (that portion of the needle placed inside the

Vacutainer holder) to prevent blood from leaking from the needle when changing from one test tube to the next.

Isolation Techniques

When a patient has an infectious or communicable disease, certain safeguards must be followed to prevent further spread of the infection to hospital personnel or to other patients. Special techniques are also needed to shield or protect infection-prone patients from pathogens and other bacteria. To ensure optimal care of these patients, laboratory personnel should follow the procedures listed below, depending on the type of illness of the patient being treated:

1. When handling patients with leukemia, severe burns, body radiation, kidney transplants, and plastic surgery, who must be protected from infection, the technologist should wear a sterile gown, cap, gloves, and mask. Shoe coverings may also be required.
2. Strict isolation is used in cases of active tuberculosis, meningococcal meningitis, rabies, diphtheria, viral encephalitis, polio, and certain infectious diseases such as measles, smallpox, and mumps. A gown should be worn by the technologist, as well as a mask and gloves when indicated.
3. When in contact with patients who have diseases spread through direct contact with a wound or discharge, such as abscesses, tetanus, gas gangrene, impetigo, and dysenteries, the technologist should wear a gown. Frequently, gloves also are necessary.
4. When in contact with patients who have venereal disease and dermatosis, it may be necessary for the technologist to wear gloves.

DISCUSSION

1. When Vacutainer techniques are employed for collecting blood, all tubes of blood from the isolated patient must be inverted and placed in a beaker of 70% alcohol and taken to the laboratory in this manner. These tubes should be the only laboratory equipment to leave the patient's room.
2. Care must always be taken in the laboratory with blood, urine, and stool specimens. Many dysenteries can be transmitted through the stool specimen. Hepatitis is also easily transmitted through blood, urine, and stool samples.

ANTICOAGULANTS

Some laboratory procedures must be performed on whole blood or plasma. Therefore, as soon as the blood is withdrawn from the patient, it is mixed with an anticoagulant to prevent coagulation. These are five anticoagulants that may be used for hematologic procedures.

1. *Ammonium oxalate and potassium oxalate* mixture, also called double oxalate, consists of six parts ammonium oxalate and four parts potassium oxalate. It is used in a concentration of 2 mg per 1 ml of whole blood. Coagulation is prevented by the removal of calcium from the blood. The sole disadvantage of using the double oxalate in routine hematologic procedures is that the blood cannot be used for the preparation of blood films. Crenation of the red blood cells, vacuoles in the granulocytes, and bizarre forms of lymphocytes and monocytes occur within a few minutes after the blood has been mixed with this anticoagulant.

2. *Heparin* may be used in a concentration of 0.2 ml of saturated heparin per 1 ml of whole blood. Coagulation is prevented for a period of approximately 24 hours by the neutralization of thrombin. Heparin is the anticoagulant of choice for the osmotic fragility test (if anticoagulated blood is used). Heparinized blood, however, has been found to be unsatisfactory for the preparation of blood smears that

are to be Wright-stained because a blue background forms on the smears when stained.

3. *EDTA* (sequestrene or versene) is the disodium or dipotassium salt of ethylenediaminotetraacetic acid. It is the most widely used anticoagulant for hematologic procedures. The dipotassium salt is more soluble than the disodium salt. EDTA is used in concentrations of 1 mg per 1 ml of blood, or 0.1 ml of a 10% solution per 10 ml of whole blood. The EDTA prevents formation of artifacts and may be used for the preparation of blood films for 2 hours after blood collection. At concentrations greater than 2 mg per 1 ml of whole blood, the hematocrit value and erythrocyte sedimentation rate will be falsely low. The hemoglobin, however, will not be affected. Blood may be stored at 4° C for 24 hours without any evidence of change in the hemoglobin, hematocrit, white blood count, or red blood count. Blood stored at room temperature for 24 hours shows an elevated hematocrit reading, whereas the remaining tests are unaffected. EDTA is excellent for the prevention of platelet clumping.

4. *Sodium citrate* is the anticoagulant of choice for coagulation studies. It is used in a concentration of one part 0.109 M sodium citrate to nine parts whole blood. It prevents coagulation by binding the calcium of the blood in a soluble complex, and it protects certain of the procoagulants.

5. *Sodium oxalate* is another anticoagulant sometimes employed in coagulation studies. It is used in a concentration of one part 0.1 M sodium oxalate to nine parts whole blood. The sodium oxalate combines with calcium in the blood to form insoluble calcium oxalate, thereby preventing coagulation.

DISCUSSION

1. When anticoagulated blood is used, the tube of blood must always be checked for clots. This may be ac-

complished by stirring two applicator sticks in the blood. If a clot is found, the blood must be discarded and a new specimen obtained.

2. The proper ratio of anticoagulant to blood should be adhered to at all times. If too much blood is added to the anticoagulant, clotting usually occurs. In hematologic testing, morphologic and cellular changes occur if an insufficient amount of blood is added. In coagulation tests, false results are obtained.

3. When a dried anticoagulant is used, care must be taken to ensure that it is mixed well with the blood to prevent coagulation. (Adequate mixing is necessary whether a liquid or dry anticoagulant is used.)

THE MICROSCOPE

The microscope used in the routine hematology department is, in simple terms, a magnifying glass. It is termed a *compound light microscope* because it contains two separate lens systems, the objective and the ocular. This microscope generally consists of an eyepiece, objective, a mechanical stage, a substage condenser system with an iris diaphragm, and a light source (Fig. 10).

EYEPIECE LENS

The conventional eyepiece lens, or ocular, has a magnification of $10\times$. ($\times$ is used to designate the units of magnification, known as diameters. If a lens has a magnification of $10\times$, this does not mean that it magnifies an object to 10 times its original size [area], but rather that the diameter of the object is magnified 10 times its original size.) A monocular microscope consists of one eyepiece; a binocular microscope, the most commonly used today, contains two eyepieces.

OBJECTIVE LENS

Most light microscopes contain three objective lenses, each with different pow-

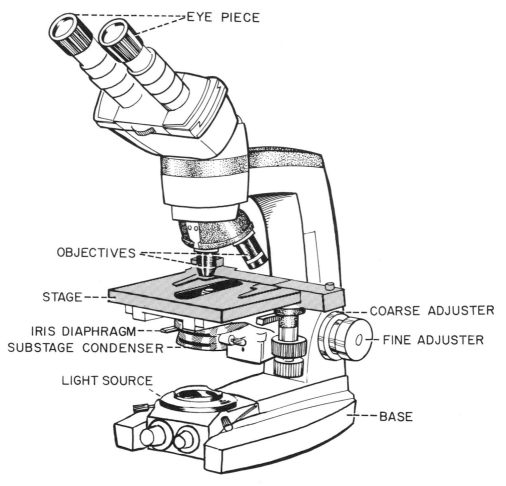

Fig. 10. Binocular microscope.

ers of magnification. The most commonly employed objectives are $10\times$ (low power), $40\times$ (high-dry), and $100\times$ (oil immersion). A fourth lens, $50\times$ (low oil immersion), may be utilized by experienced technologists for performing a differential cell count.

OPTICAL TUBE

The optical tube length is the distance between the eyepiece and objective lenses which is usually 160 mm.

STAGE

The stage holds the slide that is being examined and contains a moveable assem-

bly to facilitate the study of different parts of the slide.

SUBSTAGE CONDENSER

The most commonly used substage condenser is the Abbe condenser, which directs the beam of light from a source onto the specimen. It consists of two lenses (Fig. 11). The light is focused on the object or specimen by raising or lowering the condenser system. Lack of a substage condenser causes fuzzy rings and haloes around the object being studied.

IRIS DIAPHRAGM

The iris diaphragm contains a number of leaves that are opened or closed to in-

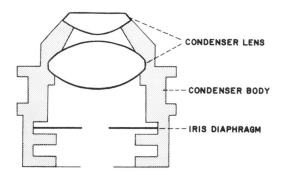

Fig. 11. Substage condenser and iris diaphragm.

crease or decrease the amount of light illuminating the object (Fig. 11).

LIGHT SOURCE

There are two different types of light sources that may be employed. The older and less commonly used illuminator consists of an outside light source. This microscope is equipped with a mirror, in front of which is placed a substage lamp or special microscope light. The mirror is then adjusted so that the rays of light from the lamp are projected upward into the condenser system. The newer microscopes contain a built-in light source at the base of the microscope. This type of light source may contain a built-in transformer to adjust the light intensity (see Fig. 10). There is also a swing-in neutral density filter present in this light source. Centering screws enable the viewer to center the light passing up through the condenser. A field iris diaphragm is present that may be opened or closed and is used to focus the microscope properly.

TOTAL MAGNIFICATION AND IMAGE

Total magnification is equal to the magnification of the eyepiece times the magnification of the objective lens. For example, using a 10× eyepiece and the 40× objective lens, the total magnification is 400×. The magnification of each system is printed on each of the appropriate parts. The image seen by the eye through a compound microscope, the virtual image, is

upside down and reversed. The right side is seen as the left end vice versa; therefore, movement of the slide is also reversed.

NUMERICAL APERTURE

The numerical aperture is a designation of the amount of light entering the objective from the microscopic field (or, as in the condenser, the amount of light entering the substage condenser from the light source). It may be thought of as a method for expressing the fraction of the wave front admitted by a lens (Fig. 12). The numerical aperture is constant for any single lens and is dependent on the radius of the lens (AC) and the focal length of the lens (PC).

$$\text{Numerical aperture} = R \times \sin u$$

u = The angle made by the one ray passing through the edge of the lens, with the other ray passing through the center of the lens

R = The refractive index of the medium between the object and the objective lens

The numerical aperture of the objective should be the same as the numerical aperture of the substage condenser. If these numerical apertures are not similar, interference effects occur.

REFRACTIVE INDEX

The refractive index of a substance is calculated as the speed with which light travels in air divided by the speed with which light travels through the substance.

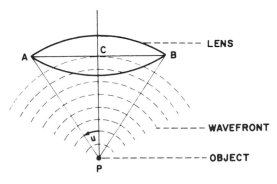

Fig. 12. Numerical aperture.

(Since light travels more slowly through immersion oil, the numerical aperture is increased by placing oil between the oil immersion objective and the object.)

RESOLVING POWER

Resolving power is the useful limit of magnification. It is the ability of the microscope, at a specific magnification, to distinguish two separate objects situated close to one another and the ability of the lens to reveal fine detail. The smaller the distance between the two specific objects that can be distinghished apart, the greater the resolving power of the microscope.

$$\text{Minimal distance between two objects (resolvable distance)} = \frac{0.612 \times \lambda}{\text{Numerical aperture}}$$

λ = The wavelength of the light

The resolving power is, therefore, dependent on the wavelength of light and the numerical aperture. The light source remains constant and so, in routine work, may be ignored. The larger the numerical aperture, the smaller the resolvable distance, and, hence, the more efficient the resolving power.

DEPTH OF FIELD

Depth of field is the capacity of the objective lens to focus in different planes at the same time. This is largely dependent on the numerical aperture. The greater the numerical aperture, the smaller the depth of field. It is possible to increase the depth of field slightly by closing the iris diaphragm (thus decreasing the numerical aperture).

ABERRATIONS

Different wavelengths of light are not bent in the same way as they pass through the lens and, therefore, are not brought to the same focus. These are called *chromatic* aberrations (Fig. 13).

With *spherical* aberrations, the light waves, as they travel through the lens, are bent differently, depending on which part of the lens they pass through. Rays passing through the peripheral portion of the lens are brought to a shorter focal point than those rays passing through the thicker part of the lens (Fig. 14).

LENSES

To compensate for aberrations, *achromatic* and *apochromatic* lenses are employed. The achromatic lens is the most commonly used lens for color correction. It brings rays of two colors to a common focus and obtains a reasonable compromise for the remaining colors. Apochromatic lenses are the finest lenses produced and correct for chromatic and spherical aberrations. This lens brings three colors (blue, yellow, and red) to a common focus. A factor that must be taken into consideration for the most effective use of the microscope lens is the medium between the objective and the object being studied. The low power ($10\times$) and high-dry objective lenses ($40\times$) use air. When the oil immersion lens is employed, a drop of oil should be used; otherwise, bending of the light waves occurs (Fig. 15*B*).

OPERATING PROCEDURE

1. With the $10\times$ objective in position, place the object to be studied (slide or counting chamber) on the microscope stage.
2. If you are using a binocular microscope, adjust the distance between the eyepieces as necessary.
3. Focus the object, using the coarse adjustment knob. Bring the object into sharp focus with the fine adjustment knob.
4. While looking through the microscope, close the field diaphragm on the light source so that the image of the leaves of the diaphragm may be seen in the field of view.
5. Focus the condenser by raising or lowering it until the leaves of the iris diaphragm are in sharp focus. (The condenser should now be left in this

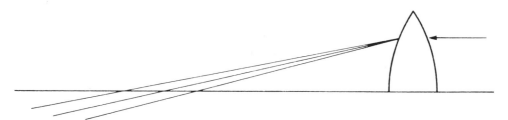

Fig. 13. Chromatic aberration.

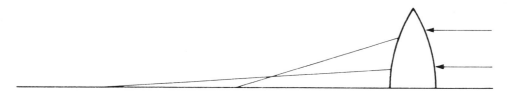

Fig. 14. Spherical aberration.

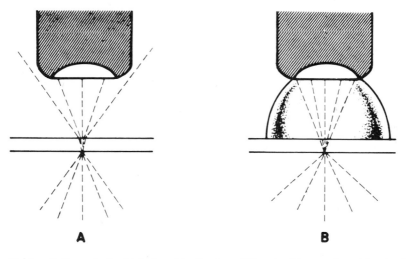

Fig. 15. Light path through the high-dry objective lens (A) and oil immersion objective lens (B).

position for use with all like objects to be studied.)

6. Center the light source by using the two centering screws (on the light source) so that the image of the field diaphragm in the field of view is in the center. Open the field diaphragm until the iris leaves just disappear from view.

7. Remove one eyepiece and, while looking through the microscope (without the eyepiece), close the condenser diaphragm. Reopen the dia-

phragm until the diaphragm leaves just disappear from view. (Further closing of the condenser diaphragm may increase contrast and depth of focus, depending on the specimen.) This procedure allows you to obtain the best resolving power for the microscope. Replace the eyepiece.

8. Generally, as you increase the magnification of the microscope (change objectives), the condenser diaphragm must be opened while the field diaphragm (light source) is fur-

ther closed. The condenser and field diaphragms should not be used to control light intensity. This is generally done by adjusting the transformer setting on the light source or by using filters.

DISCUSSION

1. When employing the high-dry or oil immersion objective, a suitable field for study should be found and focused using the low power objective (10×). A drop of oil may then be placed on the slide and the oil immersion objective swung into place. Never use oil with the high-dry objective.

2. To clean the lenses, only lens paper should be used. The paper is designed for this purpose and will not scratch the lenses, which other, more harsh paper or material might do.

3. The oil must be removed from the oil immersion lens (with lens paper) whenever it is not in use to prevent oil seepage to the inside of the lens.

4. If xylene is used to remove oil and clean the lenses, the structures holding the objective lenses may loosen in time because of the solvent qualities of xylene.

5. If the field of study is dirty, the cause may be dirt on the eyepiece. Revolve the eyepiece as you are looking through the miscroscope. If the dirt also revolves, the eyepiece needs cleaning.

Phase Microscopy

Phase microscopy is employed in hematology for the counting of platelets. Doing this on a light microscope is tedious and more liable to error because the platelets are unstained and small. Phase microscopy enables the viewer to see platelets and various structures in larger cells while they are still alive due to differences in the refractive index, shape, and absorption characteristics of the cells and cellular components.

Light travels in waves. If two sets of light waves in phase are allowed to travel through the same medium, they remain in phase (Fig. 16), and the brightness of the light is the sum of the two amplitudes (height of the peaks). If one of the two light waves (which were originally in phase) passes through an object, it is slowed down; the two waves are then out of phase (Fig. 17), and the light is diminished.

If the two light waves are out of phase by a half of a wavelength, there will be no light because the peak of one wave is cancelled by the trough of the other light wave (Fig. 18).

When rays of light pass through a slide containing cells, platelets, or living unstained organisms, those rays that pass through the cells may be retarded or slowed down but not diffracted from their pathway. These are termed direct rays.

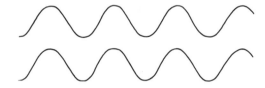

Fig. 16.   Light waves in phase.

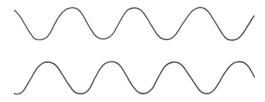

Fig. 17.   Light waves out of phase.

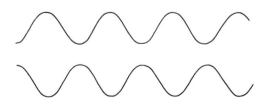

Fig. 18.   Light waves out of phase.

Other light waves may be retarded and, at the same time, diffracted. The amount of retardation of the light wave is dependent on the optical density, refractive index, and shape of the cell or cellular component.

For maximum contrast between the cell and its surroundings, the light wave should be retarded by a quarter of a wavelength. Cells and cellular components, however, are not able to retard the wavelength to this great a degree. Therefore, two additional parts are added to the light microscope to increase the small wave changes by about a quarter of a wavelength. This then becomes the phase microscope. An annular diaphragm is placed below, or in the substage condenser, and a phase-shifting element is situated in the rear focal plane of the objective. The light passes up from its source, through the clear circular area of the annular diaphragm (Fig. 19A), and through the specimen. The phase-shifting element is constructed so that light waves pass quickly through the clear areas (Fig. 19B) but are retarded by a quarter of a wavelength when going through the shaded circular area. These two components are so situated that the diffracted rays pass directly through the clear area of the phase-shifting element. All light waves that are undiffracted pass through the treated (shaded)

areas of the phase-shifting element and are, therefore, slowed by an additional quarter of a wavelength. These alterations in the phases of the rays increase the contrast and enable the viewer to get a more highly visible picture of the cells and their components.

Electron Microscopy

Magnifications greater than $1500\times$ are not practical with the light microscope due to a decreased efficiency in resolving power. For this reason, the electron microscope has come into use, where magnifications of $50,000\times$ may be obtained with a high degree of resolving power. The electron microscope employs a stream of electrons moving at a high velocity in place of a beam of light of short wavelength. The image is produced when the electrons hit a phosphorescent screen that then emits photons visible to the human eye. (This is similar to a television picture tube.)

SPECTROPHOTOMETRY

If a substance can be converted into a soluble, colored material, its concentration can then be determined by the amount of color present in the solution. The filter photometer and spectrophotometer are widely used in today's laboratory as the main instruments for this type of meas-

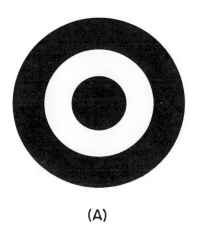

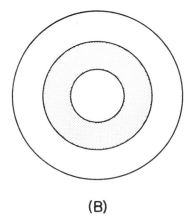

(A)   (B)

Fig. 19.   Annular diaphragm (A) and phase-shifting element (B).

urement. There are only a few tests in the field of hematology that employ spectro-photometry, unlike chemistry, in which spectrophotometry is much more widely used. This section gives the student a basic outline of this tool.

In both the filter photometer and spectrophotometer, a photoelectric cell is used to measure color intensity. This is done by measuring the amount of light from a source that passes through the colored solution. To obtain the greatest or optimal sensitivity, the light permitted to pass through the solution is of a particular wavelength. If a filter is used to determine the wavelength, the colorimeter is termed a *filter photometer*. In the *spectrophotometer*, the wavelength is selected by a prism, or diffraction grating.

As shown in Figure 20, the light from a light bulb (1) passes through a filter, prism, or diffraction grating (2). Only light of a predetermined wavelength can pass from the filter through the cuvette (3) containing the material to be measured. The amount of light passing through the solution (those light waves not absorbed by the material) comes in contact with the photoelectric cell (4), where the light energy is converted into electric energy. This electric energy is proportionally increased by the amplifier (5) and measured by the galvanometer (6). A scale located on the galvanometer is calibrated to read percent transmittance (%T) or optical density (O.D.). Most laboratories today use spectrophotometers that contain both of these scales. The percent transmittance scale measures the amount of light allowed to pass through the solution. Optical density, or absorbance, measures the amount of light absorbed by the solution. All the colors that make up light have a wavelength of a specific length measured in nanometers (nm) (Fig. 21). A blue solution is blue because all colors except blue have been absorbed by the solution. That is, that color wavelength passes through the solution.

The principle of photometry is based on the Lambert-Bouger-Bunsen-Roscoe-Beer laws, which have been combined to give what is commonly known as *Beer's law*. According to this law, the absorbance (optical density) of a solution is directly proportional to the concentration of the solute (material in solution being tested for) and the length of the light path through this solution. Since the predetermined wavelength is the same and cuvettes with a given, constant diameter are employed, the length of the light path through the solution is set, and the optical density is, therefore, directly proportional to the concentration of the solute. If the optical density and concentration of a standard are known, the unknown concentration may

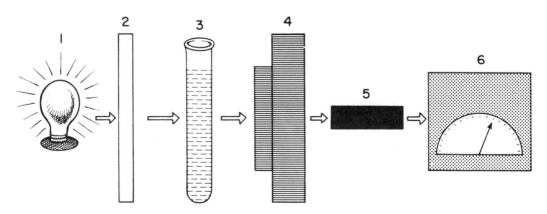

Fig. 20.   Principle of a photoelectric colorimeter or spectrophotometer.

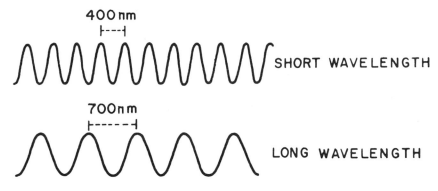

400 nm

SHORT WAVELENGTH

700 nm

LONG WAVELENGTH

Fig. 21. Measurement of wavelengths.

be calculated if its optical density is known.

$$\frac{\text{Concentration of unknown}}{\text{Concentration of standard}}$$
$$= \frac{\text{Optical density of unknown}}{\text{Optical density of standard}}$$

OPTICAL DENSITY VS. PERCENT TRANSMITTANCE

If L represents the light energy entering the solute and Lo is the light energy leaving the solute (that light hitting the photoelectric cell), then $\frac{Lo}{L}$ equals the transmittance (T) of the solute. If the energy leaving the solute is the same as the energy entering the solute, then $\frac{Lo}{L} = 1$ and, $1 \times 100 = 100\%$ transmittance, and the solution does not contain any of the material for which it is being tested. Optical density and percent transmittance are related logarithmically to each other:

$$\text{O.D.} = -\log T$$

The percent transmittance scale reads from left to right, whereas the optical density scale is read from right to left. When plotting a curve using optical density, regular graph paper is used. In plotting percent transmittance, semilog paper is employed. If solutions of varying concen-

trations are used, a straight line curve will be obtained if the test follows Beer's law. Not all solutions, however, follow Beer's law, in which case a curved line results.

DETERMINATION OF THE WAVELENGTH

To determine the optimal wavelength to be used for a specific test, an absorbance curve, reading optical density, should be plotted against the wavelength, as shown in Figure 22. Using a single concentration of the solution and the appropriate blank, take optical density readings at a series of different wavelengths. Plot the results on graph paper. Where the absorbance is at a maximum (point A), there should be maximum sensitivity, and this will, therefore, be the wavelength chosen for this test (540

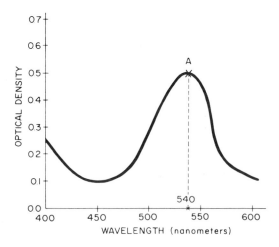

Fig. 22. Determination of wavelength.

nm). Care should be taken that (1) the solution follows Beer's law in the wavelength chosen, (2) the sensitivity is not so great as to give too many readings at the extreme ends of the scale (for the greatest accuracy, readings should be taken between 20% transmittance and 90% transmittance), and (3) interfering substances are not picked up at this wavelength.

PREPARATION OF A CURVE

To construct a curve for a specific test, various known concentrations of the substance must be used. A graph is made, plotting the concentration of the substance (on the X-axis, or abscissa) against the optical density or percent transmittance readings (on the Y-axis, or ordinate). All unknown readings from this curve should then fall in between the highest and lowest standards used in setting up the curve. The graph should be checked daily, using known controls. When new reagents or new bulbs are used, a new curve should be made up. Graphs and tables supplied with a new instrument by the manufacturer should not be used, for the obvious reason that reagents and conditions in your laboratory are not the same as those found in the manufacturer's laboratory.

DISCUSSION

1. A common problem in hospitals is variation in line voltage. For this reason, it is advisable to employ an electronic power supply, battery, or voltage regulator that will feed a constant voltage to the instrument.
2. Reagent blanks should be used with all tests and must contain all the reagents used in the unknown, with the exception of the unknown specimen.
3. Care must be taken to ensure that the cuvettes used are not scratched. It is advisable to use the same cuvette for each sample. Rinsing the cuvette between samples is unnecessary if drainage is efficient, except in cases where the unknown is much more diluted or concentrated than the previous sample. In this instance, rinse the cuvette with a small amount of the mixture to be read next.
4. The cuvette should be placed in the spectrophotometer facing in exactly the same direction for each reading. If the cuvette is turned around slightly, there may be a difference of 1.5 to 2% transmittance in the reading.
5. Spectrophotometers must be allowed time to warm up when they are first turned on. See the manufacturer's directions for the amount of time required.
6. Any turbidity present in the sample will cause false results to be obtained unless the method used is measuring only for turbidity.
7. When taking readings on more than one sample, it may be necessary to reset the reagent blank in between unknowns. This will depend on the stability of the instrument. It may be possible to read numerous samples without resetting the reagent blank.
8. Before obtaining readings for the samples, it is important to ensure that the photometer is set at 0% transmittance when the light source has been blocked from the photoelectric cell. That is, when the instrument is on and the photoelectric cell is not receiving light energy from the light source, the percent transmittance scale must read 0.

STATISTICAL TOOLS IN THE EVALUATION OF LABORATORY RESULTS

In hematology, as in other departments of the laboratory, statistical tools are used to identify and define the normal values for a test and to validate test results.

REPRODUCIBILITY VS. ACCURACY

Regardless of how good a technologist's technique is, there is a certain amount of error in all tests. This is unavoidable. An *accurate* method is one that gives values, or results, that agree closely with the known value. On the other hand, a *reproducible* method is one that gives closely similar results when multiple tests are made on the same specimen. All laboratory procedures must be both accurate and reproducible.

Determination of Normal Values

The purpose of laboratory testing is to determine whether a patient's blood contains a normal, low, or elevated amount of the substance for which it is being tested. To determine this, normal values, or values within a normal range, must be determined for each procedure so that the abnormal patient can be identified. The normal range for a test depends on several factors. Two such factors are (1) the method used by a particular laboratory and (2) the geographic location of the patients being tested.

For most laboratory procedures there are several different methods. Each of these methods may have different sensitivities. That is, method No. 1 may be only sensitive enough to react with 90% of the substance being tested for, whereas method No. 2 can pick up 99% of the substance being tested for but also reacts with 5% of interfering substances present in the specimen. Therefore, a normal range must be determined for each procedure used that is specific for that method.

Certain components in the blood vary in different geographic locations. For example, a healthy person living in mountainous regions normally has a higher hemoglobin level than a person living in lower altitudes. (There is a decreased oxygen concentration at high altitudes. To compensate for this, the blood must contain more red blood cells so that the tissues continue to receive the proper amount of oxygen.) In such a case, a normal range must be determined for this particular locale.

METHOD FOR DETERMINING NORMAL VALUES

1. Select a large number (50 to 100) of normal individuals who are not known to have any disease.
2. Determine and record the test value for each individual.
3. Construct a graph, placing the number of subjects on the abscissa (vertical axis) and the test values received for the subjects on the ordinate (horizontal axis).
4. Plot the test values on the graph. A normal frequency distribution curve for these values is shown in Figure 23.
5. Point A, or the central point, is the mean or average value for this series of tests and is contained within the *mode* (the most frequently occurring value in a frequency distribution). The curve is now described in terms of distances from the mean, using standard deviation as the unit to measure this distance. The central area of this curve from -1 standard deviation to $+1$ standard deviation contains 68% of the values received. Within ± 2 standard deviations, 95% of the values are found, and 99.7% of the test values are contained within ± 3 standard deviations. There will be 0.3% of the values outside of ± 3 standard deviations. The normal range for the particular test will be those values that fall within ± 2 standard deviations of the mean and will contain 95% of the normal population. An individual's test value that falls outside of the ± 3 standard deviation limit is said to be abnormal. If the test value falls between the second and third standard deviation limit, this may or may not be considered abnormal. The frequency distribution is termed the *gaussian curve* (Fig. 23). (Note: If the population being tested does not show a normal frequency distribution, the resulting curve will be skewed and

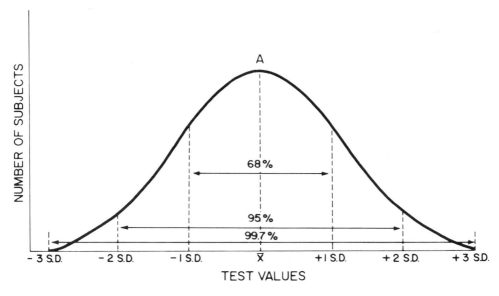

Fig. 23. Gaussian curve (normal frequency distribution curve).

not gaussian in character. In this instance, the standard deviation is not applicable because it is valid only when the frequency distribution curve is normal.)

Validation of Test Results

Standard deviation may also be used to determine the validity of test results. If certain reagents are no longer good, if the equipment used is not working well, or if the technologist running the test has made an error in the procedure, inaccuracies will appear in the results. Calculation of the standard deviation is based on the test results received from known control serum or whole blood. The specimens must be from the same pool, if pooled blood is used, or from the same lot number, if a commercial control is employed.

Procedure for Determining the Standard Deviation

1. Perform the test on the control specimen each day for a minimum of 30 days. Determination of the standard deviation for hemoglobin will be used as an example.

DATE	HEMOGLOBIN RESULT IN GRAMS PER DECILITER
9/1	13.8
9/2	13.9
9/3	14.1
9/4	14.1
9/5	13.6
9/6	14.0
9/7	14.2
9/8	14.0
9/9	13.9
9/10	13.9
9/11	14.2
9/12	13.9
9/13	14.0
9/14	14.1
9/15	14.0
9/16	13.8
9/17	14.1
9/18	14.0
9/19	14.0
9/20	13.9
9/21	14.0
9/22	13.8
9/23	14.0
9/24	14.0
9/25	14.1
9/26	13.9
9/27	14.2
9/28	13.8
9/29	14.2
9/30	14.1
	420.0

2. Calculate the average, or mean ($\overline{\overline{X}}$), by determining the sum of all the test

results (Σ), and dividing by the number of tests run (N).

$$\overline{X} = \frac{\Sigma}{N}$$

$$\overline{X} = \frac{420 \text{ g/dl}}{30}$$

$$\overline{X} = 14.0 \text{ g/dl}$$

3. Determine the difference from the average for each of the preceding test results ($\overline{X} - X$) and then square this difference ($\overline{X} - X)^2$. (The individual test result is represented by X.)

HEMOGLOBIN RESULT IN GRAMS PER DECILITER	$(\overline{X} - X)$	$(\overline{X} - X)^2$
13.8	0.2	0.04
13.9	0.1	0.01
14.1	0.1	0.01
14.1	0.1	0.01
13.6	0.4	0.16
14.0	0.0	0.00
14.2	0.2	0.04
14.0	0.0	0.00
13.9	0.1	0.01
13.9	0.1	0.01
14.2	0.2	0.04
13.9	0.1	0.01
14.0	0.0	0.00
14.1	0.1	0.01
14.0	0.0	0.00
13.8	0.2	0.04
14.1	0.1	0.01
14.0	0.0	0.00
14.0	0.0	0.00
13.9	0.1	0.01
14.0	0.0	0.00
13.8	0.2	0.04
14.0	0.0	0.00
14.0	0.0	0.00
14.1	0.1	0.01
13.9	0.1	0.01
14.2	0.2	0.04
13.8	0.2	0.04
14.2	0.2	0.04
14.1	0.1	0.01
		0.60

4. Add the squared differences and divide by one less than the number of test results (N − 1). (Σ = the sum of.)

$$\frac{\Sigma (\overline{X} - X)^2}{N - 1} = \frac{0.60}{29} = 0.0206896 \text{ or } 0.0207$$

5. Determine the standard deviation (S.D.) by calculating the square root of the preceding result. (For a review of square root calculation, see the end of this chapter.)

$$\text{S.D.} = \sqrt{0.0207} = 0.1438 \text{ or } 0.14 \text{ g/dl}$$

That is, 1 S.D. = 0.14 g/dl

2 S.D. = 2 × 0.14 g/dl
= 0.28 g/dl

3 S.D. = 3 × 0.14 g/dl
= 0.42 g/dl

The formula for standard deviation is:

$$\text{S.D.} = \sqrt{\frac{\Sigma (\overline{X} - X)^2}{N - 1}}$$

COEFFICIENT OF VARIATION (C.V.)

The coefficient of variation is the standard deviation expressed as a percent of the mean, or average. Using the previous figures from the hemoglobin calculations, the percent of variation of one standard deviation from the average or mean (C.V.) would be:

$$\text{C.V.} = \frac{\text{S.D.}}{\overline{X}} \times 100$$

$$\text{C.V.} = \frac{0.14}{14.0} \times 100 = 1.0\%$$

One standard deviation is then regarded as being 1% of the average or mean value.

DISCUSSION

1. Standard deviation, as it refers to frequency distribution, should not be confused with standard deviation as it relates to error in measurement. The standard deviation of a frequency distribution curve is calculated from single test values made on different individuals. The standard deviation used to indicate errors in measurement is calculated from multiple test values made on the same sample or specimen. Mathematically, standard deviation, as it refers

to frequency distribution, is calculated in the same way as the standard deviation that relates to errors in measurement.

2. Of the values determining the standard deviation (in error of measurement), 68% will fall within ±1 standard deviation, 95% within ±2 standard deviations, and 99.7% of the values will lie within ±3 standard deviations.

Quality Control Charts

STANDARD DEVIATION

A control blood or serum should be run each time a test is performed on unknown specimens. A quality control chart is prepared for each procedure, and these control results are plotted daily. The values for these controls should fall within ±2 standard deviations from the mean. For example, using the previous figures for a hemoglobin control, the control value received each day should be 14.0 g/dl, ± 0.28 g/dl. The test, therefore, has an acceptable range of 13.7 g/dl to 14.3 g/dl (Fig. 24). When interpreting this graph, attention must be given to several details: (1): As stated previously, 68% of the control values obtained will fall within ±1 S.D.,

95% within ±2 S.D., and the remaining 5% outside the 2 S.D. limit. Therefore, one might expect to receive a control value outside the 2 S.D. limit 5% of the time or on one of every 20 samples. Since this occurs by chance, it must be interpreted along with the preceding values. If the control is repeated at this time, the value should fall within ±2 S.D. If it does not, the chances are that the test is out of control. (2) If the control value consistently falls above (below or on) the median for 5 or 6 successive days, an out-of-control situation is most likely present, and investigative work should be done to determine the cause, even though these values fall within ±2 S.D. (Fig. 25). (3) There should be an equal scattering of values above and below the mean (Fig. 26, June 1 through 12).

Possible sources of error and reasons why control values fall outside of the allowable ±2 standard deviation limit are dirty or contaminated glassware, technical error, improper calibration of equipment, use of the wrong or deteriorated reagents, or improperly working equipment.

TWIN-PLOT CHART

When two control samples (normal and abnormal) are run, the twin-plot graph of

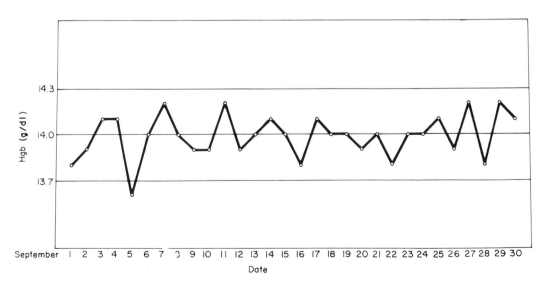

Fig. 24.   Quality control graph for hemoglobin procedure (September).

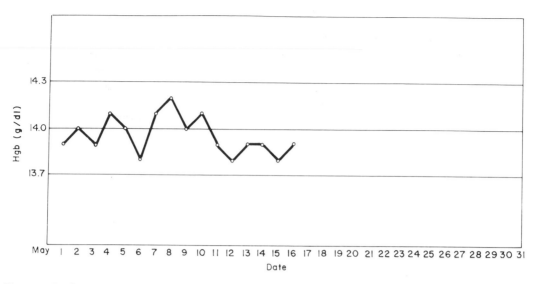

Fig. 25. Quality control graph for hemoglobin procedure (May). Note that the last six values beginning on May 11 are all below the median. By May 15 there should be concern about these values and investigation made as to their cause.

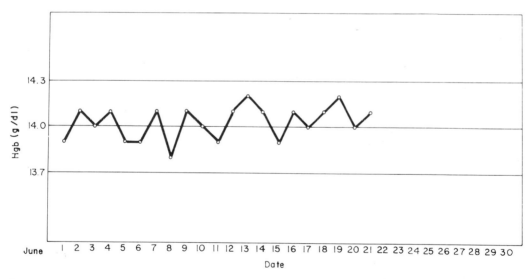

Fig. 26. Quality control graph for hemoglobin procedure (June). Beginning on June 12 there appears to be an upward trend in the control values. Even though five or six successive plots are not above the mean, the cause for this shift should be found.

Youden, modified by D.B. Tonks, may be utilized. This same graph may also be employed using two control values by the same method or one control value from each of two separate methods.

The graph is prepared by drawing on the vertical axis the mean +2 S.D., and −2 S.D. limits for the abnormal control or con-trol No. 2. On the horizontal axis, mark off the mean, +2 S.D., and −2 S.D. limits for the normal control or control No. 1. Draw a square field in the middle of the graph connecting the two S.D. limits (Fig. 27). The cross in the middle of the square denotes the mean for both control samples. The line drawn connecting the bottom left

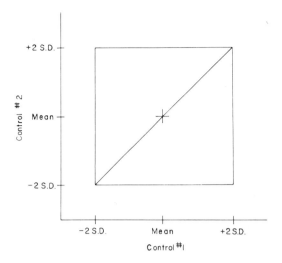

Fig. 27.   Twin-plot graph.

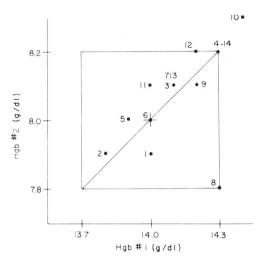

Fig. 28.   Twin-plot chart for normal and abnormal hemoglobin results (July).

corner with the top right corner denotes the line of normal distribution. Each day the control value is plotted with regard to both control results. As an example, the following results were obtained on the dates indicated and plotted as shown (Fig. 28).

DATE	NORMAL HEMOGLOBIN CONTROL (G/DL)	ABNORMAL HEMOGLOBIN CONTROL (G/DL)
July 1	14.0	7.9
2	13.8	7.9
3	14.1	8.1
4	14.3	8.2
5	13.9	8.0
6	14.0	8.0
7	14.1	8.1
8	14.3	7.8
9	14.2	8.1
10	14.4	8.3
11	14.0	8.1
12	14.2	8.2
13	14.1	8.1
14	14.3	8.2

When interpreting this graph, several details should be noted: (1) Under normal conditions, when the test procedure is in control, the plotted control values should fall along the diagonal line of normal distribution, as seen in Figure 28 for July 1 through July 7. (2) If one of the controls is high and the other control is low, something is probably wrong. Both control sam-

ples were not affected in the same manner in the procedure, and patient values may be erratic. This condition shows up in the chart by the appearance of the plotted point in the lower right or upper left corner of the square, as shown in Figure 28 for July 8. (3) The plotted values should fall along the diagonal line from the lower left corner to the top right corner. An uneven distribution in one of the two corners indicates an upward or downward shift, and, therefore, an out-of-control situation. Note that beginning with July 9, all values are in the upper right corner, indicating an upward trend (Fig. 28). (4) If, at any time, both control values fall outside the ± 2 S.D. limit, something is wrong with the procedure and the cause for these results should be found. In Figure 28, the control values for July 10 were both outside normal limits.

THE CUMULATIVE SUM (CUSUM) GRAPH

The CUSUM graph is a third method for charting control results. In this method, after the mean for the control is determined, the result is subtracted from each day's control results. The resulting value is added to the total of the previous days to give a cumulative difference from the

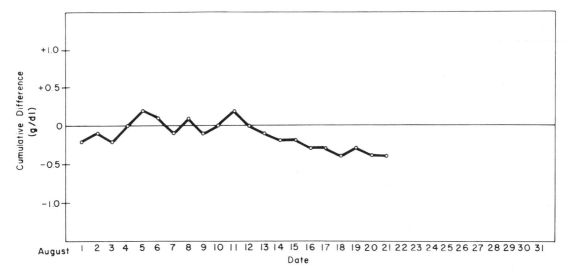

Fig. 29. Cumulative difference graph for hemoglobin (August).

mean. Each day this cumulative difference is plotted on the graph.

The CUSUM graph consists of a single line representing the mean. Negative cumulative differences are plotted below the mean line and positive differences are plotted above the line (Fig. 29). As an example, the following hemoglobin control results were obtained in the month of August, at which time the mean hemoglobin was 14.0 g/dl.

DATE		HEMOGLOBIN CONTROL RESULTS G/DL	DIFFERENCE FROM MEAN	CUMULATIVE DIFFERENCE
August	1	13.8	− 0.2	− 0.2
	2	14.1	+ 0.1	− 0.1
	3	13.9	− 0.1	− 0.2
	4	14.2	+ 0.2	0.0
	5	14.2	+ 0.2	+ 0.2
	6	13.9	− 0.1	+ 0.1
	7	13.8	− 0.2	− 0.1
	8	14.2	+ 0.2	+ 0.1
	9	13.8	− 0.2	− 0.1
	10	14.1	+ 0.1	0.0
	11	14.2	+ 0.2	+ 0.2
	12	13.8	− 0.2	0.0
	13	13.9	− 0.1	− 0.1
	14	13.9	− 0.1	− 0.2
	15	14.0	0.0	− 0.2
	16	13.9	− 0.1	− 0.3
	17	14.0	0.0	− 0.3
	18	13.9	− 0.1	− 0.4
	19	14.1	+ 0.1	− 0.3
	20	13.9	− 0.1	− 0.4
	21	14.0	0.0	− 0.4

When the test procedure is in control, the plotted graph should show a line moving back and forth close to and above and below the 0 line (Fig. 29, August 1 through August 12). If the graph begins to show a trend upward or downward, this indicates a trend toward high or low control results, respectively. Beginning on August 12, there is a downward trend of the control. Any time five or six successive plots go down or up on this graph, it is an indication that the test is out of control.

QUALITY CONTROL UTILIZING DUPLICATE SPECIMENS

A fourth method for maintaining quality control consists of charting the differences between duplicate patient samples or duplicate control samples. This method of quality control monitors the precision or reproducibility of test results. To obtain a 2 S.D. limit, 30 different specimens (patient blood or control blood) are run in duplicate. Using the following figures as an example, the 2 S.D. limit is obtained for the Activated Partial Thromboplastin Time (APTT), as shown on page 26.

DATE		PATIENT	APTT RESULT #1 (SECONDS)	APTT RESULT #2 (SECONDS)	DIFFERENCE BETWEEN PAIRS (SECONDS)	DIFFERENCE SQUARED
January	1	1	31.3	30.9	0.4	0.16
		2	36.5	35.0	1.5	2.25
	2	3	34.1	33.4	0.7	0.49
		4	33.7	33.0	0.7	0.49
		5	44.6	45.4	0.8	0.64
		6	32.0	32.9	0.9	0.81
	3	7	34.3	34.1	0.2	0.04
		8	30.2	30.6	0.4	0.16
		9	49.0	50.1	1.1	1.21
		10	33.7	33.6	0.1	0.01
	4	11	34.5	34.8	0.3	0.09
		12	32.3	32.3	0.0	0.00
		13	38.9	38.6	0.3	0.09
		14	32.4	32.9	0.5	0.25
		15	37.8	36.9	0.9	0.81
	5	16	39.0	37.9	1.1	1.21
		17	29.5	29.9	0.4	0.16
		18	44.3	43.0	1.3	1.69
		19	35.6	36.1	0.5	0.25
	6	20	37.9	38.8	0.9	0.81
		21	34.4	33.0	1.4	1.96
		22	32.1	32.0	0.1	0.01
	7	23	36.5	37.0	0.5	0.25
		24	33.4	33.9	0.5	0.25
		25	37.1	38.7	1.6	2.56
		26	34.9	35.7	0.8	0.64
	8	27	33.6	33.0	0.6	0.36
		28	37.2	37.5	0.3	0.09
	9	29	32.5	31.4	1.1	1.21
		30	33.4	32.9	0.5	0.25
						19.2

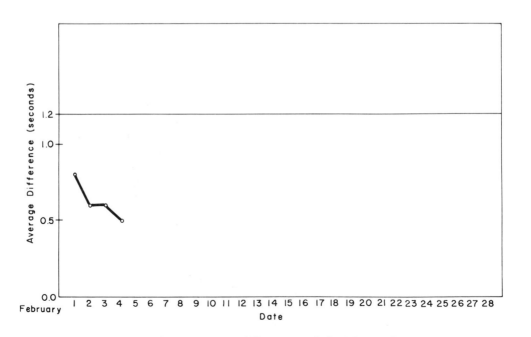

Fig. 30. Duplicate specimen difference graph for APTT (February).

$$S.D. = \sqrt{\frac{\Sigma\,d^2}{2\,N}}$$

Where:

Σ = the sum of
d = the difference between the pairs
N = the total number of specimens

$$S.D. = \sqrt{\frac{19.2}{2 \times 30}}$$
$$= \sqrt{0.32}$$

1 S.D. = 0.56 or 0.6 seconds
2 S.D. = 1.2 seconds

If control blood is used to set up the 2 S.D. limit, values should be obtained over a 30-day period rather than running a large group of controls on 1 or 2 days.

When the 2 S.D.-limit is established, a graph is set up, and the average of the differences between duplicate specimens is plotted each day. The following results are given as an example and are plotted in Figure 30.

DATE	PATIENT	APTT RESULT #1 (SECONDS)	APTT RESULT #2 (SECONDS)	DIFFERENCE BETWEEN PAIRS (SECONDS)
February 1	1	36.2	37.4	1.2
	2	31.4	30.5	0.9
	3	41.6	41.3	0.3
			Average difference =	0.8
2	4	31.2	31.1	0.1
	5	37.9	37.5	0.4
	6	49.3	50.5	1.2
			Average difference =	0.6
3	7	36.4	37.2	0.8
	8	31.4	31.0	0.4
			Average difference =	0.6
4	9	29.6	30.0	0.4
	10	41.2	42.0	0.8
	11	35.3	35.1	0.2
			Average difference =	0.5

If the average difference between duplicate specimens appear to be decreasing, a new 2 S.D. limit may be determined simply by taking the last 30 sets of duplicate specimens that were run and calculating the 2 S.D. from these values.

Calculation of Square Root

To determine the square root of 691.503:

1. Separate the numbers into pairs beginning at the decimal point and working to the left and/or right. (The answer will contain one number for each of the two numbers paired.) If the number on the far left has only one number, as shown (the 6) use this number by itself. When there is a single number to the far right, add a 0. Place the decimal point directly above the one under the square root sign.

$$\sqrt{691.5030}$$

2. Using the first number or pair of numbers on the far left, find the largest perfect square number that is smaller than this number and place it above the number, as shown.

$$\begin{array}{r} 2\ \ . \\ \sqrt{691.5030} \end{array}$$

3. Square this number (2) and place it beneath the 6. Subtract and bring down the next pair of numbers.

$$\begin{array}{r} 2\ \ . \\ \sqrt{691.5030} \\ 4 \\ \hline 291 \end{array}$$

4. Double the partial answer above the square root sign and place it on the left.

$$\begin{array}{r} 2\\[-2pt] \sqrt{691.5030}\\[-2pt] 4\\ \hline 291 \end{array}$$

4

5. Select a number which, when placed on the right of the 4, will give the closest result to 291 (must be less than 291) when this number (46) is multiplied by the number selected (6). Place this number above the square root sign over the number 91.

$$\begin{array}{r} 2\ 6.\\[-2pt] \sqrt{691.5030}\\[-2pt] 4\\ \hline 291 \end{array}$$

46 $\underline{276}$

6. Subtract this number from the number above and bring down the next pair of numbers.

$$\begin{array}{r} 2\ 6.\\[-2pt] \sqrt{691.5030}\\[-2pt] 4\\ \hline 291 \end{array}$$

46 $\underline{276}$
$15\ 50$

7. Double the partial answer, as in step 4, and bring it down to the left.

$$\begin{array}{r} 2\ 6.\\[-2pt] \sqrt{691.5030}\\[-2pt] 4\\ \hline 291 \end{array}$$

46 $\underline{276}$
$15\ 50$
52

8. Select a number which, when placed on the right of 52, will give the closest result to 1550 when this number (522) is multiplied by the number selected (2).

$$\begin{array}{r} 2\ 6.\ 2\\[-2pt] \sqrt{691.5030}\\[-2pt] 4\\ \hline 291 \end{array}$$

46 $\underline{276}$
$15\ 50$
522 $\underline{10\ 44}$
$5\ 0630$

9. Double the partial answer, as in step 4, and bring it down to the left. Select a number which, when placed on the right of 524, will give the closest result to 50630 when this number (5249) is multiplied by the number selected (9).

$$\begin{array}{r} 2\ 6.\ 2\ 9\\[-2pt] \sqrt{691.5030}\\[-2pt] 4\\ \hline 291 \end{array}$$

46 $\underline{276}$
$15\ 50$
522 $\underline{10\ 44}$
$5\ 0630$
5249 $\underline{4\ 7241}$
3389

10. This procedure may be continued to a third or fourth decimal place by adding one pair of zeros for each decimal place desired when the answer does not come out to an even number. In such cases, calculations should be carried out to one more decimal place than is needed. The number is rounded off to the desired decimal point.

$$\begin{array}{r} 2\ 6.\ 2\ 9\\[-2pt] \sqrt{691.503000}\\[-2pt] 4\\ \hline 291 \end{array}$$

46 $\underline{276}$
$15\ 50$
522 $\underline{10\ 44}$
$5\ 0630$
5249 $\underline{4\ 7241}$
338900

If it is necessary to find the square root to one decimal point, the result received (26.29) would be rounded off to 26.3. The number of significant decimal places used in laboratory calculations depends on the procedure involved. Calculations rarely have to be carried out beyond two decimal places.

2

Routine Hematology Procedures

COMPLETE BLOOD COUNT

In most hospitals, the complete blood count (CBC) consists of the white blood cell count, the hemoglobin, hematocrit, and red blood cell count. Also included are the red blood cell indices, which give the average red blood cell size and relative and absolute values for the amount of hemoglobin in the average red blood cell for each particular patient. The last test in the CBC is the differential, in which the different white blood cells present are classified, further information about the red blood cells is given, and the platelets are reviewed for number and morphologic features. The importance of the CBC cannot be underestimated. In addition to being a screening procedure, it is helpful in the diagnosis of many diseases, it is used to reflect the body's ability to fight disease, and it is employed as an indicator of the patient's progress in certain diseased states such as infection or anemia.

HEMOGLOBIN

The measurement of hemoglobin is a reasonably accurate test and, along with the hematocrit (and reticulocyte count), is used to follow the treatment of anemias.

The normal values for hemoglobin in the peripheral blood vary with the age and sex of the individual. Altitude also plays a role in that the normal hemoglobin concentration for persons at high altitudes is higher than for those individuals living at sea level. At birth, the hemoglobin concentration is normally 17 to 23 g per dl. This value decreases to 9 to 14 g per dl at about 2 months. By 10 years of age, the normal hemoglobin is 12 to 14 g per dl. Normal adult values range from 13 to 15 g per dl for women and from 14 to 17 g per dl for men. There is a slight decrease in the hemoglobin level after 50 years of age.

Cyanmethemoglobin Method

REAGENTS AND EQUIPMENT

1. Cyanmethemoglobin reagent, which contains sodium bicarbonate, potassium cyanide, and potassium ferricyanide. This reagent may be obtained commercially as cyanmethemoglobin reagent or Drabkin's reagent.
2. Test tubes, 13 × 100 mm.
3. Sahli pipets or disposable pipets, 0.02 ml.
4. Colorimeter or spectrophotometer.

SPECIMEN

Whole blood, using EDTA, heparin, or ammonium-potassium oxalate as the anticoagulant. Capillary blood may also be used.

PRINCIPLE

Whole blood is added to a solution containing potassium cyanide and potassium ferricyanide (cyanmethemoglobin re-

29

agent). The ferricyanide converts the hemoglobin iron from the ferrous state (Fe^{2+}) to the ferric state (Fe^{3+}) to form methemoglobin, which then combines with potassium cyanide to form the stable pigment, cyanmethemoglobin. The color intensity of this mixture is measured in a photometer at a wavelength of 540 nm or by using a yellow-green filter. The optical density of the solution is proportional to the concentration of hemoglobin. All forms of hemoglobin are measured with this method except sulfhemoglobin.

PROCEDURE

1. For each patient to be tested, place exactly 5.0 ml of cyanmethemoglobin reagent into an appropriately labeled test tube. Place 5.0 ml of the reagent into a test tube to be used as the blank.

2. Add 0.02 ml of well-mixed whole blood (or capillary blood) to the appropriately labeled tube. Rinse the pipet three to five times with the cyanmethemoglobin reagent until all blood is removed from the pipet.

3. Mix the preceding solutions well and allow to stand at room temperature for at least 10 minutes to allow adequate time for the formation of cyanmethemoglobin.

4. Transfer the mixture to a cuvette and read in a spectrophotometer (or colorimeter) at a wavelength of 540 nm (or with a yellow-green filter) using the cyanmethemoglobin reagent in the blank tube to set %T at 100%. Record the readings for the patient samples from the %T scale and refer to the precalibrated chart for the actual value of the hemoglobin in g per dl.

DISCUSSION

1. Before the unknown sample is read, the solution must be crystal clear. If any turbidity is present, a falsely high result is obtained. Clouding may be due to:
   A. An exceptionally high white blood cell count. (In such cases, centrifuge the mixture and use the supernatant as the test sample.)
   B. Hemoglobin S and hemoglobin C. (Dilute the mixture 1:1 with distilled water, read on the spectrophotometer, and multiply the result by 2.)
   C. Abnormal globulins. (Add 0.1 g of potassium carbonate to the cyanmethemoglobin reagent).
   D. Lipemic blood. (Add 0.02 ml of the patient's plasma to 5.0 ml of cyanmethemoglobin reagent and use this mixture for the patient blank.)

2. The concentration of anticoagulant does not affect hemoglobin results.

Preparation of a Standard Hemoglobin Curve

Using the stock solution of cyanmethemoglobin standard, set up at least four dilutions according to the directions received with the reagent or as shown in Table 1.

Using semilogarithmic graph paper, plot hemoglobin in g per dl on the abscissa (horizontal axis) against percent transmittance on the ordinate (vertical axis)—this is a straightline curve. A chart is then made to facilitate reading the test results.

Abnormal Hemoglobin Pigments

If hemoglobin is converted to an abnormal hemoglobin pigment, it is no longer capable of oxygen transport and, if this impairment is severe enough, a condition of hypoxia or cyanosis occurs. The three abnormal hemoglobin pigments of most significance are discussed briefly.

1. *Carboxyhemoglobin* is formed by the combination of hemoglobin with carbon monoxide. The hemoglobin molecule has a much greater affinity for

TABLE 1.   DILUTIONS FOR A HEMOGLOBIN CURVE

TUBE	CYANMETHEMOGLOBIN REAGENT	STOCK STANDARD	CONCENTRATION OF HEMOGLOBIN
1	0.0 ml	5.0 ml	100% of value given for the hemoglobin standard
2	1.0 ml	4.0 ml	80% of value given for the hemoglobin standard
3	2.0 ml	3.0 ml	60% of value given for the hemoglobin standard
4	3.0 ml	2.0 ml	40% of value given for the hemoglobin standard

carbon monoxide than for oxygen and, therefore, readily combines with the carbon monoxide, even when it is present in low concentrations. The formation of carboxyhemoglobin is reversible. It is found in the blood of tobacco smokers in concentrations of 2 to 10%.

2. *Methemoglobin* is a type of hemoglobin in which the ferrous ion has been oxidized to the ferric state and is, therefore, incapable of combining with or transporting the oxygen molecule that is replaced by an hydroxyl radical. Methemoglobin formation is reversible and is normally present in the blood in concentrations of 1 to 2%.

3. *Sulfhemoglobin* is not normally found in the blood. When it is present, its formation is irreversible, and it remains for the life of the carrier red blood cell. Its exact nature is unknown, but it is thought to be formed by the action of certain drugs and chemicals such as sulfonamides and aromatic amines. It is incapable of transporting oxygen.

HEMATOCRIT

When anticoagulated whole blood is centrifuged, the space occupied by the packed red blood cells is termed the *hematocrit reading* and is expressed as the percentage of red blood cells in a volume of whole blood. Because of its simplicity and reproducibility, the hematocrit is one of the more accurate hematology tests. The values for the hematocrit closely parallel the values for the hemoglobin and red blood cell count.

When whole blood is centrifuged, the

heavier particles fall to the bottom of the tube and the lighter particles precipitate out on top of them, as shown in Figure 31. When reading the hematocrit, it is important to take the reading at the top of the red blood cell layer. This is most significant in cases in which there is an extremely elevated white blood cell or platelet count.

The normal values for the hematocrit vary with the age and sex of the individual. Altitude plays a role in that the normal hematocrit for residents at high altitudes is higher than that of individuals living at sea level. At birth, the normal range for the hematocrit is 50 to 62%. This range then decreases to 31 to 39% by 1 year of age. The normal hematocrit value gradually increases to levels for adults of 36 to 46% for women and 42 to 52% for men. There is a slight decrease in the hematocrit level after 50 years of age.

Microhematocrit Method

REAGENTS AND EQUIPMENT

1. Capillary hematocrit tubes approximately 7 cm in length and having a bore of approximately 1 mm (Fig. 32). If anticoagulated whole blood is used, the capillary tube should not contain an anticoagulant. If capillary

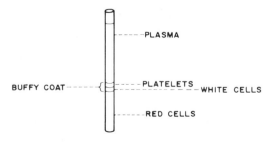

Fig. 31.   Cell layers in centrifuged whole blood.

blood is employed, the hematocrit tube should contain a proper amount of heparin.

2. Clay, to seal one end of the hematocrit tube.

3. Centrifuge capable of producing centrifugal fields ranging from 11,500 to 15,000 revolutions per minute (RPM), with an appropriate head for the capillary hematocrit tubes.

4. Microhematocrit tube reader.

SPECIMEN

Whole blood, using EDTA, heparin, or ammonium-potassium oxalate as the anticoagulant. Capillary blood may also be used.

PRINCIPLE

Whole blood is centrifuged for maximum red blood cell packing. The space occupied by the red blood cells is measured and expressed as a percentage of the whole blood volume.

PROCEDURE

1. Allow capillary or well-mixed anticoagulated whole blood to enter two capillary hematocrit tubes until they are approximately two-thirds filled with blood. (Air bubbles denote poor technique but do not affect the results of the test.)

2. Seal one end of the hematocrit tube with clay.

3. Place the two hematocrit tubes in the radial grooves of the centrifuge head

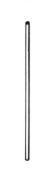

Fig. 32. Capillary hematocrit tube.

exactly opposite each other, with the sealed end away from the center of the centrifuge.

4. Centrifuge for 5 minutes.

5. Remove the hematocrit tubes as soon as the centrifuge has stopped spinning. Obtain the results for both hematocrits, using the microhematocrit tube reading device. Results should agree within ± 2%. If they do not, repeat the preceding procedure.

DISCUSSION

1. Incomplete sealing of the hematocrit tubes generally give falsely low results because, as the tubes spin, there is a greater loss of red blood cells than of plasma.

2. Inadequate centrifugation of the hematocrit tubes or allowing the tubes to stand too long after the centrifuge has stopped gives falsely elevated readings. The time and speed of centrifugation are extremely important to obtain maximum red blood cell packing.

3. If blood is overanticoagulated, the hematocrit reading will be falsely low due to shrinkage of the red blood cells.

4. Even when the hematocrit is spun for the correct time period and at the proper speed, a small amount of plasma still remains in the red blood cell portion. This is termed *trapped plasma*. When comparing spun microhematocrit results with hematocrit results obtained from an electronic cell counter (Coulter Counter, Model S), the spun hematocrit results are generally 1.3 to 3.0% higher, unless the electronic cell counter has been calibrated against spun microhematocrits uncorrected for trapped plasma. An increased amount of trapped plasma is found in macrocytic anemias, spherocytosis, thalassemia, hypochromic anemias, and sickle cell anemia (the amount of

trapped plasma increases as the percentage of affected sickle-shaped red blood cells increases).

BLOOD CELL COUNTS

The International Committee for Standardization in Hematology has recommended that all units of volume be measured in liters. Up until this time, all quantitative counts of the formed elements of the blood (white blood cells, red blood cells, and platelets) have been expressed in cubic millimeters (cu mm or mm³). Since the difference between 1 cu mm and 1 microliter (μl) (1 cu mm = 1.00003 μl) is considered to be insignificant, 1 μl will be considered to be equivalent to 1 cu mm (1 μl = 10^{-6} liters). Therefore, a white blood cell count of 6,000/cu mm = 6.0×10^3/cu mm = 6,000/μl = $6.0 \times 10^3/\mu$l = $6,000 \times 10^6$/l = 6.0×10^9/l.

In this text, the microliter (μl) will be used in place of cubic millimeters.

WHITE BLOOD CELL COUNT

The white blood cell count (WBC) denotes the number of white blood cells in 1 μl of whole blood. In a normal, healthy individual, the white count falls between 4,500 and 11,000 white blood cells per μl. This count varies with age. The white count of a newborn baby is 10,000 to 30,000 per μl at birth. It decreases to about 10,000 per μl after the first week and drops to normal levels by about 4 years of age.

The white count is a useful measurement to the physician. It is used to indicate infection and may also be employed to follow the progress of certain diseases. The white blood cell count may be elevated in bacterial infections, appendicitis, leukemia, pregnancy, hemolytic disease of the newborn, uremia, ulcers, and normally at birth. The white count may drop below normal values in viral diseases (such as measles), brucellosis, typhoid fever, infectious hepatitis, rheumatoid arthritis, cirrhosis of the liver, and lupus erythematosus. Radiation or drug therapy tends to lower the white count. In these cases, patients have white counts done while receiving therapy to ensure that the white blood cell count does not become too low. A white count above 11,000 per μl is termed *leukocytosis*; a white count below normal is known as *leukopenia*. The white count in children usually shows a greater variation during disease. For example, during infection, a child's white count reaches much higher elevations than does an adult's white count in response to a corresponding infection. An individual's normal white count is subject to variations, being slightly higher in the afternoon than in the morning. There is also an increase in the number of white blood cells following strenuous exercise, emotional stress, and anxiety.

Two methods are currently used to determine the white blood cell count. The older method is the manual, or microscopic, method. In the past several years, there has been a changeover to the electronic method of counting white blood cells. The manual white count is discussed in this section. Please refer to Chapter 7, Automation, for electronic methods of counting blood cells.

Manual White Blood Cell Count

The following procedure for the manual white count is presented in detail. The techniques outlined are the same as those employed in the manual red blood cell count, platelet count, and direct eosinophil count. Therefore, these detailed methods are presented only once. Learn and familiarize yourself with this procedure before progressing to the other manual counts outlined later in this chapter. It takes many attempts before these techniques are mastered, but do not be discouraged.

REAGENTS AND EQUIPMENT

1. White-count pipet and aspirator (Fig. 33). A Stop-it mouthpiece (Fig. 34) (obtainable from Medical Device Di-

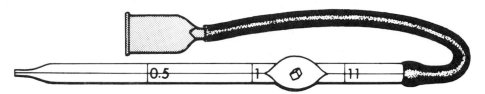

Fig. 33.   White-count pipet with aspirator.

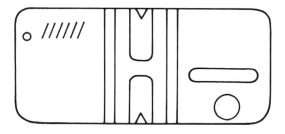

Fig. 34.   Stop-it mouthpiece and aspirator.

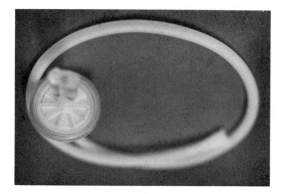

Fig. 35.   Neubauer hemocytometer.

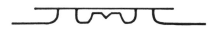

Fig. 36.   Neubauer hemocytometer (side view).

vision, Gelman Sciences, Inc., Ann Arbor, Michigan) may be used in place of the regular mouthpiece. This safety device contains a Gelman microporous membrane that will prevent the passage of aqueous liquids through it. Air passes through the membrane so that it does not interfere with pipetting. (Vapors from strong acids, bases, or solvents may penetrate the filter and make it ineffective.)

2. White-count diluting fluid. Any one of the following diluting fluids may be used:
   A. Acetic acid, 2% (v/v)
   B. Hydrochloric acid, 1% (v/v)
   C. Turk's diluting fluid
Glacial acetic acid	3 ml
Aqueous gentian violet, 1% (w/v)	1 ml
Distilled water	100 ml

3. Microscope.
4. Clean gauze or cloth.
5. Hemocytometer or counting chamber (Fig. 35), with cover glass. The hemocytometer with Neubauer ruling consists of two raised platforms. There is a raised ridge on both sides of the two platforms on which a cover glass is placed. The space between the top of the platform and the cover glass over it is 0.1 mm (Fig. 36). Each of the platforms contains a ruled area composed of nine large squares of equal size (Fig. 37). The entire ruled area of the platform (nine large squares) is 3 mm wide and 3 mm long, each large square measuring 1 mm by 1 mm. The volume of the entire ruled area on one platform is 0.9 μl. The volume of one large square is 0.1 μl. The four large corner squares, each of which is subdivided into 16 smaller squares, are labelled "W" and are the four squares used for counting white blood cells. (All hemocytometers used in the clinical laboratory must meet the specifications of the National Bureau of Standards

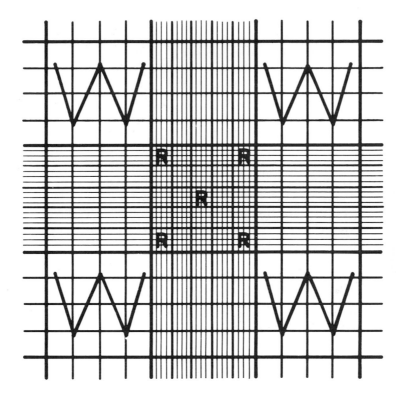

Fig. 37. Neubauer hemocytometer, counting area.

[NBS] and are identified by those initials.)

SPECIMEN

Whole blood, using EDTA, heparin, or ammonium-potassium oxalate as the anticoagulant. Capillary blood may also be used.

PRINCIPLE

Whole blood is mixed with a weak acid solution to dilute the blood and hemolyze the red blood cells.

PROCEDURE

1. Dilution of blood.
   A. Mix the specimen of blood for approximately 1 minute. Using the aspirator and white-cell pipet, draw the blood up to the 0.5 mark in the pipet. It is permissible for the blood to go slightly beyond the 0.5 mark. (If the blood is drawn up too far beyond this mark, however, the dilution is inaccurate, because a small amount of blood continues to adhere to the inside of the stem when the excess blood is withdrawn from the pipet.)
   B. Remove blood from the outside of the pipet with a clean gauze or cloth. Be careful that the material does not withdraw any blood from the stem of the pipet. Place a nonabsorbent material to the end of the pipet, bringing the blood down exactly to the 0.5 mark. (If an absorbent cloth is used to remove the excess blood from the stem, the cloth tends to absorb the liquid portion of the blood and, therefore, the blood will have a higher concentration of cells.)
   C. Holding the pipet almost verti-

cally, place the tip of the pipet into the white-count diluting fluid. Draw the diluting fluid into the pipet slowly, while gently rotating the pipet with your hand to ensure a proper amount of mixing. Aspirate the diluting fluid until the mixture reaches the 11 mark. (If the level of blood falls below the 0.5 mark at any time during this step, repeat the entire procedure, beginning with a clean pipet. Use fresh diluting fluid if any blood has dropped into the bottle, contaminating the fluid. If the pipet has not been held in a vertical position while aspirating the diluting fluid, air bubbles tend to form in the bulb. If this occurs, the dilution is inaccurate, and the procedure must be repeated, using a clean pipet. It is permissible for the level of the mixture to go slightly above or below the 11 mark.)

D. Place the pipet in a horizontal position and firmly hold the index finger of either hand over the opening in the tip of the pipet. Detach the aspirator from the other end of the pipet.

E. The dilution of blood is now complete. The white-cell pipet is divided into units or volumes: 0.5, 1.0, and 11 (Refer to the diagram of the white-cell pipet, if necessary.) The stem contains 1.0 unit and the bulb holds 10 units. The blood is drawn up into the pipet first. As the diluting fluid is aspirated, all of the blood is drawn up into the bulb. Therefore, if the blood is drawn up to the 0.5 mark and diluted to the 11 mark, there is 0.5 volumes of blood and 9.5 volumes of diluting fluid in the bulb of the pipet, for a total of 10 volumes. The stem contains the last 1.0 volume of diluting fluid

and contains no blood. The dilution of blood is, therefore, 0.5 in 10, or a 1:20 dilution.

F. Repeat the preceding procedure on the same blood sample so that there are two white-count dilutions on the same specimen of blood.

2. Clean the counting chamber and cover glass with a clean, lint-free cloth. The use of 95% (v/v) ethanol also facilitates the cleaning process. Carefully replace the cover glass on top of the ruled area of the counting chamber.

3. Mix the diluted white blood cell counts for approximately 3 minutes to ensure hemolysis of the red blood cells and adequate mixing. This may be done with a mechanical shaker. If there is no shaker available, place your thumb over the tip of the pipet and your middle finger over the other end of the pipet. Moving your hand only, mix the pipet in the direction shown in Figure 38.

4. Filling the counting chamber.

A. Hold the pipet in a vertical position with the right index finger

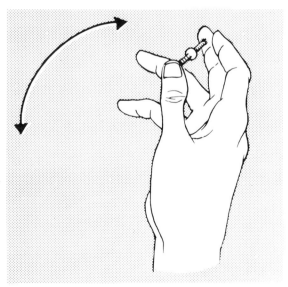

Fig. 38.   Mixing of diluted white blood cell count.

covering the top of the pipet. Discard the first four drops of the mixture onto a piece of gauze.

B. Remove any excess liquid from the outside of the pipet with a piece of gauze.

C. Using the right index finger to control the rate of flow, place the tip of the pipet on the edge of the ruled area of the counting chamber. Allow the mixture to seep under the cover glass gradually and exactly fill this area. (If the pipet is removed just before the area looks filled, the area will fill without becoming flooded.) Care should be taken not to move the cover glass. (Steps 4A, B, and C must be done quickly so that the white blood cells in the mixture do not begin to settle out. Figure 39 illustrates the proper and improper filling of the counting chamber. If the counting chamber is filled improperly, reclean the counting chamber and cover glass. If there is enough diluted blood remaining in the white-cell pipet, remix, expel three drops of the mixture, and refill the counting chamber. Otherwise, repeat the entire procedure beginning at step No. 1.)

D. Fill the opposite side of the counting chamber with the second white-count dilution.

E. When the counting chamber is filled, care should be taken that it is not jarred or the cover glass moved. The filled counting chamber should be allowed to stand for approximately 1 minute prior to performing the count to give the white blood cells time to settle.

5. Count the white blood cells.

A. Carefully, keeping the counting chamber horizontal at all times, place the hemocytometer on the stage of the microscope.

B. Using low power only ($10\times$ objective), make certain that the microscope light is adjusted properly. In proper focus, the white blood cells should look like small dark or black dots.

C. Scan the four large corner squares marked "W" on the counting chamber (Fig. 37). For accurate white counts, there should be an even distribution of cells in all four large squares, with no more than a 10-cell variation between the four squares.

D. Beginning with the upper left square, count all white blood cells in the four large corner squares and add the results together to obtain the total number of cells counted. In counting the cells that touch the outside lines of the large square, count only those that touch the left and upper outside lines (in counting chambers with double lines), dis-

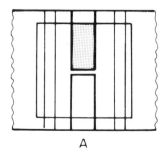 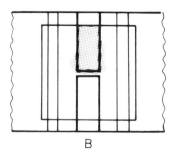

A   B

Fig. 39. Properly (A) and improperly (B) filled counting chamber.

regarding those that touch the right and lower outside margin. If the chamber has triple lines, count those cells that touch the middle of the three outside lines on two sides and disregard those touching the corresponding lines on the other two sides. (That is, count the cells touching either the right margin or the left margin and the cells on the upper margin or lower margin. Whichever you choose is immaterial, but it is important to be consistent and count the cells touching the same two lines every time.)

E. Count the cells on the opposite side of the counting chamber and record the number of cells counted in these four large squares. This total should be close to the first count. (If not, repeat entire procedure starting with step No. 1. The number of cells in each of the eight squares should not differ from each other by more than 15 cells.)

6. Calculation of the white blood cell count.

A. For each of the two white counts performed, calculate the number of white blood cells per μl, as shown below:

B. White blood cells/μl =

Number of white blood cells counted × Correction for volume × Correction for dilution

Number of white blood cells counted. The total number of white blood cells counted in four large squares of the counting chamber. For example:

Square 1	25 white cells	25
Square 2	34 white cells	34
Square 3	32 white cells	32
Square 4	31 white cells	31

Number of cells counted = 122

Correction for volume. The white blood cell count is given as the number of white blood cells in 1 μl of blood. Therefore, if the cells are counted in four large squares, the total volume counted is 4 (1.0 × 1.0 × 0.1) μl, or 0.4 μl. To obtain a volume of 1.0 μl, 0.4 is multiplied by 2.5 ($\frac{1.0}{0.4}$). The correction factor for volume is then 2.5.

Correction for dilution. Since the blood was initially diluted 1:20, the correction factor for dilution is 20.

C. Therefore:
White blood cells/μl = 122 × 2.5 × 20 = 6,100 white blood cells/μl.

D. Calculate the white blood cell count for the second white count and average the two results for the final report.

DISCUSSION

1. In certain conditions, such as leukemia, the white blood cell count may be extremely high. If the white count is above 30,000 per μl, it is advisable to employ a larger dilution of blood. Using a red-cell pipet (see the section entitled Red Blood Cell Count), the blood is drawn up to the 1.0 mark and diluted to the 101 mark with the white-count diluting fluid, thus obtaining a 1:100 dilution. If the white count is markedly elevated, as in some leukemias, in which it may be as high as 100,000 to 300,000 per μl, a 1:200 dilution is used. This is accomplished by drawing the blood up to the 0.5 mark in the red-cell pipet and diluting to the 101 mark with white-count diluting fluid. The procedure for the white count then proceeds as previously described. The correction factor for the dilution, however, changes accordingly.

2. Whenever the white count drops

below 3,000 per μl, a smaller dilution of the blood should be used to achieve a more accurate count. In this situation, the blood is drawn up to the 1.0 mark in a white-cell pipet and diluted to the 11 mark with the white-count diluting fluid for a dilution of 1:10. The white count then proceeds as previously outlined, with a correction factor of 10 for the dilution.

3. It is important that the diluting fluid remain free from contamination. Often, small amounts of blood collect in the diluting fluid, causing inaccuracies and difficulties in distinguishing and counting the white blood cells.

4. It is imperative that the counting chamber and cover glass be free from dirt and lint. This contamination may again cause inaccuracies and difficulties in counting white blood cells. (The counting chamber and cover glass should be cleaned off immediately after completion of the count.)

5. Pipets must be free of dirt and dried blood. Never leave undiluted blood in a pipet. It quickly hardens and plugs up the pipet. Draw water or diluting fluid into the pipet and place it in a container of water.

6. There is an approximate 15% error for the manual white blood cell method.

7. The diluting fluid used for the white cell count destroy or hemolyze all non-nucleated red blood cells. In certain disease states, nucleated red blood cells are present in the peripheral blood. These cells, because they contain a nucleus, cannot be distinguished from the white blood cells. Therefore, any time there are five or more nucleated red blood cells per 100 white blood cells in a differential, the white blood cell count must be corrected as follows:

$$\text{Corrected white blood cell count} = \frac{\text{Uncorrected white blood cell count} \times 100}{100 + \text{number of nucleated red blood cells per 100 white blood cells}}$$

The white count is then reported as the "corrected" white blood cell count.

8. Once the hemocytometer is filled, the counting of the cells must proceed without delay. If too much time elapses, the fluid in the chamber begins to evaporate, causing inaccuracies in the white count.

RED BLOOD CELL COUNT

The red blood cell count (RBC) is the number of red blood cells in 1 μl of whole blood.

The normal red count is 3,600,000 to 5,000,000 (or 3.6 to 5.0 million) per μl for females and 4.2 to 5.4 million per μl for males. The newborn shows a red blood cell count of 5.0 to 6.5 million per μl at birth, which gradually decreases to 3.5 ± 0.4 million per μl at 1 year of age. During childhood and adolescence, the normal values for the red blood cell count are slightly below the normal adult values. There is also a slight decrease in the red blood cell count after 50 years of age.

As in the white blood cell count, there are two methods used for counting red blood cells: the manual method and the procedure employing an electronic cell counter. The manual method for the red blood cell count is similar to that for the white count. It is suggested that the student master the white blood cell count before attempting to count red cells. For this reason, and to avoid duplication of material, the red blood cell count is not presented in as detailed a manner as the white count. When in doubt, refer to the section entitled Manual White Blood Cell Count.

REAGENTS AND EQUIPMENT

1. Red-count pipet and aspirator (Fig. 40).
2. Red-count diluting fluid. Any one of

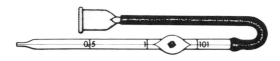

Fig. 40.   Red-count pipet with aspirator.

the following diluting fluids may be used:

A. Hayem's solution

Sodium sulfate	2.50 g
Sodium chloride	0.50 g
Mercuric chloride	0.25 g
Distilled water	100 ml

Certain conditions, such as hyperglobulinemia, cause precipitation of protein, rouleaux, and clumping of the red blood cells when Hayem's solution is used.

B. Gower's solution

Sodium sulfate	12.5 g
Glacial acetic acid	33.3 ml
Distilled water	200 ml

Gower's solution is superior to Hayem's solution in that it prevents rouleaux and clumping of the red blood cells.

C. Sodium chloride, 0.85% (w/v)

Sodium chloride	0.85 g
Distilled water	100 ml

3. Microscope.
4. Clean gauze or cloth.
5. Hemocytometer and cover glass. Referring to Figure 37 and the explanation of the hemocytometer in the section entitled Manual White Blood Cell Count, note the large middle square containing 25 smaller squares of equal size. The five small squares labeled "R" are the areas to be counted for the red blood cell count. The large center square has a volume of 0.1 μl. Therefore, the volume of each of the 25 smaller squares is 0.004 μl, or a total volume for the 5 small squares of 0.02 μl.

SPECIMEN

Whole blood, using EDTA, heparin, or ammonium-potassium oxalate as the anticoagulant. Capillary blood may also be used.

PRINCIPLE

To facilitate counting and prevent lysis of the red blood cells, whole blood is diluted with an isotonic diluting fluid.

PROCEDURE

1. Draw the blood up to exactly the 0.5 mark in the red-count pipet and dilute to the 101 mark with red-count diluting fluid, thus making a 1:200 dilution of blood. Repeat, making a second dilution on the same specimen.
2. Clean the counting chamber.
3. Shake both pipets for 3 minutes.
4. Fill the counting chamber, using both pipets (one red-count dilution filling each side of the hemocytometer). Expel the first four drops of each mixture onto a piece of gauze. Once the counting chamber is filled, allow approximatly 3 minutes for the red blood cells to settle before proceeding to step No. 5.
5. Count the red blood cells, as described in the following steps.
   A. Carefully place the filled counting chamber on the microscope stage.
   B. Using low power (10× objective), place the large center square in the middle of the field of vision. Carefully examine the entire large square for even distribution of red blood cells.
   C. Carefully change to the high-dry objective (40×).
   D. Move the counting chamber so that the small upper left corner square is completely in the field of vision. This square is further subdivided into 16 even smaller

squares. This facilitates cell counting.

E. Count all the cells in this square, remembering to count the cells on two of the outer margins but excluding those lying on the other two outside edges.

F. Some of the red blood cells may be lying on their sides and, therefore, do not appear as round as the majority of cells in the area. These cells are to be included in the count.

G. If there are any white blood cells in the area being counted, do not include these cells in your count. (The white blood cell is usually much larger than the red blood cell and does not have as smooth an appearance.)

H. Count the red blood cells on the opposite side of the counting chamber.

6. Calculate the red blood cell count for each of the red counts performed and average the two results for the final report.

Red cells/μl =

$$\frac{\text{Number of}}{\text{cells counted}} \times \frac{\text{Correction}}{\text{for volume}} \times \frac{\text{Correction}}{\text{for dilution}}$$
in five small
squares

For example:

Number of cells counted in five small squares
  = 400
Dilution = 1:200
Volume counted = five small squares
  = 0.2 cu mm
Red blood cells/μl = 400 × 200 × $\frac{1.0}{0.02}$
  = 4,000,000 red blood
    cells/μl

DISCUSSION

1. In certain conditions, such as polycythemia, the red blood cell count may be extremely high, which makes it difficult to obtain an accurate count. In this instance, make a larger dilution of blood by drawing the blood to the 0.3 mark in the red cell pipet and diluting to the 101 mark. The dilution factor is then 333.

2. For a patient who has severe anemia and in whom the red blood cell count is low, draw the blood up to the 1.0 mark and dilute to the 101 mark. The dilution factor is then 100.

3. Ensure that the diluting fluid is free from blood and other contamination.

4. Make certain that the pipets, hemocytometer, and cover glass are free from dirt, lint, and dried blood.

5. A red blood cell count takes longer to perform than a white count because of the larger number of cells. Therefore, proceed as quickly as possible once the cells have settled. Drying of the solution in the counting chamber causes inaccuracies in the final cell count.

6. If the red blood cells show agglutination when using Hayem's diluting fluid, report this to your supervisor so that the patient's doctor may be notified. This may be helpful in diagnosing the patient's condition. Proceed with the red blood cell count by diluting the blood with 0.85% (w/v) sodium chloride or Gower's solution.

7. The range of error for a manual red blood cell count usually falls within ±20%, with a minimum error of ±11% and a maximum error of ±30%.

THE BLOOD SMEAR AND WRIGHT'S STAIN

Three different types of blood smears are used in today's laboratory: (1) the cover-glass smear, (2) the wedge smear, and (3) the spun smear. The cover-glass smear is thought by many to be more satisfactory than the wedge smear. However, it is more time-consuming, and the technique is somewhat more difficult to master. The spun smear is used primarily in conjunction with automated differential counters, although it may be used in laboratories in which differentials are done manually by the technologists. Once the blood smear is made, it is stained with Wright's stain so that a differential white blood cell count and morphology study can be done. Blood smears using blood anticoagulated with EDTA should be made within 2 hours of blood collection.

Cover-Glass Method for Making Blood Smears

1. Obtain two clean cover glasses, 22 mm square and 0.13 to 0.17 mm thick (number 1 or 1.5).
2. Hold one cover glass by its two adjacent corners with the thumb and index finger of one hand.
3. Place a small drop of blood on this cover glass.
4. With the other hand, hold a second cover glass in the same manner as the first.
5. Gently place the second cover glass over the cover glass containing the drop of blood (with the drop of blood in between the two cover glasses), so that the two cover glasses, one on top of the other, form a 16-sided figure (Fig. 41). As soon as the two cover glasses come together, the blood begins to spread.
6. Just before the spreading of the blood is complete, separate the two cover

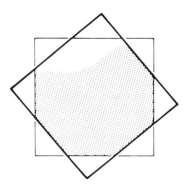

Fig. 41. Cover-glass method of making a blood smear.

glasses by a rapid, even, horizontal, lateral pull. Care should be taken to avoid squeezing together the cover glasses.
7. Allow the smears to air-dry completely.
8. The cover-glass smears are now ready for Wright staining.

DISCUSSION

1. The cover glasses must be scrupulously clean.
2. When obtaining blood from a fingertip puncture (or toe or heel), the skin must not touch the cover glass.
3. As soon as the drop of blood is placed on the cover glass, the two cover glasses should be brought together without delay. If the drop of blood sits for longer than 3 to 5 seconds, clumping of the platelets and white blood cells and rouleaux formation of the red blood cells occur.
4. Do not put too large a drop of blood on the cover glass. This results in smears too thick for accurate study.

Manual Method for Making Wedge Blood Smears

1. Obtain two clean glass slides, one spreader slide, and, if using anticoagulated blood, two applicator sticks or a plain microhematocrit tube. (The spreader slide is merely a glass slide with specially ground ends to ensure even spreading of the blood.)
2. If anticoagulated blood is used, hold two applicator sticks together and dip them into the tube of well-mixed blood (or fill a microhematocrit tube with blood). Carefully place a small drop of blood in the middle of the slide, approximately 1 cm from the end.
3. When using blood from the finger, toe, or heel, place a drop of blood on the slide as stated in the preceding description, being careful not to

touch the skin of the finger (toe or heel) with the slide.

4. Place the slide on a flat table top with the drop of blood on the right. (For left-handed people, it may be easier to reverse all techniques to the opposite hand.)

5. With the thumb and index finger of the left hand, hold the two left edges of the slide. With the right hand, hold the spreader slide with the thumb on the edge of one side and the other four fingers on the edge of the other slide (Fig. 42). Place the end of the spreader slide slightly in front of the drop of blood on the other slide. There should be an approximately 25° angle between the two slides (Fig. 43).

6. Draw the spreader slide back toward the drop of blood. As soon as the spreader slide comes in contact with the drop of blood, the blood begins to spread to the edge of the spreader slide. If this does not occur, wiggle the spreader slide a little until it does so. (Be careful that no blood gets in front of the slide.)

7. Keeping the spreader slide at a 25° angle and the edge of the spreader slide firmly against the horizontal slide, push the spreader slide rapidly over the entire length of the slide. This step should be performed at the moment when the blood has spread to within about ⅛ inch of the edges of the slide.

8. The blood smears should be dried quickly by waving them rapidly in the air. This prevents distortion of the red blood cells. The blood smears are now ready for Wright's stain.

DISCUSSION

1. The glass slides must be scrupulously clean.

2. As soon as the drop of blood is placed on the glass slide, the smear should be made without delay. Any delay whatsoever results in an abnormal distribution of the white blood cells, with many of the larger white blood cells accumulating at the thin edge of the smear. Rouleaux of the red blood cells and platelet clumping may also occur.

3. Common causes of a poor blood smear:
   A. Drop of blood too large or too small.
   B. Spreader slide pushed across the slide in a jerky manner.
   C. Failure to keep the entire edge of the spreader slide against the slide while making the smear.
   D. Failure to keep the spreader slide at a 25° angle with the slide. (Increasing the angle results in a thicker smear, whereas a smaller angle gives a thin smear.)
   E. Failure to push the spreader slide completely across the slide.

4. The Hemaprep automatic blood smearing instrument affords the technologist a semiautomated method for preparing consistently

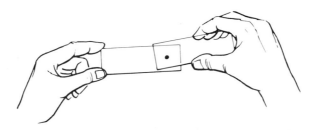

Fig. 42.   Method of holding slides for preparation of blood smear.

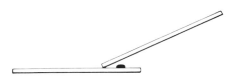

Fig. 43. Proper 25° angle for spreader slide.

good quality wedge smears. This instrument is described in Chapter 7.

Automated Spun Smear

The spun smear is prepared on an instrument called a spinner. A clean glass slide is placed on a platen, and three to four drops of blood are placed in the middle of the slide. When the top of the instrument is closed, the platen spins at high speed for a set amount of time. During this period, excess blood is thrown from the slide into a catch basin, and the resultant slide is completely covered with a thin monolayer of cells. The more sophisticated spinners contain an optical system. During spinning, a beam of light passes up through the glass slide onto a sensor. When the cells have separated the proper amount, the sensor detects this and the platen automatically stops spinning. In this way, spreading of the blood is consistent from one smear to the next, regardless of the patient's hematocrit.

Staining of Blood Smears

For best results, blood smears should be stained within 1 to 2 hours after they are made. The stain used for routine examination of blood and bone marrow smears is Wright's stain or Wright-Giemsa stain.

PRINCIPLE

Wright's stain is a polychromatic stain in that the dyes present in the stain produce multiple colors when applied to cells. Wright's stain is a mixture of methylene blue and eosin. In the manufacture of the stain, methylene blue is heated to form polychromed methylene blue. Eosin is then added to the polychromed methylene blue to form a precipitate. Addition of the precipitate to methanol then yields the commonly used Wright's stain. The quantities of polychromed methylene blue and eosin used in preparing the Wright's stain powder must be carefully controlled to yield a neutral compound dye and optimum staining results. In the staining process, when the buffer solution is added to the stain, ionization occurs, during which time the process of staining the cells takes place. The eosin ions are negatively charged and stain the basic components of the cells an orange to pink color. The acid structures of the cell are stained varying shades of blue to purple by the positively charged, basic, methylene blue ions. The neutral components of the cells are probably stained by both components of the dye. Because of the complexity of preparing the polychromed methylene blue, Wright's stain powder may vary slightly from one lot to another.

REAGENTS AND EQUIPMENT

1. Wright-Giemsa stain

Wright's stain powder	9.0 g
Giemsa stain powder	1.0 g
Glycerin	90 ml
Methanol (absolute, anhydrous, acetone-free)	2,910 ml

   (Mallinckrodt methanol is recommended for use in the Wright's stain.)

   Mix the preceding reagents in a large, tightly stoppered brown bottle. The stain should be allowed to age for approximately 30 days prior to use. During this time, the stain should be shaken once a day. Incubation at 37°C speeds the aging process. The stain must be freshly filtered before use (only filter a 1- or 2-day supply at a time).

2. Phosphate buffer (pH 6.4)

Anhydrous monobasic potassium phosphate (KH_2PO_4)	6.63 g
Anhydrous dibasic	

sodium phosphate   2.56 g
(Na$_2$HPO$_4$)

Distilled water   1,000 ml

The pH of the buffer solution should be within a pH range of 6.4 to 6.7, depending on the staining times and the Wright's stain or Wright-Giemsa stain used. If a more alkaline pH (than 6.4) is desired, it is prepared by decreasing the amount of monobasic potassium phosphate and increasing the amount of dibasic sodium phosphate. A pH of 6.7 is obtained by diluting 5.13 g of monobasic potassium phosphate and 4.12 g of dibasic sodium phosphate to 1,000 ml with distilled water. In place of the phosphate buffer, distilled water may be used. However, it is not advisable because the pH of water varies from day to day.

3. Methanol, Mallinckrodt (absolute, anhydrous, acetone-free).
4. Staining rack.

PROCEDURE

1. Place the air-dried blood smears on a level staining rack, with the smear side up.
2. Fix the smears by flooding the slides with methanol. Drain the excess methanol off the slides. (An alternative method is to dip the smears into a coplin jar containing methanol and then place the slides on the staining rack. However, the utmost care must be taken to change the methanol in the coplin jar several times a day and to keep the jar covered when not in use because methanol readily takes up water. If anhydrous copper sulfate is placed in the coplin jar, the uptake of water by the methanol is minimized.)
3. Flood the slides with Wright's stain and time for 4 minutes.
4. Without removing the Wright's stain, add an equal volume of phosphate buffer to the slide. Mix the two re-

agents on the slide by gently blowing back and forth over the solutions. A metallic green sheen should now form on top of this mixture. Time for 7 minutes.
5. Rinse the slide off thoroughly with a stream of tap water or distilled water.
6. Wipe the back of the slides with a piece of gauze to remove any stain.
7. Stand the slides up on end to air-dry. Never blot the smears dry.
8. A well-stained smear shows pink to orange red cells, dark purple nuclei in the lymphocytes and neutrophils, a lighter purple nucleus in the monocyte, bright orange granules in the eosinophil, dark blue granules in the basophil, and violet to purple platelets. The cytoplasm of the monocyte is a gray-blue with fine reddish granules. The neutrophil has a light pink cytoplasm with lilac granules, and the lymphocyte shows varying shades of blue cytoplasm.

DISCUSSION

1. Generally, when bone marrow smears are stained, the staining times must be increased.
2. The staining times for both peripheral blood and bone marrow smears vary from one laboratory to another. This is due to the Wright's stain and the pH of the buffer. Frequently, when a new lot of Wright's stain is used, it is necessary to change the staining times.
3. During staining, the phosphate buffer controls the pH of the stain. If the pH is too acid, those cells or cell parts taking up an acid dye stain well, whereas those cells that stain at a more alkaline pH appear pale. For example, eosinophils and red blood cells take up an acid dye, whereas nuclei and platelets prefer a more basic pH. Therefore, to stain all cells and cell parts well, the pH of the phosphate buffer is critical.

4. The staining rack must be exactly level to guard against uneven staining of the smear.
5. Insufficient washing of the smears when removing the stain and buffer mixture causes precipitate on the smear.
6. Leaving water on the smear after rinsing or prolonged rinsing causes the stain to fade.
7. If it is desirable to restain a slide, the original Wright's stain may be removed with methanol. Flood the smear with methanol and rinse with tap water as many times as necessary to remove the stain and then restain the slide according to the previously described procedure. This is not recommended, however. For best results, make a new smear.
8. For cover glass smears, after the stained smears have dried, mount the cover glass, blood side down, on a slide using a mounting medium.

DIFFERENTIAL CELL COUNT

The differential white blood cell count is performed to determine the relative number of each type of white blood cell present in the blood. At the same time, a study of red blood cell, white blood cell, and platelet morphology is done. A rough estimate of the platelet and white counts is also made. More information can be obtained from a detailed examination of the stained blood smear than from any other single laboratory test. In performing a complete blood count, the differential should be done last. In this way, examination of the smear may be used to double-check the white blood cell count, and a rough estimate of the hemoglobin, hematocrit, and red blood cell count may be made.

In disease states, a particular white blood cell type may show an absolute increase in number in the blood. Common diseases showing an increased number of a specified cell type are listed below.

1. Absolute increase in the number of neutrophils (neutrophilia):
   A. Appendicitis
   B. Myelogenous leukemia
   C. Bacterial infections
2. Absolute increase in the number of eosinophils (eosinophilia):
   A. Allergenic reactions
   B. Allergies
   C. Scarlet fever
   D. Parasitic infestations
   E. Eosinophilic leukemia
3. Absolute increase in the number of lymphocytes (lymphocytosis):
   A. Viral infections
   B. Whooping cough
   C. Infectious mononucleosis
   D. Lymphocytic leukemia
4. Absolute increase in the number of monocytes (monocytosis):
   A. Brucellosis
   B. Tuberculosis
   C. Monocytic leukemia
   D. Subacute bacterial endocarditis
   E. Typhoid
   F. Rickettsial infections
   G. Collagen disease
   H. Hodgkin's disease
   I. Gaucher's disease

Procedure for Examination of the Stained Blood Smear

1. Examine the blood smear using the low-power (10×) objective.
   A. The white blood cells should be evenly distributed over the smear.
   B. Estimate the white blood cell count (by noting the number of white blood cells in relation to the number of red blood cells). It should agree with the test result obtained. If it does not, the white count should be repeated.
   C. Examine the thin peripheral edge of the smear if a wedge-type smear is being used. If there is an increased number of white cells in this area, the differential cell count is inaccurate. Most of the

cells at the edge of the smear are the larger white blood cells, namely, neutrophils and monocytes. This, therefore, shows poor distribution of white blood cell types in the smear. If there are clumps of platelets in this area, the smear then shows a decrease in platelets. In such situations, the blood smear should be discarded and another made.

D. In scanning the blood smear, it is important to note anything unusual or irregular, such as large, abnormal-looking cells or rouleaux formation of the red blood cells.

E. Choose that portion of the blood smear where there is only a slight overlapping of the red blood cells. Place a drop of oil on the slide and carefully change to the oil immersion objective (100×).

2. Perform the differential cell count and examine the white blood cell morphology.

A. Begin in the thin area of the slide where the red blood cells are slightly overlapping. Gradually move the slide as shown in Figure 44. Count each white blood cell seen and record on a differential cell counter until 100 white blood cells have been counted. If any nucleated red blood cells are seen during the differential count, enumerate them on a separate counter. These cells are not to be included in the 100-cell differential count.

B. While counting the white blood cells, make a note of any abnormalities present in the cells.

3. Examine the red blood cell morphology in a thin area of the slide where the red blood cells either do not overlap or only slightly overlap. Note any variations from normal and classify them as slight, moderate, or marked (or 1+, 2+, and so on).

4. Examine the platelets on the smear for morphology and number present. Using the same fields on various parts of the smear, as in step No. 3 for the red blood cell morphology, determine the approximate number of platelets per field. A normal blood smear (normal red blood cell count and normal platelet count) should show approximately 8 to 20 platelets per field in this area. One method for reporting platelet estimates is to determine the average number of platelets per field (using 5 to 10 different fields) and to multiply this result by 20,000 (for a wedge-type smear) to obtain a rough estimate of the platelet count. If the platelet estimate is:

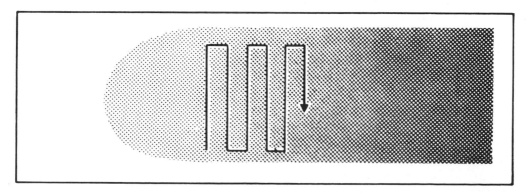

Fig. 44. Pathway for the differential cell count.

Platelet Estimate of	Report Platelet Estimate as:
0–49,000/μl	Marked decrease
50,000–99,000	Moderate decrease
100,000–149,000	Mild decrease
150,000–199,000	Low normal
200,000–399,000	Plentiful
400,000–599,000	Mild increase
600,000–800,000	Moderate increase
Above 800,000	Marked increase

A patient with a red blood cell count of 5 million per μl and a platelet count of 300,000 per μl has 30 platelets for every 500 red blood cells. This must be kept in mind when performing a platelet estimate and adjustments made when the patient's red count is greater or less than 5 million per μl. For example, if a patient's red count is 2.5 million per μl and the platelet count is 300,000 per μl, there are 30 platelets for every 250 red blood cells, or 60 platelets for every 500 red blood cells. It is, therefore, helpful to know the patient's red blood cell count when doing a platelet estimate. (If the red count is not readily available, the patient's hemoglobin or hematocrit generally suffices.)

DISCUSSION

1. The differential white count gives the relative number of each type of white blood cell. At times, however, it is helpful to know the actual number of each white blood cell type per microliter of blood. This is referred to as the absolute count and is calculated as follows:

> Absolute number of cells/μl = % of cell type in differential × white blood cell count.

The absolute white blood cell count is not used often in the laboratory. The technologist, however, should be familiar with this procedure.

2. When studying a stained smear, the following outline should be followed:
   A. White blood cells.
      1) Estimate number present.
      2) Differential count.
      3) Examine for morphologic abnormalities.
   B. Red blood cells.
      1) Examine for:
         a. Size.
         b. Shape.
         c. Relative hemoglobin content.
         d. Polychromatophilia.
         e. Inclusions.
         f. Rouleaux formation or agglutination.
   C. Platelets.
      1) Estimate number present.
      2) Examine for morphologic abnormalities.

3. When studying a stained smear, do not progress too far into the thick area of the slide. The morphologic characteristics of the cells are difficult to distinguish in this area. Also, do not use the thin edge of the smear in which the red blood cells appear completely filled with hemoglobin and show no area of central pallor. The cells in this area are generally distorted and do not show a true morphologic picture.

4. When the white count is below 1,000 per μl, it is difficult to find many white blood cells on the stained smear. In this situation, a differential is usually performed by counting 50 white blood cells. A notation on the report must then be made that only 50 white blood cells were counted.

5. In a differential showing:
   A. Over 10% eosinophils,
   B. Over 2% basophils,
   C. Over 12% monocytes, or
   D. More lymphocytes than neutrophils (except in children),
   200 white blood cells should be counted. The results are then divided by 2 and a note made on the report that 200 white blood cells were counted.

6. Before reporting platelets as being decreased, scan the slide on low

power, especially the feathered edge, for platelet clumps. Also recheck the tube of blood for a clot.

7. When the differential count is completed, the results may show the presence of immature white blood cells. This is termed *a shift to the left* and is found in leukemias and infections. A *shift to the right* refers to an increased number of hypersegmented neutrophils.

8. The technical error in the differential cell count has been described at ± 10 to $\pm 15\%$.

9. Never hesitate to ask questions concerning the morphology or the identification of cells. The differential is the most difficult laboratory test to learn. In fact, learning about cells and their morphologic features is a process that continues for as long as you perform differentials.

RED BLOOD CELL INDICES

The red blood cell indices are used to define the size and hemoglobin content of the red blood cell. They consist of the mean corpuscular volume (MCV), mean corpuscular hemoglobin (MCH), and mean corpuscular hemoglobin concentration (MCHC). The red blood cell indices are used as an aid in differentiating anemias. When these indices are combined with an examination of the red blood cells on the stained smear, a clear picture of red blood cell morphology may be obtained.

The derivation of the formulas for the calculation of red blood cell indices is given on the following pages. It is not important that the student memorize how to derive these formulas, but he should be aware of what the equations mean. The size of the individual red blood cell is small, and the amount of hemoglobin in a single cell is rather minute.

Mean Corpuscular Volume (MCV)

The MCV indicates the average volume of the red blood cells.

$$MCV = \frac{\text{Volume of red blood cells in femtoliters (fl)/}\mu\text{l of blood}}{\text{Red blood cells/}\mu\text{l of blood}}$$

If:

Hematocrit = 45% (or 0.45)

Red blood cell count = 5,000,000/μl
(or $5.0 \times 10^6/\mu$l)

$1 \mu l = 10^9$ fl

Then:

$$MCV = \frac{0.45 \times 10^9 \text{ fl/}\mu\text{l}}{5.0 \times 10^6/\mu\text{l}}$$
$$= \frac{45 \times 10 \text{ fl}}{5}$$
$$= 90 \text{ fl}$$

Therefore, the formula:

$$MCV = \frac{\text{Hematocrit} \times 10}{\text{Red blood cell count in millions}} \text{ fl}$$

Normal value for the MCV: 80–97 fl

DISCUSSION

The MCV indicates whether the red blood cells appear normocytic, microcytic, or macrocytic. If the MCV is less than 80 fl, the red blood cells are microcytic. If the MCV is greater than 97 fl, the red blood cells are macrocytic. If the MCV is within the normal range, the red blood cells are normocytic.

Mean Corpuscular Hemoglobin Concentration (MCHC)

The MCHC is an expression of the average concentration of hemoglobin in the red blood cells. It gives the ratio of the weight of hemoglobin to the volume of the red blood cell.

$$MCHC = \frac{\text{Hemoglobin in g/dl}}{\text{Hematocrit/dl}}$$
$\times 100$ (to convert to %)

If:

Hemoglobin = 15.0 g/dl
Hematocrit = 45%

Then:

$$MCHC = \frac{15.0 \text{ g/dl} \times 100}{45 \text{ volumes/dl}} \%$$
$$= 33\%$$

Therefore, the formula:

$$MCHC = \frac{Hemoglobin \times 100}{Hematocrit}\%$$

Normal value for the MCHC: 32–36%

DISCUSSION

The MCHC indicates whether the red blood cells are normochromic, hypochromic, or hyperchromic. An MCHC below 32% indicates hypochromia, an MCHC above 36% indicates hyperchromia, and red blood cells with a normal MCHC are termed normochromic. Please note that an MCHC above 38% should not occur. Such a result is usually due to incorrect calculation of the MCHC, or the patient's red blood cells may be agglutinated (cold agglutinin), thereby causing a falsely low red blood cell count (the hematocrit may also be falsely low if measured by an electronic cell counter).

Mean Corpuscular Hemoglobin (MCH)

The MCH indicates the average weight of hemoglobin in the red blood cell.

$$MCH = \frac{\text{Weight of hemoglobin in 1 } \mu l \text{ of blood}}{\text{Number of red blood cells in 1 } \mu l \text{ of blood}}$$

If:

1 g = 10^{12} pg

1 ml = 10^3 μl

Then:

Weight (in pg) of hemoglobin in 1 μl of blood

$$= \frac{Hemoglobin \times 10^{12} \text{ pg}}{100 \times 10^3 \text{ } \mu l}$$
$$= Hemoglobin \times 10^7 \text{ pg/}\mu l$$

If:

Hemoglobin = 15.0 g/dl
Red blood cell count = 5,000,000/μl

Then:

$$MCH = \frac{15 \times 10^7 \text{ pg/}\mu l}{5 \times 10^6 \text{ } \mu l}$$
$$= \frac{15 \times 10 \text{ pg}}{5}$$
$$= 30 \text{ pg}$$

Therefore, the formula:

$$MCH = \frac{Hemoglobin \times 10}{Red \text{ blood cell count in millions}} \text{ pg}$$

Normal value for the MCH: 27–31 pg

DISCUSSION

The MCH indicates the amount of hemoglobin in the red blood cell and should always correlate with the MCV and MCHC. An MCH lower than 27 pg is found in microcytic anemia and also with normocytic, hypochromic red blood cells. An elevated MCH occurs in macrocytic anemias and in some cases of spherocytosis in which hyperchromia may be present.

Examples of Red Blood Cell Indices with Corresponding Red Blood Cell Morphology

1. $MCV = \dfrac{41 \times 10}{4.5} = 91 \text{ fl}$

   $MCH = \dfrac{14.0 \times 10}{4.5} = 31 \text{ pg}$

   $MCHC = \dfrac{14.0 \times 100}{41} = 34\%$

The red blood cells are normocytic and normochromic.

2. $MCV = \dfrac{30 \times 10}{4.5} = 67 \text{ fl}$

   $MCH = \dfrac{9.8 \times 10}{4.5} = 22 \text{ pg}$

   $MCHC = \dfrac{9.8 \times 100}{30} = 33\%$

The red blood cells are microcytic and normochromic.

3. $MCV = \dfrac{30 \times 10}{4.5} = 67 \text{ fl}$

   $MCH = \dfrac{9.0 \times 10}{4.5} = 20 \text{ pg}$

   $MCHC = \dfrac{9.0 \times 100}{30} = 30\%$

The red blood cells are microcytic and hypochromic.

4. $\text{MCV} = \dfrac{45 \times 10}{4.0} = 113 \text{ fl}$

$\text{MCH} = \dfrac{15.0 \times 10}{4.0} = 38 \text{ pg}$

$\text{MCHC} = \dfrac{15.0 \times 100}{45} = 33\%$

The red blood cells are macrocytic and normochromic.

5. $\text{MCV} = \dfrac{41 \times 10}{4.5} = 91 \text{ fl}$

$\text{MCH} = \dfrac{11.8 \times 10}{4.5} = 26 \text{ pg}$

$\text{MCHC} = \dfrac{11.8 \times 100}{41} = 29\%$

The red blood cells are normocytic and hypochromic.

ERYTHROCYTE SEDIMENTATION RATE

When anticoagulated whole blood is allowed to stand for a period of time, the red blood cells settle out from the plasma. The rate at which the red blood cells fall is known as the *erythrocyte sedimentation rate* (ESR).

The ESR is affected mainly by three factors: erythrocytes, plasma, and mechanical and technical factors.

ERYTHROCYTES

A factor of chief importance in determining the rate of fall of the red blood cells is the size or mass of the falling particle. The larger the particle, the faster its rate

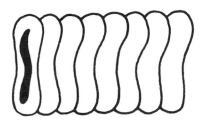

Fig. 45. Rouleaux formation of the red blood cells.

of fall. In normal blood, the red blood cells remain more or less separated from each other. They are negatively charged and, therefore, repel each other. In certain diseases, however, plasma proteins, namely fibrinogen and globulin, may be altered, causing rouleaux formation (Fig. 45). This leads to a larger mass and an increased sedimentation velocity. Agglutination of the red blood cells due to changes in the erythrocyte surface also leads to an increased red blood cell mass and a more rapid sedimentation rate. Macrocytes tend to settle more rapidly than microcytes. Red blood cells that show an alteration in their shape, such as sickle cells and spherocytes, are unable to agglutinate or form rouleaux and their sedimentation rate is decreased (normal). In severe anemia, the ESR is markedly elevated. The concentration of the erythrocytes in the blood is decreased. Therefore, they settle out more easily and rapidly. (A chart has been devised by Wintrobe and Landsberg to correct for anemia. This graph utilizes the patient's hematocrit and theoretically yields the ESR value that results when the patient is not anemic. This value is then termed the *corrected ESR*. There are, however, serious objections to this procedure, and it is not used too commonly.) In polycythemia, in which the red blood cell count is high, the ESR is normal.

PLASMA COMPOSITION

The plasma composition is the single most important factor determining the ESR. Rouleaux and aggregation of the red blood cells are affected mainly by the levels of fibrinogen, alpha-1 globulin, and alpha-2 globulin, increasing as these three plasma protein levels are increased in the blood.

MECHANICAL AND TECHNICAL FACTORS

It is important that the ESR tube be exactly perpendicular. A tilt of 3° can cause errors up to 30%. Also, the rack holding the tubes should not be subject to any movement or vibration. Minor, everyday variations in room temperature do not significantly affect the ESR. With large changes in temperature, however, the sedimentation rate increases as the temperature increases. The length and inner diameter of the ESR tube also affect the final test results.

SIGNIFICANCE OF THE ERYTHROCYTE SEDIMENTATION RATE

Children normally have a lower ESR than adults. In adults over 60 years of age, the ESR is frequently higher than the normal adult levels. The ESR reflects mainly changes in the plasma proteins that accompany most of the acute and chronic infections, tumors, and degenerative diseases. It may be used to follow the progress of certain diseases such as tuberculosis and rheumatism. The ESR represents a nonspecific response to tissue damage and denotes the presence of disease, but not its severity. An elevated ESR may be found in pregnancy (after the third month), acute and chronic infections, rheumatic fever, rheumatoid arthritis, myocardial infarction, nephrosis, acute hepatitis, menstruation, tuberculosis, macroglobulinemia, cryoglobulinemia, hypothyroidism, and hyperthyroidism.

Modified Westergren Method

REFERENCES

Gambino, R.S., DiRe, J.J., Monteleone, M., and Budd, D.C.: The Westergren sedimentation rate, using K_3EDTA, Techn. Bull. Regist. Med. Techn., 35, 1, 1965.

National Committee for Clinical Laboratory Standards: Standardized Method for the Human Erythrocyte Sedimentation Rate (ESR) Test, National Committee for Clinical Laboratory Standards, Villanova, Pa., 1977.

REAGENTS AND EQUIPMENT

1. Sodium chloride, 0.85% (w/v).
2. Westergren pipet, calibrated in millimeters (Fig. 46).
3. Westergren pipet rack.

SPECIMEN

Whole blood, 3 ml, using EDTA as the anticoagulant.

PRINCIPLE

Well-mixed, whole blood is diluted with 0.85% sodium chloride, placed in a Westergren pipet, and allowed to stand for exactly 1 hour. The number of millimeters the red blood cells fall during this timed period constitutes the ESR. The normal values for the modified Westergren ESR are 0–20 mm per hour for women, 0–15 mm per hour for men, and 0–10 mm per hour for children.

PROCEDURE

1. Mix the whole blood for at least 2 minutes on a rotator. (The blood should be at room temperature.)
2. Place 0.5 ml of 0.85% sodium chloride in a plain 13 × 100 mm test tube.
3. Add 2.0 ml of well-mixed, whole blood to the test tube.
4. Mix the tube for 2 minutes.
5. Make certain that the Westergren ESR rack is exactly level.
6. Fill the Westergren pipet to exactly the 0 mark, making certain there are no air bubbles in the blood.
7. Place the pipet in the rack. Be certain the pipet fits snugly and evenly into the grooves provided for it.
8. Allow the pipet to stand for exactly 60 minutes.
9. At the end of 60 minutes, record the number of millimeters that the red blood cells have fallen. This result is

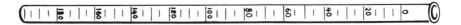

Fig. 46. Westergren pipet.

the erythrocyte sedimentation rate in millimeters per hour.

Wintrobe and Landsberg Method

REFERENCE

Davidsohn, I., and Nelson, D.A.: The blood. Sedimentation rate of erythrocytes. In: *Todd-Sanford Clinical Diagnosis by Laboratory Methods*, 15th ed., Davidsohn, I. and Henry, J.B., Eds., W.B. Saunders Co., Philadelphia, 1974 (15th ed. only).

REAGENTS AND EQUIPMENT

1. Wintrobe tube, calibrated in millimeters (Fig. 47).
2. Wintrobe pipet rack.
3. Disposable capillary pipet.

SPECIMEN

Whole blood, 1 ml, using EDTA or ammonium-potassium oxalate as the anticoagulant.

PRINCIPLE

Well-mixed, whole blood is placed in a Wintrobe tube and allowed to stand for 1 hour. The number of millimeters that the red blood cells fall during this time constitutes the ESR. In the Wintrobe and Landsberg method, normal values for women are 0–20 mm per hour and for men are 0–9 mm per hour.

PROCEDURE

1. Mix the whole blood for at least 2 minutes on a rotator. (Make certain the blood is at room temperature.)
2. With a capillary pipet, fill the Wintrobe tube to the 0 mark.
3. Place the tube in an exactly vertical position in the rack. Time for 60 minutes.
4. At the end of 60 minutes, record the level of the erythrocyte column. This

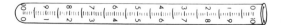

Fig. 47. Wintrobe sedimentation tube.

result is the erythrocyte sedimentation rate in millimeters per hour.

DISCUSSION

1. The sedimentation of red blood cells takes place in three stages. In the first stage, there is rouleaux formation and the sedimentation rate is slight. During the second phase, sedimentation occurs at a fairly rapid rate. In stage three, the sedimentation rate is slow because of the accumulation of red blood cells in the bottom of the tube.
2. Although care may be taken in filling the sedimentation tube to the 0 mark, occasionally the upper level of the blood may only reach the 1- or 2-mm mark. In such a case, care should be taken in reading the final result. Subtract these 1 or 2 mm from the final result. For example, if the sedimentation tube is filled to the 2-mm mark and the red blood cells fall to the 18-mm mark, the ESR is reported as 16 mm per hour. If the level of blood falls below the 5-mm mark, the test should be repeated to ensure that valid results are obtained.
3. All sedimentation racks should be equipped with leveling screws and a spirit level.
4. Sources of error:
   A. If the concentration of the anticoagulant is greater than recommended, the ESR will be falsely low.
   B. If the ESR stands for more than 60 minutes, the results will be falsely elevated. If the test is timed for less than 60 minutes, falsely low values are obtained.
   C. A marked increase (or decrease) in room temperature leads to increased (or decreased) ESR results.
   D. Tilting of the ESR tube increases the sedimentation rate.

E. Bubbles in the blood lead to false results.

F. Fibrin clots present in the blood invalidate the test results.

G. The ESR should be set up within 2 hours of blood collection. If EDTA is used as the anticoagulant, the test must be set up within 6 hours if the blood has been refrigerated.

5. The modified Westergren method is considered the more superior of the two procedures described.

6. A second type of Westergren ESR tube currently being used contains a cotton plug located at the top of the 0-mm mark. The cotton plug prevents blood from being drawn up into the tube beyond the 0 mark. In this method, an inexpensive rubber bulb is used to draw the diluted blood up into the ESR tube. The excess blood drawn up is absorbed into the cotton plug. When the pipetting bulb is removed from the tube, the blood remains in the ESR tube, being prevented from leaking out of the tube by the cotton plug at the top of the column of blood. (Based on comparative studies using the unplugged Westergren ESR tube as a standard, the cotton plug does not appear to have any effect on the ESR results.) This pipet, manufactured by Chase Instruments, Poultney, Vermont, is the same size that has been recommended by the National Committee for Clinical Laboratory Standards. It affords the technologist a quick method for setting up the ESR without the necessity of using more cumbersome pipet fillers. Also, because of the cotton plug, the chances of the blood leaking out of the ESR tube while it is standing are minimal.

7. The National Committee for Clinical Laboratory Standards has set specific dimensions for the pipets to be used for the Westergren method of determining the ESR. The pipet should be 300 mm long (± 0.5 mm), have an external diameter of 5.5 mm (± 0.5 mm), and should have an internal bore of 2.5 mm (± 0.15 mm), with the bore having a uniformity of ± 0.05 mm. The length of the graduated scale on the pipet should be 200 mm (± 0.35 mm). The internal bore and the length of the graduated scale on the pipet are critical measurements. Any tube of a different size in these two dimensions will generally give results different from those obtained using the standard-sized pipet.

8. Blood for the Westergren ESR may be collected in 0.11 M sodium citrate. If this anticoagulant is used, obtain the blood specimen and immediately mix exactly 4 volumes of whole blood with 1 volume of sodium citrate. Mix the blood well. When performing the ESR, the blood should not be mixed with the 0.85% w/v sodium chloride solution as previously described because the blood has been diluted with the sodium citrate anticoagulant.

RETICULOCYTE COUNT

The red blood cell goes through six stages of development: pronormoblast, basophilic normoblast, polychromatophilic normoblast, orthochromic normoblast, reticulocyte, and mature red blood cell. The first four stages are normally confined to the bone marrow. The reticulocyte, however, is found in both the bone marrow and peripheral blood. In the bone marrow, it spends approximately 2 days maturing and is then released into the blood, where it matures for another day before becoming a mature red blood cell.

The reticulocyte count is an important diagnostic tool. It is a relatively accurate reflection of the amount of effective red blood cell production taking place in the bone marrow. Since the life span of a red blood cell is 120 days, ± 20 days, the bone marrow replaces approximately 1% of the adult red blood cells every day. The normal values for a reticulocyte count are, therefore, 0.5 to 1.5%. The reticulocyte count is expressed as the number of reticulocytes present per 100 red blood cells (in %). A decreased reticulocyte count is found in aplastic anemia and in conditions in which the bone marrow is not producing red blood cells. Increased reticulocyte counts are found in hemolytic anemias, individuals with iron deficiency anemias receiving iron therapy, thalassemia, sideroblastic anemia, and acute and chronic blood loss.

CORRECTED RETICULOCYTE COUNT

An accurate reticulocyte count should reflect the total production of red blood cells regardless of the concentration of red blood cells in the blood (red blood cell count). As an example, compare the following two patients. Patient No. 1 has a hematocrit of 42% and a reticulocyte count of 1.0%. Patient No. 2 has a hematocrit of 21% and a reticulocyte count of 2.0%. Patient No. 2, theoretically, has half as many red blood cells as patient No. 1 but has the same number of reticulocytes as patient No. 1 because the reticulocytes are diluted by only half the number of red blood cells, as in patient No. 1. To compensate for this, a corrected reticulocyte count is calculated based on a normal hematocrit of 42% for women and 45% for men. The formula for this correction follows.

$$\begin{array}{l} \text{Corrected} \\ \text{reticulocyte} \\ \text{count in \%} \end{array} = \dfrac{\begin{array}{c}\text{Patient's}\\\text{hematocrit}\end{array}}{\begin{array}{c}\text{Normal}\\\text{hematocrit}\end{array}} \times \begin{array}{l}\text{Reticulocyte}\\\text{count in \%}\end{array}$$

In addition to correcting a reticulocyte count for an abnormally low hematocrit, consideration is also given to the presence of marrow reticulocytes present in the peripheral blood. In this circumstance, the reticulocyte production index is calculated. As previously stated, the reticulocytes spend approximately 2 days in the bone marrow before being released into the blood. In certain situations, these marrow reticulocytes are released directly into the blood prior to maturation in the bone marrow. This is detected by nucleated red blood cells and/or polychromatophilic macrocytes ("shift" cells) present in the circulating blood. To correct for this reticulocyte maturation delay, the reticulocyte production index is calculated by dividing the corrected reticulocyte count by two. In patients showing no nucleated red cells or "shift" cells, the corrected reticulocyte count is divided by one (normal reticulocyte maturation time), and the reticulocyte production index is equal to the corrected reticulocyte count.

In conditions of anemia, the bone marrow normally shows a response to this anemia by increasing red blood cell production. At the same time, the reticulocyte count in the blood also is increased. See Table 2 for the normal bone marrow response to a decreased hematocrit.

REAGENTS AND EQUIPMENT

1. Reticulocyte stain. Any of the following staining solutions may be employed:

   A. New methylene blue N solution

Sodium chloride	0.8 g
Potassium oxalate	1.4 g
New methylene blue N	0.5 g
Distilled water	100 ml

   B. Brilliant cresyl blue solution

Brilliant cresyl blue	1.0 g
Sodium chloride, 0.85% (w/v)	99 ml

   Filter both of the preceding staining solutions prior to use.

TABLE 2. NORMAL BONE MARROW RESPONSE TO ANEMIA

HEMATOCRIT	RETICULOCYTE COUNT	CORRECTED RETICULOCYTE COUNT
45	1.0%	1.0%
35	6.5%	2–3%
25	14.0%	3–5%
15	24.0%	3–5%

2. Glass slides.
3. Applicator sticks or microhematocrit tubes.
4. Microscope.

SPECIMEN

Whole blood (1 ml), using EDTA, heparin, or ammonium-potassium oxalate as the anticoagulant. Capillary blood from the finger, toe, or heel may also be used.

PRINCIPLE

After the orthochromic normoblast loses its nucleus, a small amount of RNA remains in the red blood cell, and the cell is known as a reticulocyte. To detect the presence of this RNA, the red blood cells must be stained while they are still living. This process is called *supravital staining*. After the cells have been stained by either new methylene blue N or brilliant cresyl blue, the number of reticulocytes in 1,000 red blood cells is determined. This number is divided by 10 to obtain the reticulocyte count in percent.

PROCEDURE

1. Place three drops of filtered reticulocyte stain in a small test tube.
2. Add three drops of blood to the test tube containing the stain. (Ensure that the blood specimen is well mixed.)
3. Mix the tube contents and allow to stand for about 15 minutes, or incubate the specimen at 37°C for 15 minutes. This allows the reticulocytes adequate time to take up the stain.
4. At the end of 15 minutes, mix the contents of the tube well.
5. Using applicator sticks or a microhematocrit tube, place a drop of the mixture on each of three slides and make smears.
6. Stain with Wright's stain, using the same method that was previously described for routine blood smears. (This step is not necessary and may

be omitted. See step No. 9, below, for an explanation.)
7. Allow the smears to air-dry.
8. Place the first slide on the microscope stage and, using the low-power objective (10×), find an area in the thin portion of the smear in which the red blood cells are evenly distributed and are not touching each other. Carefully change to the oil immersion objective (100×) and further locate an area in which there are approximately 100 to 200 red blood cells per oil immersion field.
9. As soon as the proper area is selected, the reticulocytes may be counted. If the smear has not been counterstained with Wright's stain, the red blood cells are a light to medium green in color. The RNA present in the reticulocytes stains a deep blue. When counterstaining with Wright's stain, the red blood cells are pink, whereas the RNA in the reticulocytes stains a deep purple. The reticulum may be abundant or sparse, depending on the cell's stage of development. The youngest reticulocyte shows a larger amount of RNA (Fig. 48A), whereas the more mature reticulocyte shows only a small amount of RNA (Fig. 48C). Count all of the red blood cells in the first field on one cell counter. At the same time, enumerate the reticulocytes (Fig. 49) in the same field with a second cell counter. Move the slide as described in the section entitled Differential Cell Count until all reticulocytes in 1,000 red cells have been counted.
10. A second technologist should repeat the reticulocyte count in the same manner as described in step 9 on the second reticulocyte smear. The two results should agree within ±20% of each other. If they do not, repeat the reticulocyte count on the third smear.
11. Average the two results and calculate

A   B   C

Fig. 48.   Stages of maturation in the reticulocyte.

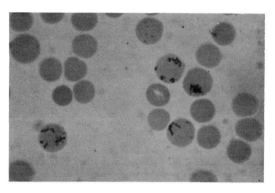

Fig. 49.   Reticulocytes. (Supravital staining of the red blood cells with new methylene blue N.) (Magnification ×1000.)

the reticulocyte count as shown below.

$$\% \text{ Reticulocytes} = \frac{\begin{array}{c}\text{Number of reticulocytes}\\\text{counted in 1,000}\\\text{red blood cells}\end{array}}{10}$$

12. Calculate the corrected reticulocyte count. If marrow reticulocytes or nucleated red blood cells are present, also calculate the reticulocyte production index.

DISCUSSION

1. There are various methods in use for mixing the stain and blood for a reticulocyte count: (1) A microhematocrit tube is one-third filled with blood, to which is added an equal amount of stain. This mixture is rotated back and forth in the hematocrit tube, allowed to stand for 15 minutes, remixed, placed on slides, and smears are made. (2) Blood is drawn up to the 1.0 mark in the white-cell pipet. Wipe off the outside of the pipet and, to have a space at the tip of the pipet, allow the blood to run up a short distance into the pipet bulb. Draw stain up to the 1.0 mark. Remove the tip of the pipet from the bottle of stain and draw the stain up into the bulb of the pipet to mix with the blood. (The bulb of the pipet is not full, but contains an equal volume each of blood and stain.) Mix the contents of the pipet, allow to stand for 15 minutes, remix, and make smears.

2. The blood-to-stain ratio does not have to be exactly equal. For best results, a larger proportion of blood should be added to the stain when the patient's hematocrit is low. Add a smaller amount of blood to the stain when the patient has an unusually high hematocrit.

3. The time allowed for staining of the reticulocyte is not critical. It should, however, never be less than 5 minutes.

4. It is extremely important that the blood and stain be mixed well prior to making smears. The reticulocytes have a lower specific gravity than mature red blood cells and, therefore, settle on top of the red blood cells in the mixture.

5. Each clinical laboratory may show slight alterations in the reticulocyte method, but all are based on the same general principles as described here. Also, corrections for the hematocrit are not carried out in all laboratories.

6. Red blood cells are frequently noted on the reticulocyte smear that contain areas which are highly refractile.

These cells should not be confused with reticulocytes. This condition is probably due to moisture in the air and poor drying of the smear.

7. The presence of high concentrations of glucose in the blood causes the reticulocytes to be poorly stained.

8. New methylene blue N is preferred to brilliant cresyl blue as a reticulocyte stain because of the inconsistent staining properties of the latter.

9. The range of error in the reticulocyte count varies, depending on the number of reticulocytes counted. Using the previously outlined procedure, there is an error of approximately ±25% in the reticulocyte counts within the normal range. This decreases to ±10% in a reticulocyte count of 5% and decreases even further as the uncorrected reticulocyte count increases.

10. There are several methods of counting reticulocytes once the smears have been made: (1) One procedure utilizes the Miller disk, which is placed inside the microscope eyepiece. This disk consists of two squares, as shown in Figure 51. The area of the smaller square (B) is one ninth that of square A. When employing this method to count reticulocytes, the red blood cells in square B are counted in successive fields on the slide until a total of 500 red blood cells have been counted. At the same time, the reticulocytes in square A are enumerated. At the completion of the count, theoretically, the reticulocytes contained in 4,500 red blood cells have been counted. The number of reticulocytes obtained in this way is divided by 45, to obtain the percentage of reticulocytes present in the blood. The count is also performed in duplicate, using a second smear, and the results are averaged to obtain the test value. This method is somewhat time-consuming. (2) Place a small "window" in the eyepiece of the microscope. This makes the field smaller and the counting of cells easier. (Cut out a round piece of paper the same diameter as the eyepiece and cut a square hole in the center. Unscrew the top lens of the eyepiece, insert the paper, and replace the top lens.) (3) For reticulocyte counts less than 10%, count at least 100 reticulocytes (except in extremely low counts where this would not be practical). Instead of counting the number of red blood cells in every field, count the red blood cells in every 8 to 10 fields and also keep track of the number of fields examined. Calculate the reticulocyte count as follows:

$$\frac{\text{Total number of RBCs counted}}{\text{Number of fields in which RBCs were counted}} \times \frac{\text{Total number}}{\text{of fields}} = \frac{\text{Total number}}{\text{of RBCs}}$$
$$\text{examined} \qquad \text{examined}$$

$$\% \text{ Reticulocytes} = \frac{\text{Number of reticulocytes counted}}{\text{Total number of RBCs examined}} \times 100$$

(4) Use of 15× eyepieces (instead of 10×) makes the field smaller and, at

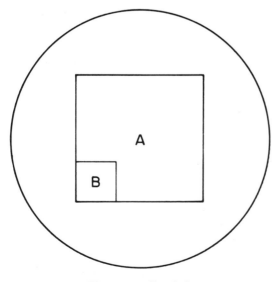

Fig. 51. Miller disk.

the same time, enables the technologist to see the reticulocytes much more clearly.

11. There are several red blood cell inclusions that are stained by the new methylene blue N and brilliant cresyl blue stains, in addition to the RNA of the reticulocytes. Howell-Jolly bodies appear as one, sometimes two, round, deep-purple-staining structures. Heinz bodies stain a light blue-green and are usually present at the peripheral edge of the red blood cell (Fig. 50). Pappenheimer bodies are most often confused with reticulocytes and are the most difficult to distinguish from reticulocytes. These purple-staining iron deposits generally appear as several granules in a small cluster. If Pappenheimer bodies are suspected, a Wright-stained smear may be examined to verify their presence.

PLATELET COUNT

Platelet counts are of great importance in helping to diagnose bleeding disorders. As stated previously, platelets function primarily in hemostasis (the stoppage of bleeding) and in maintaining capillary integrity (injuries to capillary walls are plugged by the platelets to inhibit bleeding and to maintain the sealing function of the capillary walls).

The normal range for the platelet count is 150,000 to 400,000 per μl. An increased platelet count, *thrombocytosis*, is found in polycythemia vera, idiopathic thrombocythemia, chronic myelogenous leukemia, and following a splenectomy. A decreased platelet count, *thrombocytopenia*, occurs in thrombocytopenia purpura, aplastic anemia, acute leukemia, Gaucher's disease, pernicious anemia, and sometimes following chemotherapy and radiation therapy. Prolonged bleeding time and poor clot retraction are found when there is marked thrombocytopenia.

Platelets are difficult to count. They are small, disintegrate easily, and are hard to distinguish from dirt. They readily adhere to each other (aggregation) and also become easily attached to any foreign body (adhesiveness). The use of EDTA as an anticoagulant helps to decrease the clumping of platelets. Although fingertip (or toe or heel) blood may be used, the results are generally less satisfactory and significantly lower than platelet counts performed on venous blood.

Direct Methods for Platelet Counts

There are three general methods for the direct counting of platelets. The Rees and Ecker method employs the use of the standard light microscope. The phase microscope is employed in the Brecker-Cronkite method, and an electronic cell counter is the third procedure for counting platelets.

Rees and Ecker Method

REFERENCE

Davidsohn, I., and Nelson, D.A.: The blood. Platelet count. In: *Todd-Sanford Clinical Diagnosis by Laboratory Methods*, 15th ed., Davidsohn, I., and Henry, J.B., Eds., W.B. Saunders Company, Philadelphia, 1974 (15th ed. only).

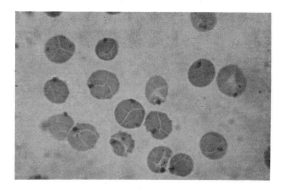

Fig. 50. Heinz bodies. (Supravital staining of red blood cells with new methylene blue N. Compare with reticulocytes stained similarly.) (Magnification ×1000.)

REAGENTS AND EQUIPMENT

1. Platelet diluting fluid

Sodium citrate	3.8 g
Brilliant cresyl blue	0.1 g
Formaldehyde, 40%	0.2 ml
Distilled water	100 ml

   Filter before use.
2. Red-count pipets.
3. Hemocytometer.
4. Glass slides.
5. Wright's stain and buffer.
6. Bright-light microscope.
7. Petri dish.
8. Filter paper.

SPECIMEN

Whole blood, using EDTA as the anticoagulant, is recommended. Fingertip, heel, or toe blood may be used if it is not feasible to obtain venous blood.

PRINCIPLE

Whole blood is diluted with a solution containing brilliant cresyl blue, which stains the platelets a light bluish color. The platelets are then counted using the standard hemocytometer. Results are double-checked by examining the platelets on a Wright-stained smear.

PROCEDURE

1. Gently mix the blood for approximately 2 minutes.
2. Prepare a blood smear and Wright's stain.
3. Using two red-cell pipets, draw blood to exactly the 0.5 mark and dilute to the 101 mark with the diluting fluid (1:200 dilution). From this point, the platelet count should be completed within 30 minutes to ensure against platelet disintegration.
4. Gently mix the pipets for 3 to 5 minutes.
5. Clean the hemocytometer thoroughly and make certain it is completely free of all dirt and lint. The use of 95% (v/v) ethyl alcohol and a lint-free

cloth is recommended for this process.

6. Prepare a moist chamber as follows: obtain a Petri dish and a piece of filter paper of approximately the same diameter as the Petri plate (either the top or the bottom of the Petri dish may be used). Thoroughly moisten the filter paper. Shake off excess moisture and place the filter paper in the top of the Petri dish so that it adheres to the dish.
7. Discard the first four drops from the red-cell pipet and fill one side of the hemocytometer. Repeat, using the second pipet, and fill the opposite side of the hemocytometer.
8. Place the moist chamber over the hemocytometer, and allow the preparation to stand for 15 minutes. This permits the platelets to settle, and the moist chamber prevents evaporation of the fluid in the counting chamber.
9. Place the hemocytometer on the microscope stage. Focus the hemocytometer under low power (10× objective) and carefully change to the high-dry objective (40×) to count the platelets. Count all platelets in two of the large corner squares, on both sides of the counting chamber. (A total of four large squares have thus been counted.) The diluting fluid used will not hemolyze the red blood cells. The platelets are much smaller than the red blood cells and appear as round, oval, or elongated particles that are highly refractile and stain a light bluish color. The utmost care must be taken not to confuse the platelets with dirt or debris.
10. Calculate the number of platelets per μl, as shown below:

    Platelets/μl =

    $$\begin{matrix} \text{Number of} \\ \text{platelets} \\ \text{counted} \end{matrix} \times \begin{matrix} \text{Correction} \\ \text{for dilution} \end{matrix} \times \begin{matrix} \text{Correction} \\ \text{for volume} \end{matrix}$$

11. A second technologist should scan a

Wright-stained smear and make a platelet estimate. If the platelet count does not reasonably agree with the platelet estimate, the platelet count should be repeated. (If the platelets do not show even distribution on the smear, a second smear and platelet estimate may be made before repeating the count.)

DISCUSSION

1. If clumps of platelets are noted in the platelet count, the procedure should be repeated. This may be due to inadequate mixing of the blood or to poor technique in obtaining the specimen of blood.
2. As in the red and white blood cell counts, there should be an even distribution of platelets in the counting chamber.
3. Thorough cleaning of the hemocytometer is extremely important in this procedure. Pipets must also be scrupulously clean and the diluting fluid freshly filtered.
4. The counting of platelets is relatively tedious, and some practice is necessary before proficiency in the technique is obtained.
5. If the platelet count is markedly decreased, make a 1:100 dilution and count four or more large squares on each side of the counting chamber. If a smaller dilution of the blood is made, the number of red blood cells present is too numerous in the counting chamber for an accurate platelet count.
6. In the event of an extremely high platelet count, make a larger dilution of the blood (blood to the 0.2 mark and diluted to the 101 mark in a red-count pipet). An alternative method is to count the platelets in 10 of the small squares (in the large middle square) on both sides of the counting chamber.

7. The range of error for the platelet count is estimated to be 16 to 25%.
8. Once the diluted count has been removed from the shaker, it should not stand for more than 8 to 10 seconds without being remixed.
9. The blood should be diluted and smears made within 5 hours of blood collection or within 24 hours if the blood has been refrigerated.

Brecker-Cronkite Method

REFERENCE

Brecker, G., and Cronkite, E.P.: Morphology and enumeration of human blood platelets. J. Appl. Physiol., 3,365, 1950.

REAGENTS AND EQUIPMENT

1. Ammonium oxalate, 1% (w/v). Store in refrigerator and filter before use.
2. Red-count pipets.
3. Phase (flat-bottomed) hemocytometer. (The hemocytometer used on a light microscope has a concave area on the underside, beneath the platform counting areas.) A thin disposable coverslip (No. 1 or 1½) should be used rather than the thick standard hemocytometer cover glass.
4. Glass slides.
5. Wright's stain and buffer.
6. Phase microscope.
7. Petri dish.
8. Filter paper.
9. Pipet rotator.

SPECIMEN

Whole blood, using EDTA as the anticoagulant, is recommended. Fingertip, heel, or toe blood may be used if it is not feasible to obtain venous blood.

PRINCIPLE

Whole blood is diluted with 1% ammonium oxalate, which completely hemolyzes the red cells. The platelets are then counted, using the phase hemocytometer and phase microscopy. Results are double-checked by examination of the platelets on a Wright-stained smear.

PROCEDURE

1. Gently mix blood for approximately 2 minutes.
2. Prepare a blood smear and Wright's stain.
3. Using two red-cell pipets, draw blood to exactly the 1.0 mark and dilute to the 101 mark with 1% ammonium oxalate (1:100 dilution).
4. Place the pipets on a blood mixer for 10 to 15 minutes. This ensures proper mixing and complete hemolysis of the red blood cells.
5. Clean the hemocytometer thoroughly and make certain it is completely free of all dirt and lint. The use of 95% (v/v) ethyl alcohol and a lint-free cloth is recommended for this process.
6. Prepare a moist chamber as follows: obtain a Petri dish and a piece of filter paper of approximately the same diameter as the Petri plate. (Either the top or the bottom of the Petri dish may be used.) Thoroughly moisten and place the filter paper in the top of the Petri dish so that it adheres to the dish.
7. When the pipets are adequately mixed, fill the counting chamber. Discard the first four drops from the red-cell pipet and fill one side of the hemocytometer. Repeat, using the second pipet and fill the opposite side of the hemocytometer.
8. Place the moist chamber over the hemocytometer and allow the preparation to stand for 15 to 30 minutes. This allows the platelets to settle and prevents evaporation of the fluid in the counting chamber.
9. Place the hemocytometer on the phase microscope stage. Focus the large middle square of the hemocytometer under low power (10×). The background appears black, with the white blood cells, platelets, debris, and markings of the hemocytometer giving an illuminated appearance. Carefully change to the 43× phase objective. The platelets appear as round or oval bodies with a light purplish sheen. When focusing up and down with the fine adjuster, the platelets may be seen to have one or more fine processes. Dirt and debris are distinguishable because of their high refractility. The platelets in 10 of the 25 small squares in the large central square are counted. The suggested squares to use are those labeled with a P, as in Figure 52. Enumerate the platelets in the same area on both sides of the counting chamber. The total number of platelets counted on each side should agree with each other by ±10 when the platelet count is in the normal range. Add the two counts together and divide by two to determine the average number of platelets counted.
10. Calculate the number of platelets per µl, as shown below:

Platelets/µl =

$$\begin{array}{c}\text{Average} \\ \text{number of} \\ \text{platelets} \\ \text{counted}\end{array} \times \begin{array}{c}\text{Correction} \\ \text{for dilution}\end{array} \times \begin{array}{c}\text{Correction} \\ \text{for volume}\end{array}$$

11. A second technologist should scan a Wright-stained smear and make a platelet estimate. If the platelet count

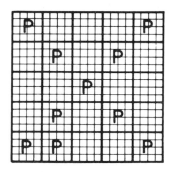

Fig. 52. Suggested squares to use for the platelet count.

does not reasonably agree with the platelet estimate, the count should be repeated. (If the platelets do not show even distribution on the smear, a second smear and platelet estimate may be made before repeating the count.)

DISCUSSION

1. If clumps of platelets are noted in the platelet count, the procedure should be repeated. This may be due to inadequate mixing or poor technique in obtaining the blood sample.

2. There should always be an even distribution of platelets in the counting chamber.

3. It is imperative that the hemocytometer and pipets be scrupulously clean and the diluting fluid be freshly filtered.

4. If fewer than 80 platelets are counted in the 10 small squares, all of the platelets in the large central square (25 small squares) on both sides of the hemocytometer should be counted. Then, if fewer than 50 platelets are counted per side, the platelet count should be repeated, diluting the original blood sample 1:20 in a white-count pipet.

5. If the platelet count is extremely high, a dilution of 1:200 or greater should be made, using the red-count pipet.

6. With experience, it is possible to perform platelet counts by phase microscopy with an error of ± 8 to 10%.

7. Once the blood has been diluted with 1% ammonium oxalate, the dilution is stable for at least 8 hours.

8. As soon as the platelet count has been removed from the shaker, it cannot stand for more than 8 to 10 seconds without being remixed.

9. The blood should be diluted and smears made within 5 hours of blood collection or within 24 hours if the blood has been refrigerated.

10. The use of 15× eyepieces on the phase microscope greatly facilitates the counting of platelets.

EOSINOPHIL COUNT

Although the relative number of eosinophils in the blood may be determined by the differential white count, it is sometimes necessary to determine more accurately the total number of eosinophils per µl of blood. Therefore, a direct method for counting eosinophils has been devised that is similar to the method used for the white blood cell and red blood cell counts.

The normal values for the eosinophil count are 150 to 300 eosinophils per µl of whole blood. A low eosinophil count (eosinopenia) is found in hyperadrenalism (Cushing's disease), shock, and following the administration of adrenocorticotropic hormone (ACTH). Increased numbers of eosinophils (eosinophilia) occur in allergic reactions, parasitic infestations, brucellosis, and certain leukemias.

There are two general methods for counting eosinophils: the indirect method and the direct method. The ideal procedure is to perform the eosinophil count by the direct method and double-check these results using the indirect method. This procedure is outlined here.

Direct Method

REFERENCE

Randolph, T.G.: Differentiation and enumeration of eosinophils in the counting chamber with a glycol stain: A valuable technique in appraising ACTH dosage. J. Lab. Clin. Med., 34,1696, 1949.

REAGENTS AND EQUIPMENT

1. Any one of the following diluting fluids may be employed:

A. Phyloxine diluting fluid

Propylene glycol	50 ml
Distilled water	40 ml
Water solution of phyloxine, 1% (w/v)	10 ml
Water solution of	1 ml

sodium carbonate, 10% (w/v)

Mix, filter, and store at room temperature. This diluting fluid is stable for a month.

B. Pilot's solution

Propylene glycol	50 ml
Distilled water	40 ml
Water solution of phyloxine, 1% (w/v)	10 ml
Water solution of sodium carbonate, 10% (w/v)	1 ml
Heparin	100 units

Mix, filter, and store at room temperature. This solution is stable for a month.

C. Randolph's stain

Solution 1

Methylene blue, 0.1% (w/v) in propylene glycol	50 ml
Distilled water	50 ml

Solution 2

Phyloxine, 0.1% (w/v) in methylene blue	50 ml
Distilled water	50 ml

Store solutions 1 and 2 at room temperature. Prior to use, mix equal volumes of solutions 1 and 2 together. This mixture is stable for 4 hours.

2. White-count pipets.
3. Counting chamber. There are three different types of counting chambers available for use in the eosinophil count.

A. Hemocytometer with Neubauer ruling. This is the counting chamber previously described in the section entitled White Blood Cell Count. This hemocytometer, however, is not recommended for the eosinophil count because of its relatively small volume.

B. Fuchs-Rosenthal hemocytometer (Fig. 53). The Fuchs-Rosenthal counting chamber consists of two platforms, or counting areas. The chamber is 0.2 mm deep. Each

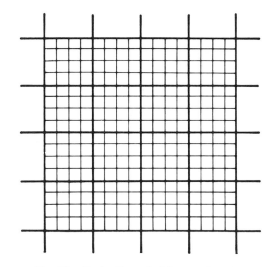

Fig. 53.   Fuchs-Rosenthal hemocytometer.

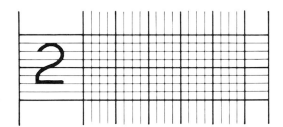

Fig. 54.   Speirs-Levy hemocytometer.

ruled counting area consists of one large square, 4 mm × 4 mm × 0.2 mm, or 3.2 µl in volume. This large square is divided into 16 smaller squares, each of which is 1 mm long and 1 mm wide. Each of these squares is further subdivided into 16 smaller squares.

C. Speirs-Levy hemocytometer (Fig. 54). The Speirs-Levy counting chamber consists of four platforms, or counting areas. The chamber is 0.2 mm deep. Each counting area consists of 10 squares, 1 mm long and 1 mm wide, arranged in two horizontal rows of 5 squares each. Each of these 10 squares is further subdivided into 16 smaller squares. The volume of one counting area is 2 mm × 5 mm × 0.2 mm, or 2.0 µl.

4. Microscope.
5. Moist chamber.
6. Glass slides.
7. Wright's stain and buffer.

SPECIMEN

Collect 1 ml of whole blood using EDTA, heparin, or ammonium-potassium oxalate as the anticoagulant. Capillary blood from the heel, toe, or finger may also be used.

PRINCIPLE

Whole blood is diluted with the staining solution. The phyloxine present in the diluting fluid serves to stain the eosinophils red; the sodium carbonate and water help to lyse the white blood cells (except the eosinophils); and the red blood cells are lysed by the propylene glycol. Heparin, if present in the diluting fluid, prevents clumping of the white blood cells. The sodium carbonate also enhances the staining of the eosinophil granules.

PROCEDURE

1. Using a white-count pipet, draw the blood up to exactly the 1.0 mark. Wipe off the outside of the pipet carefully.
2. Draw the eosinophil diluting fluid up to the 11 mark (1:10 dilution).
3. Repeat steps 1 and 2, making a second dilution on the same specimen.
4. Mix both pipets for approximately 2 minutes.
5. Expel the first four drops of the mixture from the first pipet and fill one side of the counting chamber. Repeat, using the second pipet, and fill the opposite side of the hemocytometer. (If the Speirs-Levy counting chamber is used, fill both counting areas on one side with the first pipet and the two opposite counting areas with the second pipet.)
6. Place a moist chamber (a Petri dish with a piece of wet filter paper in the top) over the filled counting chamber.
7. Allow 15 minutes for the cells to settle. Lysis of the red blood cells and staining of the eosinophils also take place during this time.
8. Using the low-power objective (10×), count the eosinophils, which are stained red. Count the following areas, depending on which hemocytometer is used:
   A. Hemocytometer with Neubauer ruling: count the entire ruled area on both sides of the counting chamber. This gives a total volume counted of 1.8 µl.
   B. Fuchs-Rosenthal hemocytometer: count the entire ruled area on both sides of the counting chamber. This gives a total volume counted of 6.4 µl.
   C. Speirs-Levy hemocytometer: count the entire ruled area on two platforms, one on each side of the counting chamber. This gives a total volume counted of 4 µl.
9. Calculate the number of eosinophils per µl as shown below:

Eosinophils/µl =

$$\text{Eosinophils counted} \times \text{Correction for dilution} \times \text{Correction for volume of chamber counted}$$

10. As a means of double-checking the preceding results, the indirect method for the eosinophil count should now be performed.
    A. Perform a white blood cell count on the specimen of blood. Make two blood smears and Wright's stain.
    B. Perform a differential white count on the blood smear.
    C. Calculate the indirect eosinophil count as follows:

$$\text{Eosinophils/µl} = \text{\% of eosinophils in differential} \times \text{White cell count}$$

D. The results obtained should correlate with the eosinophil count by the direct method. If there is too large a variation, repeat the preceding procedures for the direct and indirect eosinophil counts.

DISCUSSION

1. A single eosinophil count may be ordered on a patient or the eosinophil counts may be ordered in conjunction with the *Thorn test* for adrenal cortical function. In the performance of the Thorn test, a fasting eosinophil count is done. The patient is then given an injection of ACTH. A second eosinophil count is performed 4 hours after this injection. Normally, the second eosinophil count shows a decrease of 50% or more over the fasting eosinophil count. In hypoadrenalism (Addison's disease), the second eosinophil count will be approximately the same as the fasting eosinophil count before ACTH administration.

2. The indirect method for counting eosinophils is not as accurate as the direct method. Therefore, a close correlation between the results of the two methods is not always possible.

3. If oxalated blood is used, the blood should be diluted with the eosinophil-staining solution within 4 hours after blood collection.

4. The approximate error in the eosinophil count is ±30% when the hemocytometer with Neubauer ruling is used. Errors of approximately ±20% are found when the Speirs-Levy or Fuchs-Rosenthal counting chambers are employed.

SICKLE CELL EXAMINATION

Sickle-shaped red blood cells are found under certain conditions in the peripheral blood of people who have sickle cell anemia. This sickling phenomenon may also be demonstrated in the laboratory on patients with the sickle cell trait. The anemia and the trait are inherited and are usually confined to blacks. They are discussed in more detail in the sections on Hemoglobinopathies and Sickle Cell Anemia in Chapter 6.

Sickle cell anemia and the sickle cell trait are caused by an abnormal hemoglobin, hemoglobin S. In the presence of hemoglobin S, the red blood cells take on a sicklelike shape when the oxygen supply to the red blood cell is decreased. The degree of sickling depends on the concentration of hemoglobin S in the red blood cell. When the concentration of hemoglobin S is 80 to 100% (as in sickle cell anemia), sickling of the red blood cell occurs readily at only slightly reduced oxygen concentrations. When the concentration of hemoglobin S is only 20 to 40% (as in the sickle cell trait), oxygen concentrations must be much lower before sickling occurs.

Sodium Metabisulfite Method
(Daland and Castle Method)

REFERENCE

Daland, G.A., and Castle, W.B.: A simple and rapid method for demonstrating sickling of the red blood cells: The use of reducing agents. J. Lab. Clin. Med., 33,1082, 1948.

REAGENTS AND EQUIPMENT

1. Sodium metabisulfite, 2% (w/v)
   Sodium metabisulfite   0.2 g
   Distilled water   10 ml
2. Syringe (5 ml) filled with petroleum jelly.
3. Hypodermic needle, 19 gauge.
4. Glass slides.
5. Cover glass.
6. Microscope.

SPECIMEN

Whole blood, using EDTA, heparin, or ammonium-potassium oxalate as the anticoagulant. Capillary blood from finger, toe, or heel may also be used.

PRINCIPLE

Whole blood is mixed with sodium metabisulfite, a strong reducing agent that deoxygenates the hemoglobin. Sickle-shaped red blood cells are formed in the presence of hemoglobin S.

PROCEDURE

1. Place one drop of the blood to be tested on a glass slide.
2. Add one to two drops of 2% sodium metabisulfite to the drop of blood (two drops if the hemoglobin is normal, a single drop if anemia is present).
3. Mix well with an applicator stick.
4. Cover the mixture with a cover glass and press down lightly on it to remove any excess blood-sodium metabisulfite mixture and air bubbles.
5. Using the syringe and 19-gauge needle, carefully rim the cover glass with the petroleum jelly, completely sealing in the mixture under the coverslip.
6. Examine the preparation for the presence of sickle cells after 30 minutes, using the high-dry objective (40×). (Take care that when the objective is changed to high-dry, it does not become contaminated with the petroleum jelly.) In some instances, the red blood cells may take on more of a "holly-leaf" form, as shown in Figure 55. This form is often found in the sickle cell trait, and the test is reported as positive.
7. If there is no sickling present at the end of 30 minutes, allow the preparation to stand at room temperature for 24 hours and reexamine at that time.
8. When sickle cells or the "holly-leaf" form of the red blood cells are present, the results are reported as posi-

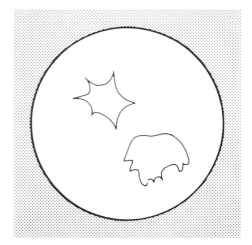

Fig. 55. Holly-leaf-shaped red blood cells.

tive. Normal-looking red blood cells or slightly crenated red blood cells are reported as negative.

DISCUSSION

1. The important characteristic of sickle cells or the "holly-leaf" form of the cell is that the cell must come to a point or points. Elongated cells with a rounded end must not be confused with sickle cells.
2. Sickling of the red blood cells is maximal at 37°C and decreases as the temperature decreases. Sickling also occurs more readily at a decreased pH.
3. With this method, it is difficult to distinguish the sickle cell trait from sickle cell anemia. (In sickle cell anemia, the sickling reaction occurs more rapidly than in sickle cell trait. This, however, is a poor tool to rely on.) If the sickle cell preparation is positive, it is advisable to perform a hemoglobin electrophoresis to differentiate the trait from the anemia.
4. Either sodium metabisulfite or sodium bisulfite may be used in this procedure.
5. Fresh reagent should be prepared every 8 hours. It is also advantageous to run a positive control each time

this test is performed in case the reagent has deteriorated.

Dithionite Tube Test Method

REFERENCES

Diggs, L.W.: Laboratory tests in the diagnosis of sickle cell disease: Part III, *Hematology*, Produced by the National Committee for Careers in the Medical Laboratory of the American Society of Clinical Pathologists and the College of American Pathologists, p. 75, 1973.

Nalbandian, R.M., Nichols, B.M., Camp, F.R., Jr., Lusher, J.M., Conte, N.F., Henry, R.L., and Wolf, P.L.: Dithionite tube test—a rapid, inexpensive technique for the detection of hemoglobin. Clin. Chem., *17*, 1028, 1971.

Schmidt, R., and Brosious E.: *Basic Laboratory Methods of Hemoglobinopathy Detection*, U.S. Department of Health, Education and Welfare, HEW Pub. No. (CDC) 74-8266, Atlanta, p. 74, 1974.

REAGENTS AND EQUIPMENT

1. Stock buffer. Place approximately 350 ml of distilled water in a 500-ml volumetric flask. Add 140.94 g of anhydrous dibasic potassium phosphate (K_2HPO_4). Mix until completely in solution. Place beaker on magnetic stirrer and slowly, over a 15-minute period, add 80.24 g of monobasic potassium phosphate crystals (KH_2PO_4). Mix until completely in solution.
2. 1% Saponin. Place 0.5 g of saponin (Fisher) in a 50-ml volumetric flask. Dilute to 50 ml with distilled water.
3. Working solution. Place 400 ml of stock buffer solution in a 500-ml volumetric flask. Add 10 g of sodium hydrosulfite (sodium dithionite) ($Na_2S_2O_4$). Mix until completely in solution. Add 30 ml of 1% saponin. Mix and dilute to 500 ml with distilled water. (This solution remains stable for a month under refrigeration.)
4. Test tubes, 12 × 75 mm.
5. Lined reader scale. (This may be prepared from a piece of white cardboard containing parallel black lines.)
6. Pipets, 20 μl.

SPECIMEN

Whole blood, using EDTA, heparin, or sodium citrate as the anticoagulant.

PRINCIPLE

When whole blood is added to the working dithionite solution, the red blood cells immediately lyse due to the saponin present. Hemoglobin S (and non-S sickling hemoglobins) in the reduced state in a concentrated buffer solution forms liquid crystals and gives a turbid appearance to the solution.

PROCEDURE

1. Add 20 μl of whole blood to 2.0 ml of dithionite working solution in a 12 × 75-mm test tube. Mix.
2. Allow tube to stand at room temperature for 6 minutes.
3. Place the tube approximately 1 inch in front of the lined reader scale. If there is no hemoglobin S or non-S sickling hemoglobin present, the solution will be clear and the lines on the reader scale will be visible through the solution. If hemoglobin S or non-S sickling hemoglobin is present, the solution will be turbid and the scale will not be visible through the solution (Fig. 56).
4. If the lines on the reader scale are visible through the test solution, report the results as negative. Failure to see these lines because of turbidity should be reported as a positive test.

DISCUSSION

1. If the dithionite tube test is positive, a hemoglobin electrophoresis should be performed on the specimen.
2. Hemoglobin electrophoresis results

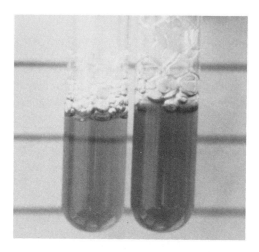

Fig. 56. Sodium dithionite tube test. (Negative results are indicated by the clear solution, where the black lines on the reader scale are visible through the test solution. Positive results are shown as a turbid solution, where the reader scale is not visible through the test solution.)

showing the presence of hemoglobin S should be verified by a positive sodium dithionite tube test.

3. The purity of the saponin reagent is important. I have found Fisher saponin to be good in this procedure. Also, care should be taken in handling the anhydrous dibasic potassium phosphate. This reagent absorbs moisture upon excessive exposure to air.

4. The size of the test tubes is important. Use of 10 × 75-mm test tubes may result in a false-negative result.

5. Two other anticoagulants, sodium citrate or heparin, may also be used in collecting the blood specimens.

6. Fresh blood specimens are not necessary for this test. Reliable results have been obtained on specimens up to 20 days old.

7. The dithionite tube test and urea-dithionite test may be adapted to the automated method and performed on the AutoAnalyzer. The reader is referred to: Nalbandian, R.M., Nichols, B.M., Camp, F.R., Jr., Lusher, J.M., Conte, N.F., Henry, R.L., and Wolf,

P.L.: Automated dithionite test for rapid, inexpensive detection of hemoglobin S and non-S sickling hemoglobinopathies. Clin. Chem., *17*, 1033, 1971.

8. The dithionite test is probably more sensitive to hemoglobin S than the sodium metabisulfite method.

9. In situations in which a patient's hemoglobin is less than 7 g/dl, a false-negative result may occur. To correct for this, double the amount of whole blood added to the working solution (add 40 µl of whole blood). Other causes of false-negative results include following multiple transfusions, at birth, or holding the sample tube too close to the lined reader scale.

10. A positive sodium dithionite tube test may be found in hemoglobin Bart's, hemoglobin C_{Harlem}, and in the presence of certain abnormal proteins and in hyperproteinemia. In cases of an extremely high hemoglobin or when too much blood has been added to the working solution, a false-positive results occurs.

11. Deterioration of reagents is an important factor in causing false-negative and false-positive results. It is, therefore, advisable to use positive and negative controls when this procedure is performed. (These control bloods may be obtained from previous patient samples that have been found to have hemoglobin S or hemoglobin A by the electrophoresis procedure.)

12. If the patient sample tubes are allowed to sit for approximately 24 hours, or overnight, it is often possible to discern whether the patient has sickle cell anemia or sickle cell trait. After 24 hours, normal blood (hemoglobin AA) remains a purplish-red color with fine flocculation. Blood heterozygous for hemoglobin S (hemoglobin AS) shows the

insoluble hemoglobin S particles on the top of the solution. The lower portion of the tube shows a clear purplish-pinkish color. A sample tube containing homozygous S hemoglobin (hemoglobin SS) shows a large amount of hemoglobin particles on top of a clear, almost colorless solution. This method should never be used in place of the hemoglobin electrophoresis confirmation procedure.

13. This test is commercially available from a number of companies. The cost per test, however, is quite a bit higher than the previously outlined procedure and reagents.

THE UNOPETTE SYSTEM

The Unopette affords the technologist a fast and accurate method for collecting and diluting blood for cell counts and hemoglobin determinations. The Unopette (Fig. 57) consists of the following elements:

1. The *reservoir* contains a premeasured volume of diluting fluid and is sealed by a thin covering of plastic *(diaphragm)* located in the neck of the reservoir.
2. The *pipet* is self-filling and is available in various sizes, depending on

the procedure to be performed. The end opposite the pipet tip is termed the *overflow chamber.*

3. The *pipet shield* protects the pipet and is also utilized to puncture the reservoir diaphragm just prior to use.

PROCEDURE

1. Immediately before use, remove the pipet from the pipet shield. Using the pointed end of the pipet shield, pierce the reservoir diaphragm firmly, inserting the shield as far as possible to obtain an opening large enough for the pipet.
2. Holding the pipet almost horizontally (about a 15° angle above the horizontal), touch the tip of the pipet to the blood sample. The pipet fills automatically by capillary action. When the sample reaches the neck of the pipet, no more blood will enter. (If the pipet is tilted too low or below the horizontal, it overfills.) Carefully wipe excess blood from the outside of the pipet without removing any blood from inside the pipet tip. Place your index finger firmly on the top of the overflow chamber.
3. Squeeze the reservoir slightly (do not lose any liquid) with your other

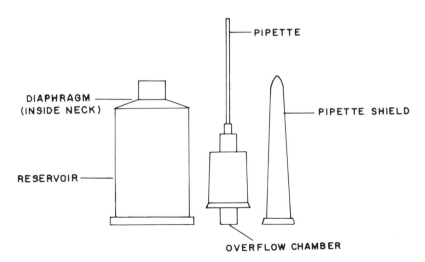

Fig. 57. Unopette.

hand. With the pipet in a vertical position (finger covering the overflow chamber), carefully place the pipet into the reservoir and seat it firmly in the neck of the reservoir.

4. Release the pressure on the reservoir and your finger from the overflow chamber. The sample is drawn from the pipet into the diluting fluid. Squeeze and release the reservoir several times to remove all blood from the pipet. (This must be done carefully to prevent the diluted sample from escaping through the overflow chamber.)

5. Place your finger over the overflow chamber and invert the reservoir several times to mix the dilution completely.

6. Immediately prior to performing the test, carefully mix the dilution by inverting the reservoir several times. Either of two methods may be used to remove the diluted sample for cell counting: (1) As soon as the sample is well mixed, squeeze the reservoir, forcing the diluted sample up into (but not out of) the overflow chamber. Place your finger over the pipet and remove from the reservoir. The sample will drain from the pipet upon removal or partial removal of your finger. (2) Convert the reservoir to a dropper assembly by removing the pipet and replacing it in the reservoir in a reverse position with the overflow chamber seated firmly in the neck of the reservoir.

DISCUSSION

1. If desired, the diluted sample may be completely removed from the reservoir by converting the reservoir to a dropper assembly as described above. Squeeze the reservoir carefully to expel the entire contents.

2. Specific Unopettes are available for the following manual procedures: red blood cell count, white blood cell count, platelet count, hemoglobin, reticulocyte count, eosinophil count, and the red blood cell fragility test. Unopettes are also available for automated counting: red blood cell count and white blood cell count (Coulter Counter Models A, B, F, Fn, and ZBI and the Fisher Autocytometer), platelet count (Coulter Counter Models F, Fn, ZBI, and Thrombocounter and the Technicon Autocounter System), and for microdilutions on the Coulter Counter S and the Coulter Counter S Plus.

3

Hematopoiesis

There are three types of cellular elements present in the blood: red blood cells (erythrocytes), white blood cells (leukocytes), and platelets (thrombocytes) (Fig. 58). (In actuality, the platelet is not considered to be a true cell in that it does not contain a nucleus.) Each of these cells has its own function, differs morphologically from the others, and has a life span characteristic for that particular cell type. In health, the destruction and production of cells is balanced, and, therefore, the number of cells present in the blood at any particular time is relatively constant. *Hematopoiesis* is a term used to signify the production of blood cells.

In the same way that a person goes through various stages until he becomes an adult, the blood cells must also go through certain stages before they mature and are thus able to carry out their intended functions. In a healthy person, only the mature adult cells are found in the blood, whereas in many diseases, the immature and abnormal forms of the cells may be present. For this reason, it is im-perative that the student of medical technology be able to identify the immature and abnormal cell forms.

In the fetus, hematopoiesis takes place at various intervals in the liver, spleen, thymus, bone marrow, and lymph nodes (Fig. 59). Within 2 weeks of embryonic life, primitive red blood cells are produced. By the second month, granulocytes and megakaryocytes begin to appear. Lymphocyte production starts at approximately the fourth month, and monocytes are produced by the fifth month.

At birth, and continuing into adulthood, major blood cell production is confined to the bone marrow. In the child, hematopoietic bone marrow (red marrow) is located in the flat bones of the skull, clavicle, sternum, ribs, vertebrae, and pelvis and also in the long bones of the arms and legs. By 18 years of age and for the remainder of the adult life, the red marrow is normally confined to the flat bones only.

ORIGIN AND INTERRELATIONSHIP OF BLOOD CELLS

In the past, one of the more perplexing and controversial problems in hematology

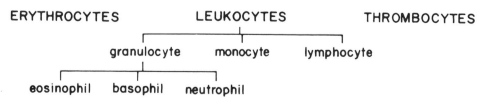

Fig. 58. Cells of the peripheral blood.

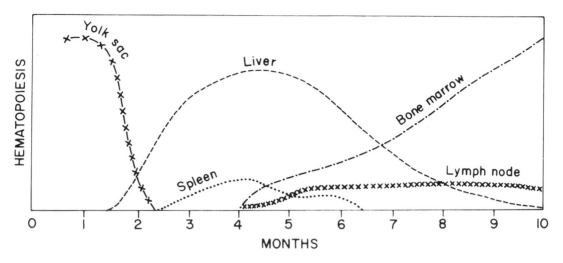

Fig. 59. Hematopoiesis in the fetus. (Modified from Wintrobe, M.M.: *Clinical Hematology*, 8th Edition, Lea & Febiger, Philadelphia, 1981.)

has concerned the origin of the blood cells and their relationship to one another. Today, as shown in Fig. 60, it is now believed that granulocytes, erythrocytes, platelets (megakaryocytes), and monocytes originate from a common stem cell, termed the *pluripotential stem cell*. The totipotential stem cell gives rise to the lymphocytes and the pluripotential stem cell. The plasma cell is thought to be derived from antigenic stimulation of a class of lymphocytes.

As stated previously, the destruction and production of cells must be balanced. This balance is thought to be maintained within the stem cell pool or compartment. In the hematopoietic system, the stem cells must have the capacity for self-renewal and differentiation (and maturation). Therefore, when a stem cell divides,

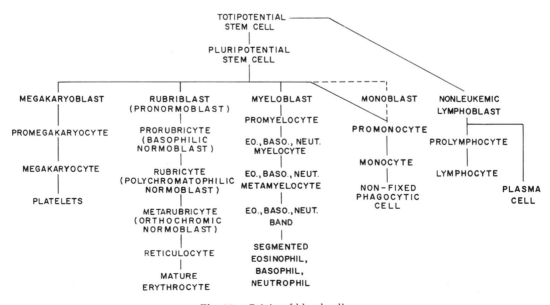

Fig. 60. Origin of blood cells.

the (daughter) cells resulting from this cellular division should be identical in appearance and potential to the mother cell. It is thought that one of these (daughter) cells remains in the stem cell pool to replace the (mother) cell, whereas the second cell leaves the pool by differentiating into a cell line. A second method of self-renewal and differentiation suggests that when a stem cell is stimulated to differentiate and, therefore, leave the stem cell pool, a second stem cell will divide, leaving both (daughter) cells in the stem cell pool.

CELL STRUCTURE

As an aid in the proper identification of cells, it is important to know their basic structure and composition. One should also have a basic understanding of the function of these cellular components.

The *plasma membrane* surrounds the outer limits of the cell and is composed of three distinct layers: a middle lipid layer located between two layers of protein (Fig. 61). The "head" of the phospholipid molecules (adjacent to each protein layer) is the water-soluble portion and is positively charged. The inner ends of the lipids, or "feet," repel water (are water insoluble). Also present in the cell membrane are small pores through which substances pass.

The *cytoplasm* of the cell is contained within the plasma membrane and is composed of a variety of organelles (Fig. 62). Among these organelles are the *mitochondria*, which are rod-shaped structures.

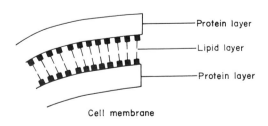

Protein layer
Lipid layer
Protein layer

Cell membrane

Fig. 61. Hypothetical diagram of a portion of a cell membrane.

Their membrane wall is composed of two layers. The inner layer juts out into the cavity and forms projections within the structure. The mitochondria supply a large portion of the cell's respiration and energy requirements. These structures do not stain with Wright's stain.

The *Golgi apparatus* is located in the cytoplasm of the cell near the nucleus. It is here that the cytoplasmic granules of the monocyte and granulocyte are formed. From studies performed on rabbits, it was found that azurophilic granule formation takes place on the inner Golgi membranes (closest to the nucleus). These granules contain enzymes and are also termed lysosomes. The specific granules are formed on the outer membranes (near the cytoplasm) of the Golgi apparatus. The enzymes made within the Golgi membranes become concentrated at the ends and ultimately pinch off from the membrane and form granules. These granules then move off and scatter throughout the cytoplasm.

The *endoplasmic reticulum* is composed of tubules contained within a membrane. One system of tubules is termed *rough-surfaced endoplasmic reticulum* and possesses *ribosomes* adhering to the membrane. The *smooth-surfaced endoplasmic reticulum* contains none of these ribosome granules. These ribosomes contain ribonucleic acid (RNA) and are active in protein synthesis. There are also small groups of RNA molecules in the cytoplasm that form *polyribosomes*. The RNA present in the cytoplasm stains blue with Wright's stain.

The *nucleus* of the cell consists primarily of deoxyribonucleic acid (DNA). This chromosomal material stains a dark purple color with Wright's stain and is called the *nuclear chromatin*. Light or unstained areas within the nucleus are termed the *parachromatin*. Located within the nucleus (of generally immature cells) is the *nucleolus*. (There may be more than one nucleolus present in a nucleus.) The nucleolus stains a bluish color with Wright's

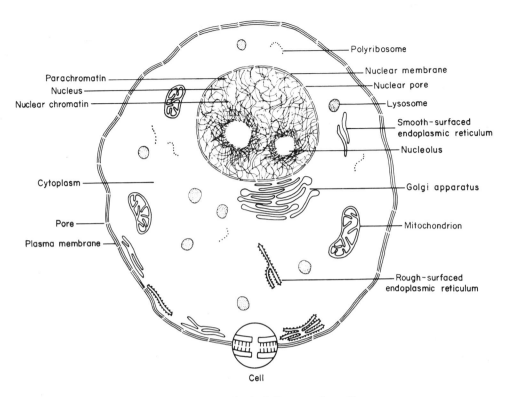

Fig. 62. Hypothetical diagram of a cell.

stain and is composed of RNA. There is a double nuclear membrane separating the nucleus from the cytoplasm. This membrane contains small holes, or pores, through which the RNA of the nucleolus is thought to carry messages from the DNA template to the cytoplasm.

NORMAL CELL MATURATION

Blood cells go through several stages of development. On the following pages the maturation of the cells is described and illustrated. Progression from one stage to the next is not abrupt. It is important to keep this fact in mind because many times the cell being studied may be in between the two stages described. (When this occurs, the cell is generally given the name of the more mature stage.) As a cell is transformed from the primitive blast stage to the mature form found in the blood, there are changes in the cytoplasm, nucleus, and cell size. Normally, all three of

these changes occur gradually and at the same time. In some disease states, these changes may take place at different rates. For example, the cytoplasm may mature more quickly than the nucleus. This occurrence is termed *asynchronism*. For convenience, these cellular changes are described individually.

CYTOPLASMIC MATURATION

The immature cytoplasm generally stains a deep blue color (basophilic) because of the high content of RNA present. As the cell matures, there is a gradual loss of cytoplasmic RNA and, therefore, a lessening of the blue color. In certain of the cells (for example, the myeloid cells), granules appear in the cytoplasm as the cell matures. At first, these granules are few and relatively nonspecific. As the cell matures further, these granules increase in number and take on specific characteristics and functions. The amount of cytoplasm, in relationship to the rest of the cell, usually increases as the cell matures.

NUCLEAR MATURATION

The nucleus of the immature cell is round or oval and is large in proportion to the rest of the cell. As the cell matures, the nucleus decreases in relative size and may take on various shapes. The nuclear chromatin transforms from a fine, delicate pattern to become more coarse and clumped in the mature form, and the staining properties change from a reddish purple to a bluish purple. Nucleoli present in the early stages of cell development gradually disappear as the cell ages.

CELL SIZE

As a cell matures, it usually becomes smaller in size. (For the new student, this change may be difficult to detect. The normal mature red blood cells or small lymphocytes are usually of relatively constant size and are used as a guide for comparison.) It is important that the student know the relative size of each cell type.

Identification of Cells

In identifying a cell, the technologist should think in the following terms:
1. What is the size of the cell?
   A. Small.
   B. Medium.
   C. Large.
2. What are the characteristics of the nucleus?
   A. Shape.
   B. Relative size.
   C. Chromatin pattern: smooth or coarse.
   D. Presence of nucleoli.
3. What are the characteristics of the cytoplasm?
   A. Granular or nongranular: specific or nonspecific granules.
   B. Color (staining properties).
   C. Relative amount.

When attempting to identify a cell, it is important also to note the degree to which the cells take up the stain. For example, if all cells seem bluer than usual, the staining technique may be poor, and cell identification must be made accordingly.

Unless otherwise stated, all cells in this text are described as they appear in Wright-stained smears.

RED BLOOD CELLS

The red blood cells are produced in the bone marrow.

Pronormoblast (Rubriblast) (Fig. 63.)

Size: 14 to 18 μm in diameter.

Cytoplasm: Deeply basophilic.
Relatively small amount, appearing as a band around the nucleus.
May show a lighter-staining area around the nucleus (perinuclear halo).

Nucleus: Relatively large.
Round or slightly oval.
Reddish purple in color.
Fine chromatin pattern.
Usually one to two nucleoli.
Nucleoli are larger than those found in the myeloblast and may stain with a slightly bluish tint.

Basophilic Normoblast (Prorubricyte) (Fig. 64.)

Size: 10 to 15 μm in diameter.

Cytoplasm: Intensely basophilic.
At times there is only a small increase in the relative amount of cytoplasm.

Nucleus: Relatively large.
Round or slightly oval.
Chromatin pattern is slightly coarser than in

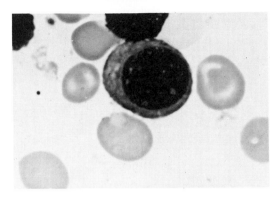

Fig. 63. Pronormoblast (center).

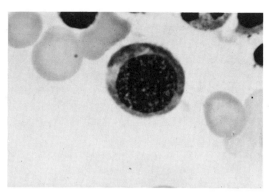

Fig. 64. Basophilic normoblast (center).

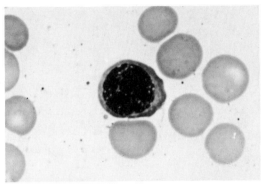

Fig. 65. Polychromatic normoblast.

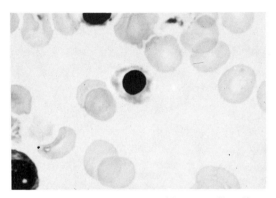

Fig. 66. Orthochromic normoblast (small cell in center).

(The above photographs have been enlarged in an attempt to show details of the nuclear chromatin pattern and the cytoplasmic consistency.)

the previous stage (pronormoblast). Nucleoli are usually absent.

Polychromatophilic Normoblast (Rubricyte) (Fig. 65.)

Size: 8 to 14 μm in diameter.

Cytoplasm: Blue-gray to pink-gray (shows a large range in the color) due to the start of hemoglobin production in the cell. A slight increase in relative amount.

Nucleus: Round. Smaller than previous stage.

More condensed. The chromatin pattern is coarse and clumped. Stains a deeper blue-purple.

Orthochromic Normoblast (Metarubricyte) (Fig. 66.)

Size: 7 to 10 μm in diameter.

Cytoplasm: Pinker than previous stage. Increased in amount compared to previous stage.

Nucleus: Pyknotic nucleus (a homogeneous blue-black mass with no structure). This is the main difference between the rubricyte and the meta-rubricytes.

Reticulocyte

Size: Approximately the same size or slightly larger than the mature red blood cell.

Cytoplasm: Pink to a slight pinkish gray. Contains a fine basophilic reticulum of RNA, which only stains with a supravital stain (see the section entitled Reticulocyte Count in Chapter 2).

Nucleus: None present.

Mature Red Blood Cell

Size: 6.7 to 7.7 μm in diameter.

Cytoplasm: Pink in color. The mature red blood cell is a non-nucleated, round, biconcave cell (Fig. 67).

Erythrocyte Structure

The normal, mature red blood cell may be described as a "biconcave disk." This distinctive shape allows the red blood cell to have a maximum membrane surface area for its size, which facilitates the transfer of gases in and out of the cell. In addition, it enables the red blood cell to undergo easily the changes in shape necessary for its travel through such areas as the microvasculature. The red blood cell membrane is composed of protein, lipid,

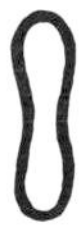

Fig. 67. Cross section of the mature red blood cell.

and a small amount of carbohydrate and can be penetrated by most solutes.

Erythropoiesis

The main function of the red blood cell is to carry hemoglobin, which transports oxygen to the tissues. The metabolic activity of the red blood cell also is capable of maintaining the hemoglobin molecule in a functional state. Normally, the rate of production of red blood cells determines the hemoglobin level or red blood cell count in the peripheral blood and shows little variation among normal individuals.

During maturation of the erythroid cell, three to five mitotic divisions occur between the pronormoblast and the polychromatophilic normoblast stages. It takes from 2 to 7 days for the pronormoblast to develop into the orthochromic normoblast. When the cell reaches the orthochromic normoblast stage, the nucleus is extremely condensed and the cell is incapable of further mitosis. After approximately 1 more day, the nucleus is extruded and the cell becomes a reticulocyte. The reticulocyte is slightly larger than the normal mature red blood cell and is slightly adhesive, appearing to be coated with a globulin, part of which may be transferrin. This characteristic may be responsible for keeping it in the bone marrow for an additional 2 to 3 days before it is released into the peripheral blood as a more mature reticulocyte. The number of reticulocytes in the bone marrow is about equal to the number of nucleated red blood cells in the marrow. The reticulocytes in the peripheral blood are slightly less in number than the marrow reticulocytes. The red blood cells of the circulating blood have a life span of approximately 120 days, ±20 days. Production of red blood cells (erythropoiesis) is initiated by a hormone, called *erythropoietin*, which is produced by the kidney and found in the plasma. When a person's hemoglobin level is below normal, his tissues do not receive an adequate supply of oxygen and a state of hypoxia is said to exist. This condition stimulates the kidneys to increase their production of erythropoietin, which activates the stem cells of the bone marrow to differentiate into pronormoblasts. An increased number of red blood cells are then produced. In addition, the rate of mitosis and of the maturation process of the red blood cells in the bone marrow increase. Hemoglobin is manufactured more quickly, and the reticulocytes are not delayed as long before they are released into the peripheral blood. As a result, the immature reticulocytes prematurely released appear somewhat larger than the normal circulating red blood cells (generally 20 to 25% larger) and are polychromatophilic (staining gray to blue-gray in color). These cells are frequently termed *shift cells* and may be indicative of increased red blood cell production. Also, this red blood cell population has a relatively short life span.

Hemoglobin Structure and Synthesis

Hemoglobin is composed of heme and the protein, globin. The synthesis of heme begins in the mitochondria with the formation of delta-aminolevulinic acid from glycine and succinyl-coenzyme A in the presence of pyridoxal phosphate (vitamin B_6) and delta-aminolevulinic acid synthetase (Fig. 68). The process continues in the cytoplasm of the cell, where two molecules of delta-aminolevulinic acid combine in the presence of delta-aminolevulinic acid dehydrase to form porphobilinogen. Four molecules of porphobilinogen combine to form uroporphyrinogen III in the presence of uroporphyrinogen III cosynthetase. Coproporphyrinogen III is then formed by the action of uroporphyrinogen decarboxylase, which removes four carboxyl groups from the acetic acid side chains. Heme is again produced in the mitochondria, where protoporphyrinogen IX is formed by the action of coproporphyrinogen oxidase. Protoporphyrin IX is formed in the presence of protoporphyrinogen oxidase, and iron is then incorpo-

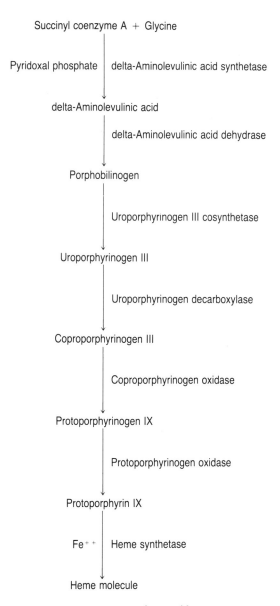

Fig. 68. Biosynthesis of heme.

rated into the molecule in the presence of heme synthetase to form the heme molecule. The atom of iron is located in the center of the structure. In the ferrous state (Fe^{++}), it binds oxygen. Iron is delivered to the red blood cell for incorporation into the protoporphyrin III molecule by a specific transport protein, transferrin (also termed *siderophilin*). Each molecule of transferrin can bind two molecules of iron. The transferrin attaches to the red blood cell, and the iron passes through the membrane and into the red blood cells. The major portion of this iron is utilized in heme synthesis. Upon insertion into the red blood cell, it proceeds to the mitochondria, where it enters the protoporphyrin III molecule. Some of this iron not used for heme production may accumulate in the cytoplasm of the red blood cell as ferritin aggregates. (This may be demonstrated by the Prussian-blue stain.) While the heme molecule is being synthesized, the globin portion of the hemoglobin is produced on specific ribosomes in the cytoplasm of the red blood cells. The globin portion of each hemoglobin molecule consists of four polypeptide chains that determine the type of hemoglobin formed. (In the normal adult, three hemoglobin types are present: hemoglobins A, F, and A_2, with hemoglobin A having a concentration of approximately 98%.) The polypeptide chains are composed of amino acids arranged in a specific sequence. Each chain is bent and coiled and forms a three-dimensional structure. The type and number of amino acids and their sequence are dependent on the type of chain being formed and are determined by

Fig. 69. Heme molecule.

the DNA molecules in the nucleus of the cell. This information in the nucleus of the cell is transferred to the cytoplasmic ribosomes by messenger RNA. Once the ribosome receives this information, it can function, without further messages from the nucleus, to synthesize the polypeptide chains. Hemoglobin A is composed of four polypeptide chains, two termed alpha (α) and two termed beta (β). Hemoglobin F is made up of two α chains and two gamma (γ) chains, whereas hemoglobin A_2 is composed, again, of two α chains and two delta (δ) chains. Using hemoglobin A as an example, when the individual α and β chains are produced, one α and one β chain combine to form a dimer. These dimers are now free in the cytoplasm of the cell, where they combine with the heme molecule and form the tetrad hemoglobin molecule consisting of two α chains, two β chains, and four heme groups. One heme group is attached to each polypeptide chain by a linkage from the iron, in the heme group, to a specific amino acid (histidine) in each α and β chain. When globin production is decreased (as is found in impaired synthesis of protoporphyrin III or porphyrin), there is no corresponding decrease in iron uptake by the red blood cell. As a result, the excess iron may accumulate in the cytoplasm of the red blood cell as ferritin aggregates or may build up in the mitochondria and may be seen around the nucleus of the immature red blood cell (ringed sideroblast). The production of heme and globin begins in the polychromatophilic normoblast stage and ends in the reticulocyte. No hemoglobin synthesis takes place in the mature red blood cell.

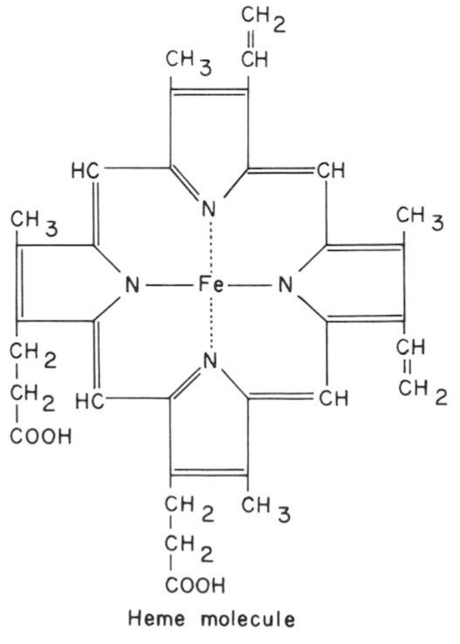

Biochemistry of the Red Blood Cell

The mature red blood cell consists primarily of hemoglobin (about 90% of the dry weight). The membrane is composed of lipids and proteins. In addition, there are numerous enzymes present that are necessary for oxygen transport and cell viability. The red blood cell derives its energy from the breakdown of glucose. About 90% of the glycolysis in the red blood cell follows the Embden-Meyerhof pathway (Fig. 70). In this way, 2 moles of adenosine triphosphate (ATP) are generated for every glucose molecule broken down to lactic acid. ATP is used to control the flow of sodium and potassium into and out of the red blood cell, maintain the biconcave shape of the cell, and protect the membrane lipids. The remaining 10% of the glucose molecules follow the hexose monophosphate shunt (Fig. 70), where re-

duced glutathione is made available to prevent oxidative denaturation of hemoglobin. When the red blood cell is exposed to an oxidant drug, the activity of the pentose phosphate pathway increases to maintain the hemoglobin molecule in its reduced state. Decreased activity of an enzyme in this pathway, results in oxidized hemoglobin, which denatures and precipitates as Heinz bodies. The methemoglobin reductase pathway (Fig. 70) maintains the iron present in the hemoglobin molecule in a functional state (Fe^{++}). The Ra-

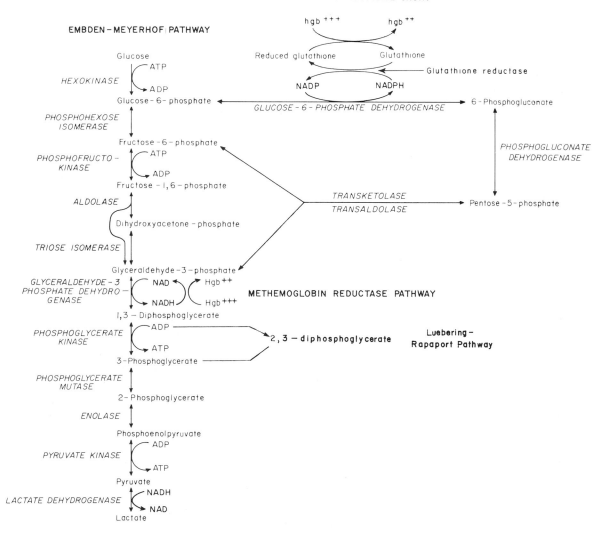

Fig. 70. Glycolytic pathways in the red blood cell.

paport-Leubering pathway allows for the production of 2,3 diphosphoglycerate (2,3 DPG), which affects the affinity of the hemoglobin molecule for oxygen. The 2,3 DPG combines reversibly with the deoxygenated hemoglobin, decreasing the affinity of hemoglobin for oxygen. DNA and RNA present in the early stages of the maturing red blood cell are absent in the mature cell.

Function of the Red Blood Cell

The red blood cell functions primarily to supply oxygen to the tissues and remove carbon dioxide. It is the hemoglobin molecule within the red blood cell that is responsible for supplying the tissues with oxygen. The normal hemoglobin molecule has an attraction (affinity) for oxygen (which binds to the iron). As soon as one atom of iron binds oxygen, the remaining three atoms of iron more readily bind oxygen. In other words, the affinity of hemoglobin for oxygen increases as the molecule binds more oxygen. This characteristic has been termed *heme-heme interaction*. The amount of oxygen that the hemoglobin molecule binds varies in relationship to the amount of oxygen in the blood. For example, when the oxygen tension in arterial blood is high (about 95 mm Hg), the hemoglobin molecule is about 95% staturated with oxygen. In the veins and tissues, the oxygen tension is lower. The hemoglobin molecule picks up and binds oxygen while in the capillary system of the lungs. As this hemoglobin travels through the tissue capillaries, in which the oxygen concentration is decreased, it releases this oxygen to the tissues. The affinity of hemoglobin for oxygen is represented graphically by the *oxygen dissociation curve* (Fig. 71), in which pO_2 represents the partial pressure of oxygen. P_{50} represents hemoglobin's affinity for oxygen and is used to designate the partial pressure of oxygen at which the hemoglobin molecule is 50% saturated with oxygen. The normal oxygen dissociation

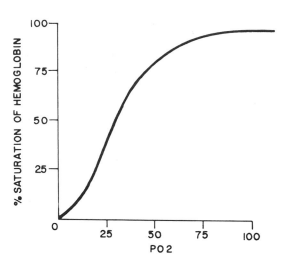

Fig. 71. Oxygen dissociation curve of hemoglobin.

curve is sigmoidal in shape and shows its steepest slope at the pO_2 levels that are generally found in the tissues. In this area of the curve, hemoglobin gives up and binds oxygen with relatively small changes in pO_2. A decreased affinity of the hemoglobin molecule for oxygen shifts this curve to the right, and hemoglobin then gives up oxygen readily. If this curve shifts to the left, hemoglobin has an increased affinity for oxygen, that is, it binds oxygen readily but does not release it to the tissues easily. The P_{50}, therefore, increases as the curve shifts to the right and decreases with a shift to the left. The normal position of the oxygen dissociation curve is dependent on carbon dioxide, hydrogen ions, and 2,3 DPG. Hemoglobin's affinity for oxygen is also influenced by the pH. This has been termed the *Bohr effect*. As the pH becomes more acid, hemoglobin's affinity for oxygen decreases. In the tissues, due to the presence of carbon dioxide, the pH is more acid, and hemoglobin is further influenced to release oxygen to the tissues. The organic phosphate 2,3 DPG also affects hemoglobin's affinity for oxygen. It binds with deoxygenated hemoglobin, thereby having an inhibitory effect on hemoglobin binding with oxygen. Hemoglobin gives up more oxygen to the tissues with increased concentrations of 2,3 DPG in the blood, and the oxygen dissociation curve is shifted to the right. The major portion of carbon dioxide is transported from the tissues by the red blood cell. Carbon dioxide reacts with water to form carbonic acid (H_2CO_3). Hydrogen ions, liberated from the H_2CO_3 (leaving $H_2CO_3^-$), are free to combine with deoxygenated hemoglobin, further decreasing the affinity of the hemoglobin molecule for oxygen. (Deoxygenated hemoglobin has more affinity for hydrogen ions because oxygenated hemoglobin is the stronger acid of the two.) Some of the carbon dioxide remaining in the tissues combines with the amino acid groups of deoxygenated hemoglobin to form carbaminohemoglobin. A small amount of carbon dioxide is removed from the tissues by the plasma in solution.

Breakdown of the Red Blood Cell

As a red blood cell ages, there is a decrease in its enzymes, a decrease in ATP, a decrease in size, and an increase in density. Approximately 1% of the red blood cells leave the circulation each day and are broken down. Destruction of the red blood cell most commonly occurs in the spleen, through phagocytosis by the reticuloendothelial cells. As soon as this occurs, there is a breakdown of the hemoglobin. The iron is freed for reuse by new red blood cells, and the amino acids from the globin are returned to the amino acid pool. The protoporphyrin ring is broken at one of the methene bridges, and biliverdin is formed. Biliverdin is reduced to bilirubin, which is carried by the plasma albumin to the liver for eventual excretion (Fig. 72). If hemoglobin is released directly into the blood, it becomes attached to *haptoglobin* (a globulin), taken to the reticuloendothelial cell, and processed in the normal way. If the plasma haptoglobin becomes depleted, the hemoglobin (dimers) are converted to *hemosiderin*. If free hemoglobin is present in the blood, it may be oxidized to *methemoglobin*. The heme groups are then released and taken up by *hemopexin*, a protein, leave the circulation, and are catabolized. If there is an excess of heme groups, they combine with albumin to form *methemalbumin* until hemopexin is available.

MEGALOBLASTIC ERYTHROPOIESIS

A nuclear maturation defect occurs in vitamin B_{12} and folic acid deficiencies. As a result, the red blood cell and its precursors are much larger in size than normal. Thus, the term *megaloblast* is used, "megalo" meaning large. The maturation of the megaloblast proceeds through the same stages of development as the normal red blood cell. Because of the defect in nuclear development (abnormal DNA synthesis), however, maturation of the nucleus takes longer than the cytoplasm, which matures at a more normal rate. Cell division is delayed because of the nuclear defect, whereas development of the cytoplasm continues. As a result, the cytoplasm appears to have matured to one stage, whereas the nucleus appears much more immature (asynchronism).

Promegaloblast (Fig. 73.)

Size:	19 to 28 μm in diameter.
Cytoplasm:	More abundant than in the pronormoblast. Deeply basophilic.
Nucleus:	Fine chromatin pattern. Chromatin pattern is more open than in the pronormoblast. Three to five nucleoli.

Basophilic Megaloblast (Fig. 74.)

Size:	17 to 24 μm in diameter.
Cytoplasm:	Deeply basophilic.
Nucleus:	No nucleoli are present. Chromatin pattern is more open than in the basophilic normoblast.

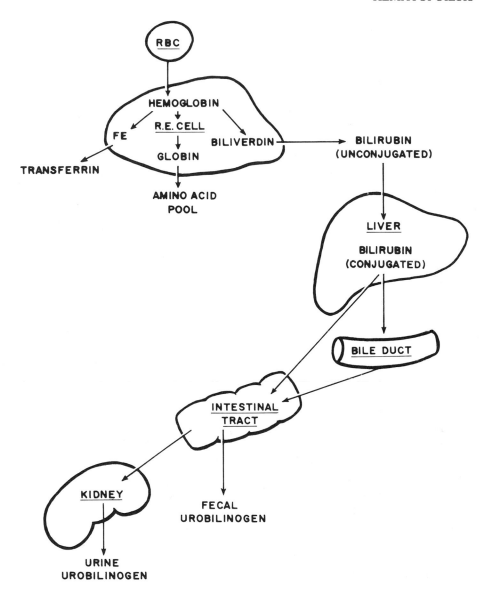

Fig. 72. Breakdown of hemoglobin.

Polychromatophilic Megaloblast (Fig. 75.)

Size:	15 to 20 μm in diameter.
Cytoplasm:	Blue-gray to pink-gray. May contain Howell-Jolly bodies (see the following section entitled Red Blood Cell Morphology).
Nucleus:	Chromatin pattern is more open than in the polychromatophilic normoblast. There may be a breaking up of the nucleus (*karyorrhexis*).

Orthochromic Megaloblast (Fig. 76.)

Size:	10 to 15 μm in diameter.
Cytoplasm:	Almost pink in color.

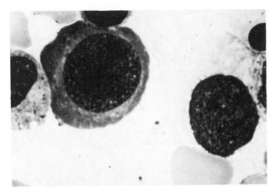

Fig. 73. Promegaloblast (large cell in center).

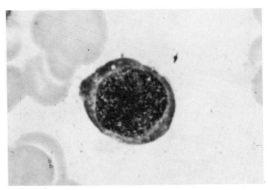

Fig. 74. Basophilic megaloblast.

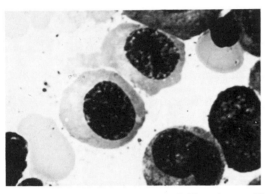

Fig. 75. Polychromatophilic megaloblast (large cell in center).

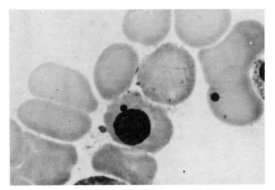

Fig. 76. Orthochromic megaloblast (center).

(The above photographs have been enlarged in an attempt to show details of the nuclear chromatin pattern and the cytoplasmic consistency.)

More abundant than is found in the orthochromic normoblast.

Nucleus: Chromatin may be clumped but is much less condensed than the normal orthochromic normoblast.

Macrocyte

Size: 9 to 12 μm in diameter.

The macrocyte may appear oval on the stained blood film.

RED BLOOD CELL MORPHOLOGY

In various anemias and other diseases, the mature red blood cells of the peripheral blood may show certain significant changes. The terms applied to each of these abnormalities are defined and illustrated here and on the following pages.

Normal red blood cells (discocytes), Fig-

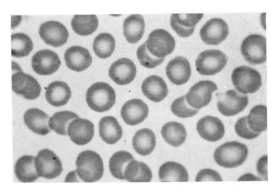

Fig. 77. Normal red blood cells. (Magnification ×1000)

ures 77 and 84A, are round, have a small area of central pallor, and show only slight variation in size.

Microcytes, Figure 78, show a decrease in the size of the red blood cell and are found in thalassemia and in a variety of anemias.

Macrocytes, Figure 79, show an increase in the size of red blood cell. These cells may be found in liver disease. When associated with vitamin B_{12} or folic acid deficiency, the macrocytes appear slightly oval in shape.

Hypochromia, Figure 80, denotes red blood cells with a large area of central pallor and is due to a decreased concentration of hemoglobin. Hypochromia is characteristically present in iron deficiency anemia

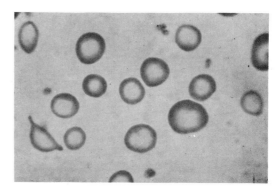

Fig. 80. Hypochromic red blood cells. (Magnification ×1000)

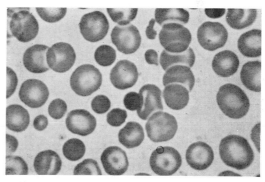

Fig. 81. Spherocytes. (Note the group of three spherocytes in the center of the illustration that show no area of central pallor. There are several more spherocytes also present.) (Magnification ×1000)

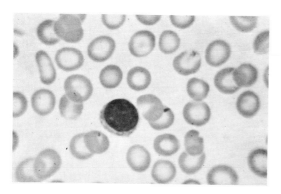

Fig. 78. Microcytes (compare red blood cell size with the size of the lymphocyte nucleus). (Magnification ×1000)

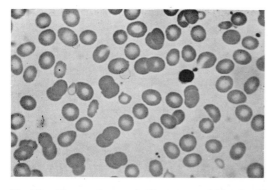

Fig. 79. Macrocytes, oval. (Compare red blood cell size with the size of the lymphocyte nucleus.) (Magnification ×500)

but is also present in other forms of anemia.

Spherocytes, Figures 81 and 84B, are not biconcave and do not have the central area of pallor that a normal red blood cell shows. The spherocyte has a smaller surface area for the cell size. These cells are associated with hemolytic anemia and hereditary spherocytosis. In some hereditary red blood cell enzyme deficiencies, the spherocytes may have many fine needlelike projections on the surface of the cell.

Spheroidocytes, Figures 82 and 84C, are thicker than normal red blood cells and show a small area of pallor that is usually off center.

Target cells (leptocytes), Figures 83 and

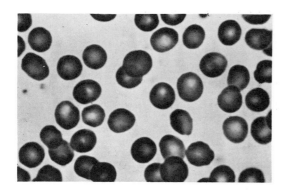

Fig. 82. Spheroidocytes. (Note the red blood cells showing only a small off-center area of pallor.) (Magnification ×1000)

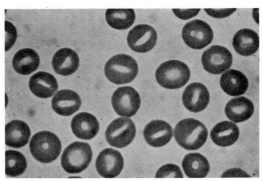

Fig. 85. Stomatocytes. (Note the oval-shaped area of central pallor in the red blood cells as compared to the round area in normal red blood cells.) (Magnification ×1000)

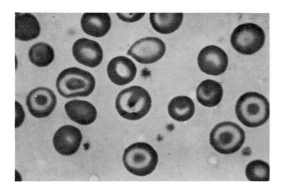

Fig. 83. Target cells. (Magnification ×1000)

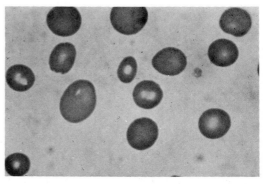

Fig. 86. Red blood cells showing anisocytosis. (Magnification ×1000)

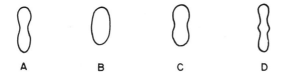

Fig. 84. Cross section of A, the normal red blood cell; B, the spherocyte; C, the spheroidocyte; and D, the target cell.

84D, show a centrally stained area and are associated with liver disease and certain hemoglobinopathies (abnormal hemoglobins): hemoglobin SC disease, hemoglobin C disease, and sickle cell anemia.

Stomatocytes, Figure 85, show an oval or rectangular area of central pallor. These cells have lost the indentation on one side and may be found in liver disease, elec-

trolyte imbalance, and hereditary stomatocytosis.

Anisocytosis, Figure 86, indicates a variation in the size of the red blood cell.

Poikilocytosis, Figure 87, indicates a variation in the shape of the red blood cell.

Sickle cells (drepanocytes), Figure 88, are red blood cells in the shape of a sickle or crescent. To be considered as sickle cells, they must come to a point at one end. These cells are associated with hemoglobin S and are found in sickle cell anemia and hemoglobin SC disease.

Ovalocytes, Figures 89 and 90, are oval-shaped red blood cells. *Elliptocytes,* more oval than ovalocytes, are cigar-shaped.

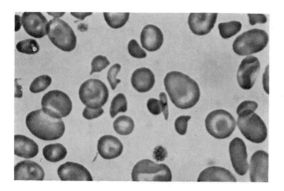

Fig. 87. Poikilocytosis of the red blood cells. Small red blood cell fragments, or schistocytes, are also present. (Magnification ×1000)

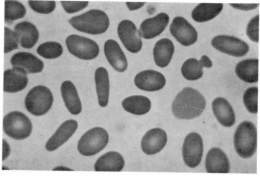

Fig. 90. Ovalocytes and elliptocytes. Note the *pincer cell* (red blood cell, shown in the upper right, which appears as if it has been pinched). (Magnification ×1000)

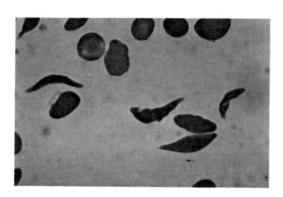

Fig. 88. Sickled red blood cells. (Magnification ×1000)

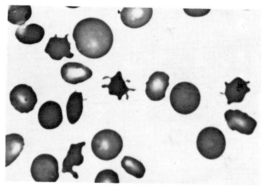

Fig. 91. Acanthocyte (center). (Magnification ×1000)

Both of these cells are found in hereditary elliptocytosis in large numbers. They are also present in various anemias but at a much lower concentration, no more than 6 to 10% of the mature red blood cell population. (These cells show normal shape in the nucleated and reticulocyte stages.)

Acanthocytes, Figure 91, are red blood cells with irregularly spaced projections. These spicules vary in width but usually contain a bulbous, rounded end. These cells have a decreased survival time and are found in abetalipoproteinemia and certain liver disorders.

Burr cells, Figures 92 and 93, are red blood cells with uniformly spaced, pointed projections on their outer edges. These cells

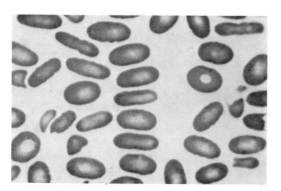

Fig. 89. Numerous ovalocytes and elliptocytes. (Magnification ×1000)

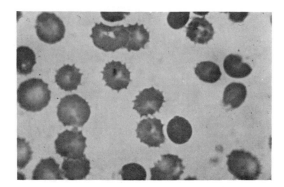

Fig. 92. Burr cells. (Magnification ×1000)

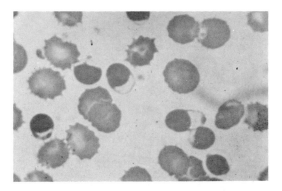

Fig. 93. Blister cells and burr cells. (Magnification ×1000)

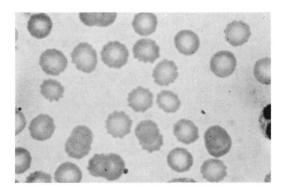

Fig. 94. Crenated red blood cells. (Note that the projections on the surface of the red blood cells are rounded, not pointed as in the burr cell.) (Magnification ×1000)

occur in uremia, acute blood loss, cancer of the stomach, and pyruvate kinase deficiency.

Crenated red blood cells (echinocytes),

Figure 94, have blunt spicules evenly distributed over the surface of the red blood cell and are usually due to faulty drying of the blood smear.

Schistocytes, Figure 87, are red blood cell fragments and may occur in microangiopathic hemolytic anemia, uremia, and hemolytic anemias caused by physical agents, as in disseminated intravascular coagulation (DIC).

Crescent bodies are faintly staining bodies in the shape of a quarter moon. They are probably ruptured red blood cells.

Basophilic stippling, Figure 95, is present as many coarse or fine, purple-staining granules in the red blood cell. The granules result from aggregation of ribosomes and are found in lead poisoning, anemias with impaired hemolgobin synthesis, alcoholism, and megaloblastic anemias.

Siderocytes are deposits of iron in the red blood cell. They are generally seen near the periphery of the cell and may appear as a single granule or as multiple granules. When present on a Wright-stained smear, the granules appear less vividly stained than Howell-Jolly bodies and are termed *Pappenheimer bodies* (Fig. 96). In contrast, when the iron deposits are stained only by iron stains, as in the Prussian-blue reaction, the cells are termed *siderocytes*.

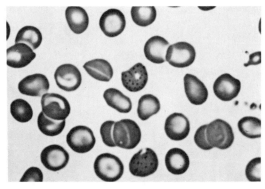

Fig. 95. Basophilic stippling (note the stippling in the red blood cell having a flattened side). (Magnification ×1000)

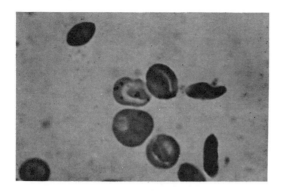

Fig. 96. Pappenheimer bodies (present in the red blood cell located in the middle of the illustration). (Magnification ×1000)

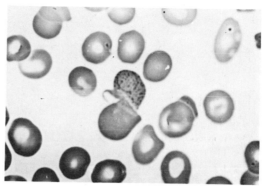

Fig. 98. Cabot ring. (Note the red blood cell in the center containing basophilic stippling and partially covered by another red blood cell. The cabot ring appears as a faintly stained circle within the red blood cell.) (Magnification ×1000)

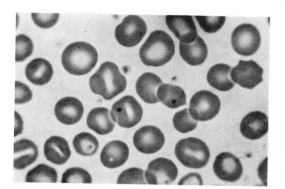

Fig. 97. Howell-Jolly bodies (one Howell-Jolly body is located in each of the two red blood cells shown in the center of the illustration). (Magnification ×1000)

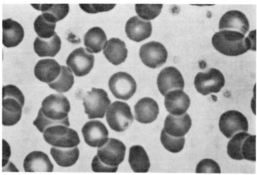

Fig. 99. Note the platelet on top of the red blood cell. When seen, there is generally a halo or clear-staining area in the red blood cell surrounding the platelet. (Magnification ×1000)

These iron-staining granules are present in sideroblastic and megaloblastic anemias, alcoholism, following splenectomy, and in some hemoglobinopathies.

Howell-Jolly bodies, Figure 97, are round, purple-staining nuclear fragments in the red blood cell. They generally appear singly in hemolytic anemia and following splenectomy. Multiple Howell-Jolly bodies in one red blood cell occur in megaloblastic anemia and in other forms of nuclear maturation defects.

Cabot rings, Figure 98, are purple-staining, threadlike filaments in the shape of a ring in the red blood cell. They are thought to be nuclear remnants or denatured pro-

tein and are seen rarely in pernicious anemia and lead poisoning.

Platelets on top of red blood cells, Figure 99, should not be confused with a red blood cell inclusion body. Compare the platelet with platelets in the surrounding field. Also, there is generally a nonstaining halo surrounding the platelet when it is positioned on top of the red blood cell.

Rouleaux formation, Figures 100 and 101, shows red blood cells arranged in rolls or stacks. This may be due to an artifact as a result of not preparing the blood smear soon enough after placing the blood on the slide. This formation of the red blood cells

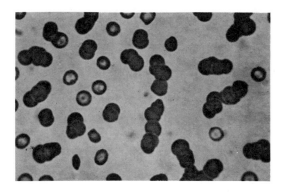

Fig. 100.   Rouleaux formation of the red blood cells. (Magnification ×500)

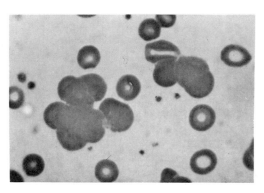

Fig. 102.   Agglutination of the red blood cells. (Magnification ×1000)

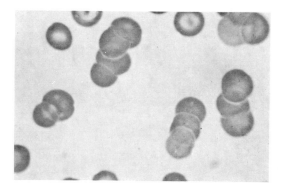

Fig. 101.   Rouleaux formation of the red blood cells. (Magnification ×1000)

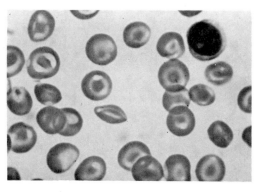

Fig. 103.   Note the *pocketbook-shaped* red blood cell located near the center of the illustration. Target cells are also present. (Magnification ×1000)

is also found in multiple myeloma and macroglobulinemia.

Polychromatophilia indicates red blood cells containing RNA. They stain a pinkish gray to pinkish blue color (Plate III).

Agglutination of the red blood cells, Figure 102, is found in patients who have a cold autoagglutinin (antibody). Note the clumping of the red blood cells rather than the stacking that is found in rouleaux. When agglutination of the red blood cells is seen on a blood smear, routine automated methods of red blood cell counting and sizing should not be utilized.

Hemoglobin C crystals, Figures 104 and 105, may be found in patients with homozygous hemoglobin C disease and char-

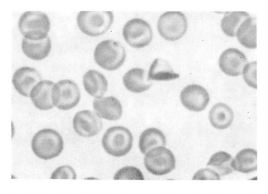

Fig. 104.   Hemoglobin C crystal. Target cells are also present. (Magnification ×1000)

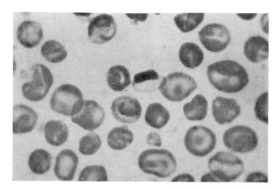

Fig. 105. Hemoglobin C crystal. Target cells are also present. (Magnification ×1000)

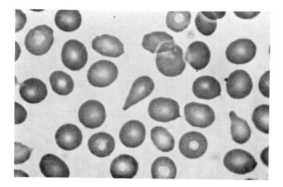

Fig. 106. Teardrop-shaped red blood cell (center of illustration). (Magnification ×1000)

acteristically in patients with hemoglobin SC disease.

Teardrop-shaped red blood cells, Figure 106, are found most notably in myelofibrosis, pernicious anemia, myeloid metaplasia, thalassemia, and some hemolytic anemias.

When examining a blood smear, any of the preceding red blood cell changes should be noted. An occasional crescent body, however, may be ignored, and crenated red blood cells need not be reported since this is generally due to poor technique. Whenever possible, a red blood cell abnormality should be described in as much detail as possible. For example, when poikilocytosis is present, the type(s) of irregularly shaped cells should be noted. Also, the generally accepted meth-

ods of reporting red blood cell irregularities include commenting on the amount of variability present. This may be accomplished by the use of adjectives (few, moderate, marked) or numerical scaling (1+, 2+, 3+, 4+). Regardless of the method chosen, it should be used on a consistent basis for each laboratory. Because the reporting of red blood cell morphology may vary among technologists, it is also helpful for each laboratory to have a uniform grading system. For example, using the 1+, 2+, 3+, 4+ system, the presence of one to five spherocytes per oil immersion field may constitute a rank of 1+ spherocytosis, 6 to 10 spherocytes, a 2+, 11 to 20 spherocytes, a 3+, and more than 20 spherocytes per field, a 4+. The grading depends on the abnormality present and is consistent for each red blood cell irregularity, or it depends on the numbers of cells per field. An example of this is to grade spherocytes in the preceding manner, classifying Howell-Jolly bodies as 1+ when there are zero to one per field, 2+ with one to two per field, 3+ with three to four per field, and 4+ with five or more per field. It is also important to select the proper area of the smear when determining red blood cell morphology. When studying wedge or coverslip smears, the area of the smear in which some red blood cells begin to overlap is generally used to determine red blood cell morphology.

WHITE BLOOD CELLS

Myelogenous (Granulocytic) Cells

There are three types of mature granulocytes: the neutrophil, eosinophil, and basophil. These three cell types are distinguishable from each other by the presence of specific granules that appear in the myelocyte stage. As the cell line progresses from the myeloblast stage to the promyelocyte, nonspecific granules form. These granules stain blue to reddish purple. As the cell matures, the formation of nonspecific granules stops, and the cell begins to form specific granules. The cell does not produce both types of granules at the same time, although both types may be seen in the myelocyte stage.

The granulocytic series of white blood cells is normally formed in the bone marrow.

Myeloblast (Figs. 107 and 115.)

Size: 15 to 20 μm in diameter.

Cytoplasm: Small amount in relation to the rest of the cell. Usually a moderate blue. Texture is smooth and usually nongranular.

Nucleus: Round or slightly oval. Occupies about four fifths of the cell. Extremely fine chromatin pattern. Reddish purple in color. Contains two to three nucleoli.

Promyelocyte (Figs. 108 and 115.)

Size: 15 to 21 μm in diameter.

Cytoplasm: Pale blue. Contains a few to many, blue to purple-staining, nonspecific granules.

Nucleus: Occupies half or more of the cell. Oval or round. Chromatin pattern may become a little coarser, although it will still be relatively fine. Two or three nucleoli present.

Myelocyte—this is the last stage capable of cell division (Figs. 109 and 115.)

Size: 12 to 18 μm in diameter.

Cytoplasm: Moderate amount. May contain a few patches of blue.

Few to moderate number of nonspecific granules. Specific granules begin to appear at this stage. Neutrophilic myelocyte: the pink specific granules may be seen as pinkish or lighter staining areas in the cytoplasm, usually appearing near the nucleus first. Eosinophilic myelocyte: the specific granules first appear as dirty orange to blue. These granules are larger than the nonspecific granules and are larger than the specific granules of the neutrophil. Basophilic myelocyte: the specific granules are few, large, and stain a dark blue-purple.

Nucleus: Oval or round. Chromatin pattern becomes coarser. Generally shows no nucleoli. Nucleus may be centrally located or eccentric.

Metamyelocyte (Figs. 110 and 115.)

Size: 10 to 15 μm in diameter.

Cytoplasm: Moderate to abundant amount. A few nonspecific granules. Full complement of specific granules. Neutrophilic metamyelocyte; the granules are pinker and more numerous. Eosinophilic metamyelocyte: the granules are a

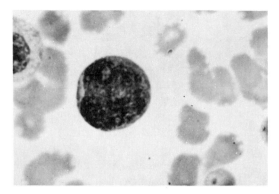

Fig. 107. Myeloblast (center).

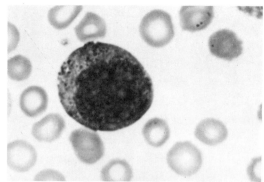

Fig. 108. Promyelocyte (center).

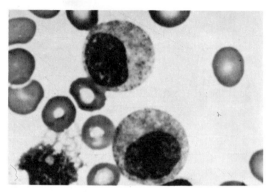

Fig. 109. Myelocytes, two.

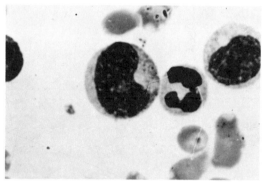

Fig. 110. Metamyelocyte and neutrophil.

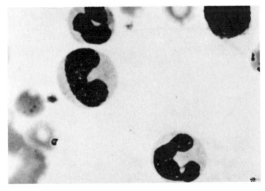

Fig. 111. Neutrophilic band.

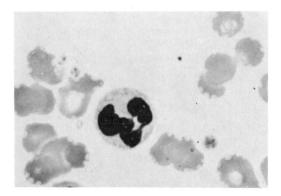

Fig. 112. Neutrophil (center).

(The above photographs have been enlarged in an attempt to show more nuclear and cytoplasmic detail.)

brighter orange-red and are more numerous. Basophilic metamyelocyte: the dark purple granules are more numerous.

Nucleus: Indented or kidney-shaped.

Chromatin pattern is coarse and clumped.

Band (Figs. 111 and 115.)

Size: 9 to 15 μm in diameter.

Cytoplasm: Same as the metamyelocyte.

Nucleus: Rod- or band-shaped.
              Thinner than in the
                  metamyelocyte.
              Chromatin pattern is
                  coarse and clumped.

Segmented Neutrophil (Figs. 110, 112, and 115.)

Size: 9 to 15 μm in diameter.

Cytoplasm: Full complement of pink
                  to rose-violet specific
                  granules.
              Abundant amount.
              Few nonspecific granules
                  are present.

Nucleus: Normally two to five
                  lobes.
              Coarse, clumped chroma-
                  tin pattern.

Eosinophil (Fig. 113.)

Size: 9 to 15 μm in diameter.

Cytoplasm: Contains the full comple-
                  ment of large, reddish-
                  orange granules.

Nucleus: Usually has two lobes.
              Coarse, clumped chroma-
                  tin pattern.

Basophil (Fig. 114.)

Size: 9 to 15 μm in diameter.

Cytoplasm: Stains slightly pink to
                  colorless.
              Contains specific dark
                  purple granules.
              There are fewer granules
                  present than are found
                  in the eosinophil. The
                  granules are water-sol-
                  uble and tend to wash
                  out when stained.

Nucleus: Does not appear as coarse
                  as in the neutrophil
                  and eosinophil.
              Generally has two to four
                  lobes.

When differentiating white blood cells, it should be noted that, except in unusual circumstances, the different stages of the eosinophil or basophil are not identified. The cells are denoted merely as eosinophils or basophils. The neutrophil stages are always differentiated. Identification of the neutrophil band varies from one laboratory to another. In this text, a neutrophil is considered to be mature if the nucleus is indented by greater than one half of its diameter.

FORMATION AND LIFE SPAN OF THE NEUTROPHILIC GRANULOCYTE

Neutrophil production and maturation occur in the bone marrow. The life cycle of the neutrophil takes place in the bone marrow, blood, and tissues. As the myeloblast develops into the mature segmented neutrophil, the myeloblast, promyelocyte, and myelocyte undergo cell division. Once the cell reaches the metamyelocyte stage, it is no longer capable of mitosis and spends its time in maturation (see Fig. 116). In the mitotic pool, the myeloblast, promyelocyte, and myelocyte will generally undergo a total of four to five cell divisions and will remain in this pool for approximately 4.5 days. For the next approximately 6.5 days the cell continues to mature and is found in the storage pool. These cells are then ready for release into the peripheral blood. This release of marrow cells into the peripheral blood is only partially understood and is most probably based on a selective type of release of mature cells rather than a random release. When the mature neutrophils leave the storage pool, they enter the peripheral blood, where approximately 50% of the neutrophils circulate freely *(circulating pool)* and the remaining 50% adhere to the walls of the blood vessels *(marginal pool)*. A small percentage of bands are also normally released to the peripheral blood along with these mature neutrophils. The neutrophils and bands in the marginal pool are not included in the white blood

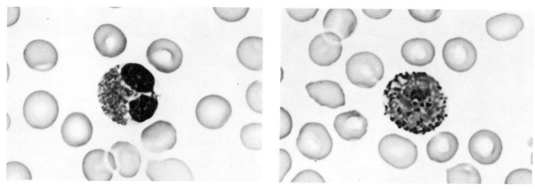

Fig. 113. Eosinophil.　　　　**Fig. 114.** Basophil.

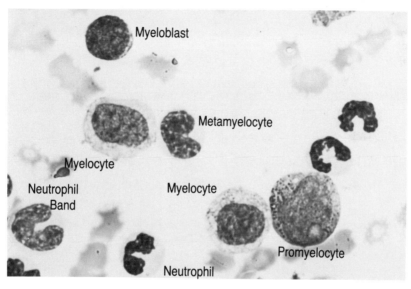

Fig. 115. Myeloblast, promyelocyte, myelocytes (2), metamyelocyte, neutrophilic band, neutrophils. Note the coarsening of the nuclear chromatin as the cell matures.

(The above photographs have been enlarged in an attempt to show more nuclear and cytoplasmic detail.)

cell count. Therefore, in a blood sample, the number of neutrophils counted in a white blood cell count and differential represents only half the amount of this cell type actually present in the peripheral blood. The neutrophils are continually changing back and forth between the marginal and circulating pools. From the marginal pool, the neutrophils randomly enter the tissues and body cavities in which they carry out their major functions. The cells leave the peripheral blood randomly, regardless of the age of the cell or the length of time it has been in the marginal or cir-

culating pool. Mathematically, the average time the neutrophil spends in the peripheral blood is considered to be about 10 hours. According to this figure, the neutrophils in the peripheral blood are completely replaced by neutrophils from the bone marrow almost 2.5 times every 24 hours. The neutrophils generally do not return to the bone marrow once they enter the peripheral blood. The number of bands and segmented neutrophils in the storage pool is about 15 times the number in the peripheral blood (the mitotic pool is approximately half the size of the storage

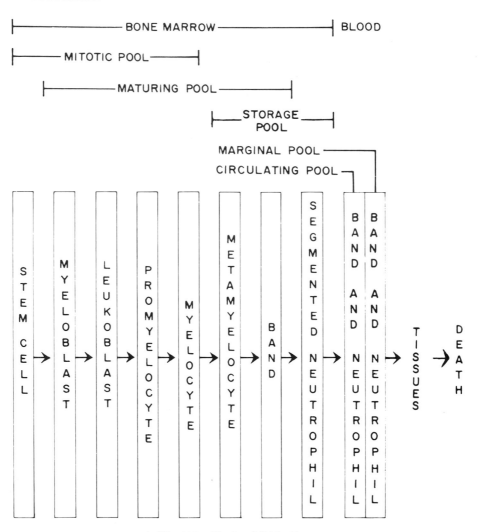

Fig. 116. Neutrophil kinetics.

pool). Normally, the neutrophils enter the tissues at the same rate as other neutrophils leave the storage pool and enter the peripheral blood. The segmented neutrophil is generally released to the peripheral blood first, before the band. When the demand for neutrophils in the peripheral blood increases, as soon as the numbers of segmented neutrophils in the storage pool become depleted, the number of bands entering the peripheral blood from the storage pool increases. This is reflected by an increased percentage of bands in the white blood cell differential count. Once the neutrophil has entered the tissues, it is uti-

lized to fight infection, or it leaves the body via excretions from the intestinal tract, the urinary tract, the lungs, or the salivary glands. It might also be destroyed by the reticuloendothelial system within 4 or 5 days.

PHYSIOLOGY AND FUNCTION OF THE NEUTROPHIL

Neutrophils are metabolically active. They are capable of both aerobic and anaerobic glycolysis. The major function of the neutrophils is to stop or retard the action of foreign material or infectious agents by means of phagocytosis and digestion of this material. The neutrophils also have a secretory function in that they release various substances into their environment. The primary (nonspecific) and secondary (specific) granules of the neutrophil are packaged and released from the Golgi apparatus. In the mature neutrophil, the ratio of specific granules to nonspecific granules is about 2 or 3:1. The primary granules are membrane-bound lysosomes and contain acid phosphatase, peroxidase, esterase, sulfated mucosubstance, β-glucuronidase, β-galactosidase, aryl-sulfatase, lysozyme, and other basic proteins. The secondary granules contain aminopeptidase, collagenase, muramidase, lactoferrin, lysozyme, and a number of basic proteins. It is not known exactly whether alkaline phosphatase is contained in the specific granules or possibly in a subpopulation of specific granules. The neutrophil is capable of random and directed locomotion (chemotaxis). The cells in the marginal pool move through the unruptured walls of the blood vessels (diapedesis) and travel to the tissues and body cavities. It is thought that in the presence of infection, inflammation, or a foreign substance the neutrophils in the marginal pool (in the area of the foreign matter) quickly move, within minutes, by diapedesis to the damaged or infected area. This directed locomotion, chemotaxis, may be brought about by cytotaxigens or cytotaxins. Cytotaxigens generate chemotactic factor when interacting with such substances as complement component, serum, or plasma. Examples of cytotaxigens are antigen-antibody complexes, lysosomes from the neutrophil, and certain bacteria. Cytotaxins are substances that have a direct action on the neutrophil itself. By some unknown method, the neutrophils are able to distinguish foreign particles and damaged cells. This is of utmost importance to its function of phagocytosis. Opsonins (specific antibodies, complement, and so on) enhance phagocytosis and increase chemo-

taxis. They act on the foreign particles and not the neutrophil. When the neutrophil phagocytizes the foreign particle, the cell membrane moves inward and encloses the material, forming a phagocytic vacuole (phagosome), the walls of which had been the outer membrane of the neutrophil before phagocytosis (Fig. 117). During phagocytosis, a number of metabolic changes take place, a few of which are: increased glycolysis and monophosphate shunt activity, a decrease in pH within the phagosome, increased oxygen consumption, and an increased formation of hydrogen peroxide. The specific neutrophil granules will then fuse with the phagosome membrane, emptying their contents into the phagosome. Following this, the nonspecific granules release their contents into the phagosome. Myeloperoxidase from the primary granules in combination with the hydrogen peroxide generated and an intracellular halide is one effective way the neutrophil is able to kill bacteria, viruses, and fungi. When the bacteria has been killed, this phagosome is known as a secondary lysosome. The cell may then expel the digested residue (exocytosis). The neutrophil is also capable of pinocytosis (ingestion of small amounts of liquid). The combination of phagocytosis and pinocytosis is termed endocytosis. In the presence of an inflammatory process, the neutrophils continually move into the infected area, phagocytize, die, and are, in turn, phagocytized by macrophages. The neutrophils are generally the first phagocytic cell to reach infected areas and are followed by the monocyte. These two cells continue their migration to the area until all of the foreign material has been phagocytized.

NEUTROPHILIA

(1) Extreme exercise and also the administration of certain drugs cause a decrease in the proportion of neutrophils in the marginal pool. These cells become part of the circulating pool and are reflected by

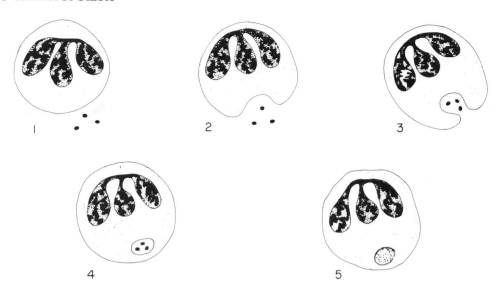

Fig. 117. Phagocytosis of bacteria by the neutrophil.

an increased white blood cell count and an increased percentage of neutrophils in the differential count. (2) In the presence of infection, an increased number of neutrophils are present in the marginal pool. These cells then enter the tissues at a faster rate. The influx of neutrophils from the storage pool increases until the rate of outflow to the tissues is exceeded by the rate of inflow from the storage pool in the bone marrow. (3) In chronic infection, the high rate of influx of neutrophils into the peripheral blood and the corresponding increased outflow may remain unchanged and a steady state of neutrophilia is maintained.

NEUTROPENIA

(1) Certain drugs cause an increased number of neutrophils to enter the marginal pool, resulting in a lower percentage of neutrophils in the circulating pool. (2) In a severe infection, the outflow of cells to the tissues may exceed the input from the bone marrow storage pool. (3) Decreased production in the bone marrow gives rise to decreased numbers of neutrophils available to the peripheral blood. (4) An increased loss of white blood cells (as might occur with splenomegaly), whereby the spleen sequesters (removes from the blood and holds) and destroys the cells, may also lead to neutropenia.

PHYSIOLOGY AND FUNCTION OF THE EOSINOPHIL

The eosinophils are produced only in the bone marrow, where they go through a maturation process similar to that of the neutrophil. The eosinophilic granules contain myeloperoxidase, several cationic proteins, β-glucuronidase, acid β-glycerophosphatase, and aryl-sulfatase. The myeloperoxidase, however, differs from that found in the neutrophils and exhibits very intense staining characteristics. Unlike the neutrophil, the eosinophilic granules do not contain lysozyme or alkaline phosphatase. Eosinophils appear at sites where foreign protein and parasites are found and in association with allergic reactions. The number of eosinophils in the blood is increased in these conditions. Little is known of their actual function and physiology. Because they are present in such small numbers, eosinophils have been difficult to study. They are actively phagocytic for antigen-antibody complexes and for microorganisms. They are less phagocytic for bacteria, however, and less bactericidal than neutrophils. Their numbers in the blood decrease during emotional stress and increase following exercise. Adrenal steroids and ACTH will normally produce an eosinopenia. There is a substantial bone marrow reserve of eosinophils, which will appear on demand.

PHYSIOLOGY AND FUNCTION OF THE BASOPHIL

The basophil is produced in the bone marrow in a manner similar to that of eosinophils and neutrophils. It exhibits chemotaxis and some phagocytic activity. In contrast to the neutrophil, the basophil has a sluggish motility, during which the nucleus advances and is in a forward position within the cell. In the neutrophil and eosinophil, the cytoplasm advances during locomotion. The basophil generally has a two- or three-lobed nucleus. The granules are water-soluble and most probably contain all of the blood histamine. They are peroxidase-positive and also contain a slow-reacting substance of anaphylaxis, platelet activating factor, kallikrein, and eosinophil chemotactic factor, and large amounts of heparin. The basophil has a secretory function in that it releases its granule contents to the outside of the cell (exocytosis) following exposure to various stimuli. They have also been shown to migrate to areas where foreign protein is present. Little is known of the function of the basophil, but it apparently participates in allergic reactions. The basophils increase in the peripheral blood in chronic myelogenous leukemia, myelofibrosis, and polycythemia vera.

MAST CELL (TISSUE BASOPHIL)

The mast cell is found in the bone marrow and in the tissues. It is not normally found in the peripheral blood. It is somewhat similar in appearance to the basophil but differs in several respects. The cell is usually larger than the basophil, and the granules are smaller, more numerous, and are not water-soluble. The granules contain heparin, histamine, hydrolytic enzymes, 5-hydroxytryptamine, and serotonin. Mast cells appear to discharge their granules outside the cell (exoplasmosis). An increase in mast cells in the bone marrow is found in aplastic anemia, chronic blood loss, and various tumors involving the bone marrow.

Lymphocytes

Lymphocytes are produced by the lymph nodes, spleen, thymus, and bone marrow.

Lymphoblast (nonleukemic lymphoblast) (Fig. 118.)

Size:	10 to 18 μm in diameter.
Cytoplasm:	No granules are present. Appears smooth. Moderate to dark blue. May stain deep blue at the periphery and a lighter blue near the nucleus. More abundant than in the myeloblast.
Nucleus:	Chromatin pattern is somewhat coarse. Round or oval in shape. Generally contains one to two distinct nucleoli.

Prolymphocyte

Size:	May be the same size as the lymphoblast or smaller.
Cytoplasm:	Moderate to dark blue. Usually nongranular. More abundant than in the lymphoblast.
Nucleus:	Round, oval, or slightly indented. Chromatin pattern is more clumped than in the lymphoblast.

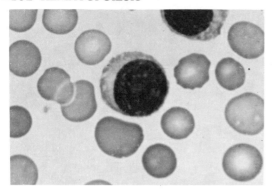

Fig. 118. Immature lymphocyte (center).

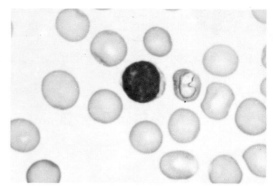

Fig. 119. Small mature lymphocyte.

(The above photographs have been enlarged in an attempt to show more nuclear and cytoplasmic detail.)

Nucleolus may or may not be visible.

Mature Lymphocyte

The lymphocytes found in the peripheral blood occur in varying sizes. For purposes of description, they are divided into three categories: small, medium, and large, with a size variation of 8 to 16 μm in diameter. In addition to differing in size, the relative amount of cytoplasm varies. Generally, the larger the lymphocyte, the more abundant the cytoplasm.

Small Lymphocyte (Fig. 119.)

Size: 8 to 10 μm in diameter.

Cytoplasm: Usually forms a thin rim around the nucleus. Moderate to dark blue.

Nucleus: Chromatin pattern is dense and clumped. Round or oval in shape and may be slightly indented. No nucleoli are visible.

Medium Lymphocyte

Size: 10 to 12 μm in diameter.

Cytoplasm: More abundant than in the small lymphocyte. Pale to moderately blue. May or may not contain a few nonspecific azurophilic granules.

Nucleus: Round or oval in shape and may be slightly indented. Chromatin pattern is clumped but not as dense-looking as in the small lymphocyte. No nucleoli are visible.

Large Lymphocyte

Size: 12 to 16 μm in diameter.

Cytoplasm: Abundant. Very pale blue. May or may not contain a few nonspecific azurophilic granules.

Nucleus: Round or oval in shape and may be slightly indented. Chromatin pattern is coarse. No nucleoli are visible. May be eccentrically located.

BIOLOGY AND PHYSIOLOGY OF THE LYMPHOCYTE

The lymphocytes are vital to the immune system. They function in the production of circulating antibodies and in

COLOR PLATES

PLATE I

Normoblasts and megaloblasts contrasted (photomicrographs. × 1000; Wright's stain).

A, B, C, D, E, Normoblasts: A, pronormoblast; B, basophilic normoblast; C, early; D, late, polychromatophilic normoblasts; E, orthochromatic normoblast with stippling.
F—O. Various stages of megaloblasts (pernicious anemia): F, Promegaloblast (left) and basophilic megaloblast (right); G, H, I, J, K, mainly polychromatophilic megaloblasts; L, M, N, O, mainly orthochromatic megaloblasts, O being from the blood. All the other cells are from the bone marrow.

PLATE I

(Legend on opposite page)

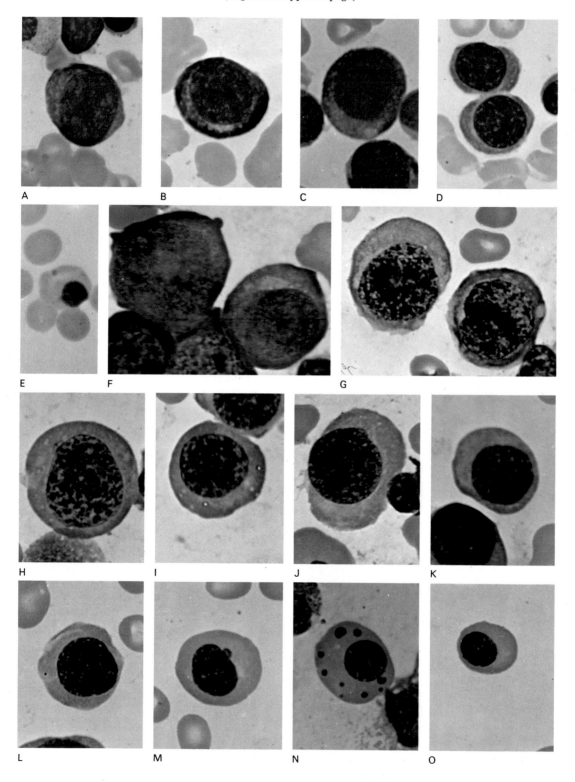

A   B   C   D

E   F   G

H   I   J   K

L   M   N   O

PLATE II

Normal leukocytes from bone marrow and blood (photomicrographs, × 1000 [approx.]; *Wright's stain*).

A, Myeloblast; B, Myeloblast, with myelocyte and late metamyelocyte; C, Two promyelocytes; D, Promyelocyte; E, Late promyelocyte or myelocyte; F, Myelocyte; G, Myelocyte; H, Late myelocyte or early metamyelocyte; I, Metamyelocyte; J, Band neutrophil; K, Band neutrophil; L, Polymorphonuclear neutrophil; M, Polymorphonuclear neutrophil; N, Polymorphonuclear neutrophil; O, Eosinophil; P, Basophil; Q, Monocyte; R, Monocyte.

PLATE II

(Legend on opposite page)

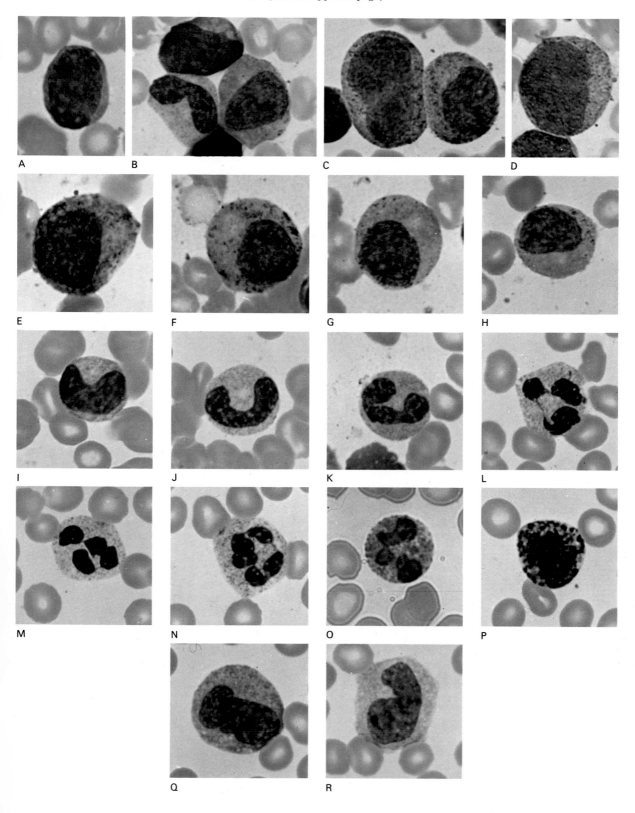

PLATE III

Immature and mature white blood cells, red blood cells, megakaryocytes and platelets. (Wright's stain. Magnification × 1000.)

A, Leukemic lymphoblast; B, Prolymphocyte (larger cell) and normal lymphocyte; C, Small lymphocyte; D, Medium-sized lymphocyte; E, Large lymphocyte; F, Blast (acute monocytic leukemia); G, Promonocyte; H, Monocyte; I, Macrophage; J, Myeloblast; K, Rubriblast (bone marrow); L, Promegaloblast (bone marrow); M, Megakaryoblast (bone marrow); N, Megakaryocyte (bone marrow) (450 ×); O, Giant platelet; P, Abnormal platelet; Q, Vacuolated monocyte; R, Vacuolated neutrophil.

PLATE III

(Legend on opposite page)

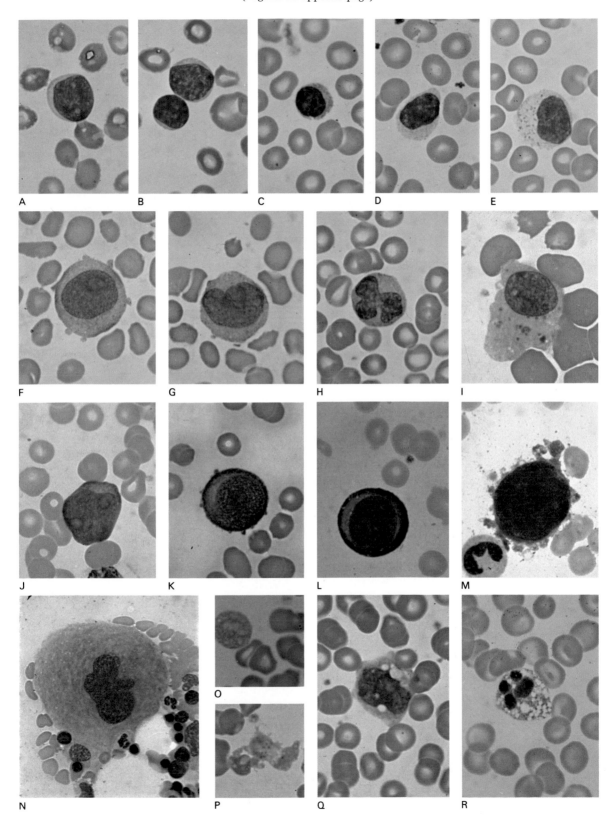

PLATE IV

Heinz bodies, reticulocytes, white blood cell morphology, and abnormal white blood cells. (Wright's stain, except where indicated. Magnification × 1000.)

A, Neutrophilic band showing toxic granulation; B, Neutrophil containing Döhle body; C, Hypersegmented neutrophil; D, Neutrophil showing a Barr body; E, Neutrophil with a pyknotic nucleus; F, Neutrophil and lymphocyte from a patient with Alder Reilly anomaly; G, Reticulocytes (new methylene blue N stain); H, Heinz bodies (new methylene blue N stain); I, Mitotic figure; J, Basket cell; K, Smudge cell; L, Plasma cell; M, Lymphosarcoma cell; N, Micromegakaryoblast; O, Reed-Sternberg cell; P, Lipid histiocyte from a patient with Gaucher's disease; Q, Lipid histiocyte from a patient with Niemann-Pick disease.

PLATE IV

(Legend on opposite page)

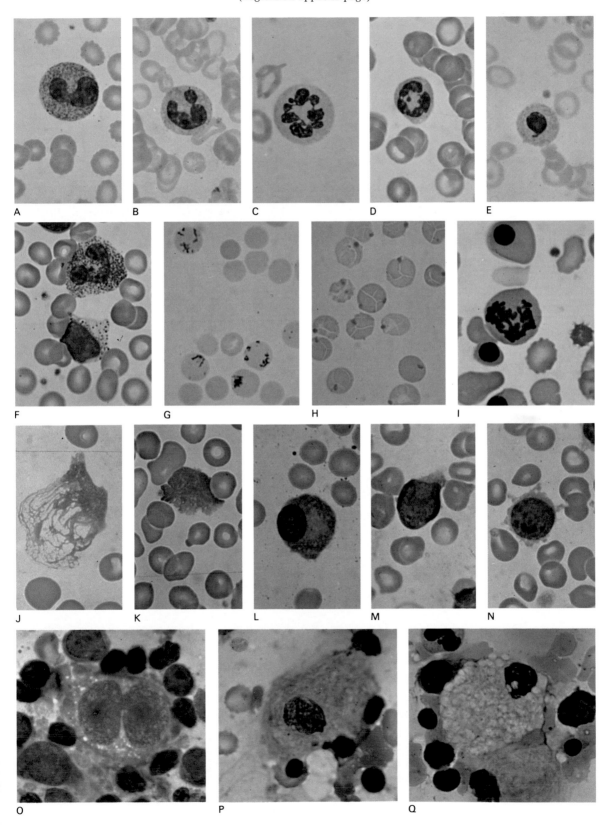

A

B

C

D

E

F

G

H

I

J

K

L

M

N

O

P

Q

PLATE V

Red blood cell and white blood cell morphology and malaria. (Wright's stain. Magnification × 403.)

A, Neutrophil from a patient with Chédiak-Higashi anomaly; B, Lymphocyte from a patient with Chédiak-Higashi anomaly; C, D, L. E. cell; E–G, Neutrophil from a patient with Pelger-Huët anomaly; H, Myeloblast containing an Auer rod; I, Plasma cells containing crystals; J, Red blood cells showing polychromatophilia; K–N, Various stages of malaria parasites; O, Platelet on top of a red blood cell (compare with malaria parasites in photographs L, M, N).

PLATE V
(Legend on opposite page)

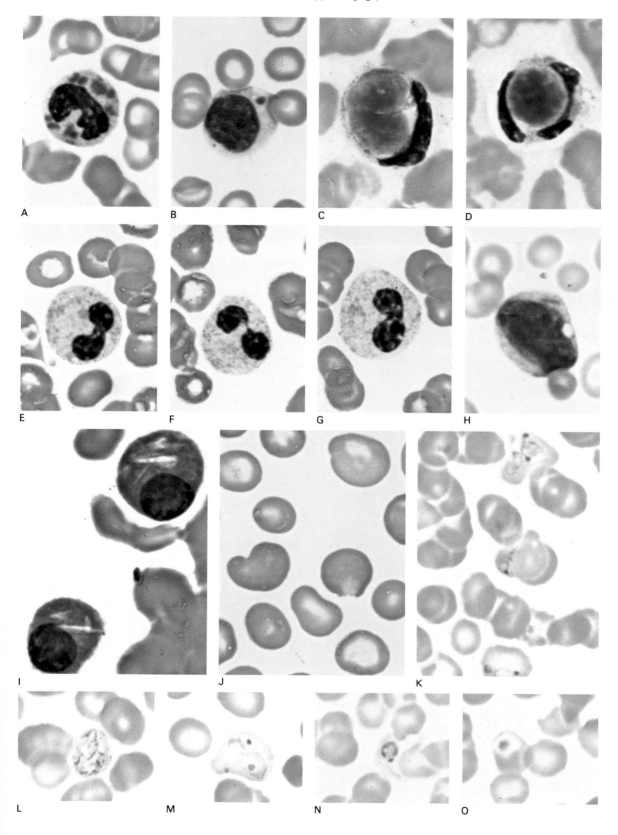

A

B

C

D

E

F

G

H

I

J

K

L

M

N

O

PLATE VI

(Legend on opposite page)

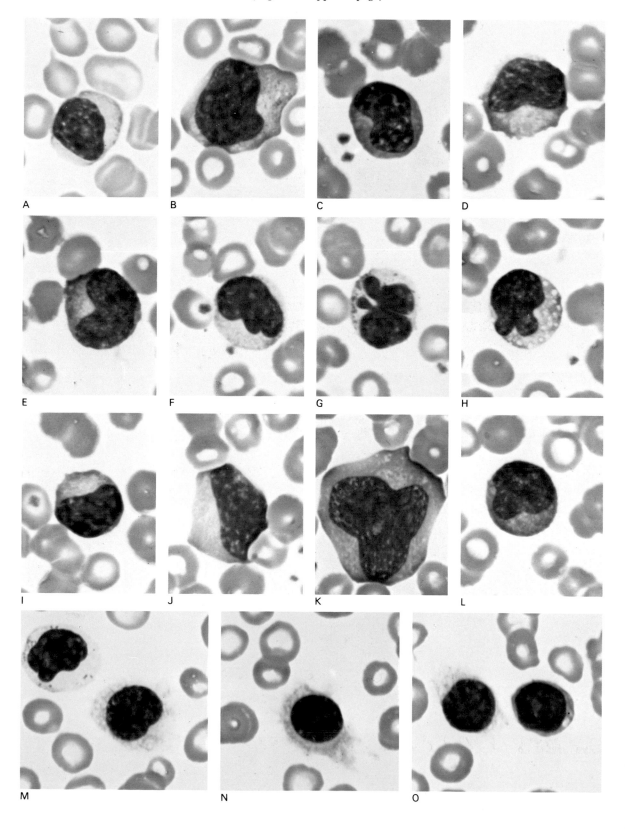

the expression of cellular immunity. The mature lymphocyte has little or no endoplasmic reticulum, only a small Golgi apparatus, and few mitochondria, and the ribosomes usually do not form clusters. Using special staining procedures, the lymphocyte is negative for chloroacetate esterase, alkaline phosphatase, and peroxidase and is positive for acid phosphatase. The lymphocyte is actively motile and, during locomotion, has the appearance of a hand mirror. When moving, the nucleus is at the leading end of the cell with the cytoplasm trailing behind, appearing as the handle of the hand mirror. Some lymphocytes (the T lymphocyte, in particular, which is described in the following paragraphs of this section) may exhibit inconspicuous, small, blunt pseudopods (uropods), which are thought to serve as a means of attachment to another lymphocyte or macrophage. The nucleus of the lymphocyte usually contains a nucleolus, which, because of denseness of the nucleus, is generally not visible under light microscopy.

THE LYMPHOCYTIC SYSTEM

The lymphocytic system in the adult is comprised of the primary lymphopoietic organs, made up of the bone marrow and thymus, and the secondary, or peripheral, lymphatic system, which includes the lymph nodes, spleen, gut-associated lymphoid tissues (lymph nodules of the intestines, which are also termed Peyer's patches, and tonsils), and the blood. The lymph tissue is composed of lymphatic vessels that form a dense network in most of the tissues of the body. The smaller vessels unite with each other to form larger vessels until all of the lymphatic vessels come together and form two main trunks: the right lymphatic duct and the thoracic duct. These two main vessels open into the veins of the neck. Lymph nodes are located along these lymphatic vessels. The contents of the vessels pass through the lymph nodes on their way to the thoracic and lymphatic ducts.

The bone marrow is the body's largest lymphopoietic mass. The source of lymphocyte replacement is the stem cell compartment in the bone marrow. The production of lymphocytes in the bone marrow and thymus is independent of antigenic stimulation and events occurring in other areas of the lymphoid system. These two organs provide the peripheral lymph system with a supply of lymphocytes that can become immunocompetent when stimulated by an antigen. The fate of the lymphocytes produced in the bone marrow varies. Some of these cells may serve as lymphocyte stem cells. Some lymphocytes may migrate to the peripheral lymphatic system. Most of the marrow lymphocytes, however, probably die randomly in the bone marrow and serve as building blocks for future generations of lymphocytes. In the thymus, most of the lymphocytes are replaced every 3 to 4 days. A few of these lymphocytes will migrate to thymus-dependent areas of the spleen and lymph nodes, whereas the remainder will die in the thymus or migrate out of the thymus and die elsewhere.

LYMPHOCYTE SUBPOPULATIONS

There are possibly four subpopulations of lymphocytes: B lymphocytes, T lymphocytes, null lymphocytes, and K (killer) lymphocytes. These cells are morphologically similar and cannot be distinguished from each other on a Wright-stained smear. The B lymphocyte is derived from the bone marrow and was so named because it was previously discovered in birds, where it was programmed by the organ called the bursa of Fabricius. The equivalent organ in the human is now felt to be the bone marrow. The B lymphocyte is primarily responsible for the production of antibodies. The T lymphocyte resides in the thymus for a short period of time, where it is acted on by this organ (possibly by hormone action) before taking on the characteristics of the T (thymus-dependent) lymphocyte, which functions primarily in cellular immune response. The null lymphocyte has neither T nor B lymphocyte characteristics. These cells may represent a separate class of lymphocytes or may represent a transition stage in the development of the B and T lymphocyte. K (killer) lymphocytes contain receptors on the surface of their cell membrane that bind specific antibodies to target cell antigens that form antigen-antibody complexes and have a cytotoxic effect on the target.

B AND T LYMPHOCYTES

B LYMPHOCYTES

B lymphocytes are generally short-lived and constitute about 20% of the lymphocytes in the peripheral blood. As the B lymphocytes mature in the bone marrow, they acquire a specific B cell antigen, termed MBLA. During further maturation, light chain components of immunoglobulins appear on the surface of the B lymphocyte. This is followed by fully developed immunoglobulins (primarily IgM). F_c receptors (receptors that bind the F_c portion of the immunoglobulin) also develop on the surface of the cell, along with receptors for complement. When the B lymphocyte leaves the bone marrow, the development of the F_c and complement receptors and immunoglobulins increases. Ultimately, the B lymphocytes transform into plasma cells and produce and secrete specific antibodies, some of which are found in the cell membrane and act as receptors for antigens. These are termed surface-bound immunoglobulins (S Ig) and are primarily IgM, IgD, IgG, and IgA. Some B lymphocytes also have been shown to have receptors for the Epstein-Barr virus.

T LYMPHOCYTES

It is thought that T lymphocytes have antigens attached to their outside surface. These antigens have been identified and named by the use of antibodies. For example, immature T lymphocytes have been found to react with monoclonal antibodies that are termed *anti-T9* and *anti-T10*. These cells are, therefore, termed $T9^+$ and $T10^+$. As these cells mature, they lose the $T9^+$ antigen, remaining positive for T10. They then acquire antigens T4, T5, and T6. When the lymphocyte becomes mature, the T6 antigen is lost, and the cells take on T1 and T3 antigens. They now show two different subsets of T lymphocytes, containing either the T4 or T5 antigen, but never both. When the T lymphocyte leaves the thymus, it no longer carries the T10 antigen. Of the peripheral circulating T lymphocytes, 55 to 65% function as T helper cells and are $T1^+$, $T3^+$, and $T4^+$; 20 to 30% of the T lymphocytes have cytotoxic and suppressor-cell functions and are $T1^+$, $T3^+$, and $T5^+$. Additional cell surface markers subdivide the T lymphocytes further: $T\mu$ cells have a receptor for IgM and $T\gamma$ cells have a receptor for IgG. T null lymphocytes have no receptors for immunoglobulins.

HLA ANTIGENS

In addition to the above surface antigens, the lymphocyte also contains a number of antigenic substances of chromosomal origin on its surface. These antigens were first determined by histocompatibility testing and have been termed *HLA-A, HLA-B, HLA-C, HLA-D,* and *HLA-DR.* The latter, HLA-DR, is the strongest on B lymphocytes but is also present to a lesser extent on T lymphocytes.

LIFE SPAN, CIRCULATION, AND RECIRCULATION OF LYMPHOCYTES

The majority of lymphocytes are long-lived, with a life span of about 4 years. Some lymphocytes, however, may live as long as 20 years. The remaining lymphocytes, about 15%, are short-lived, lasting 3 to 4 days.

Those lymphocytes present in the peripheral blood are generally in transit from one lymphoid tissue to another or to sites of inflammation. The lymphocytes have two basic patterns of circulation: (1) Immature lymphocytes will travel from the bone marrow to the thymus and from there to the peripheral or secondary lymphoid organs. (2) There is a recirculation of the mature, differentiated lymphocytes continually moving from one area of the lymphatic system to another. Immature lymphocytes steadily migrate from the bone marrow to the thymus, where they mature and are acted on by this organ. These cells then migrate to thymus-dependent areas in the peripheral lymphatic system and most probably become the long-lived T lymphocytes. These cells make up most of the recirculating pool of lymphocytes, although both B and T lymphocytes are able to recirculate and will travel back and forth between the blood, bone marrow, and peripheral lymphoid tissue. They will enter the thymus, however, only from the bone marrow. It is thought that T lymphocytes have their own patterns of recirculation in that some T lymphocytes travel only to the lymph nodes, whereas other T lymphocytes only recirculate to the gut area. Antigenic stimulation will convert short-lived, noncirculating lymphocytes into long-lived, recirculating cells, and during an immune response, the rate of blood flow through the lymph nodes may increase as much as fourfold. Also, the major factor that appears to affect the total number of lymphocytes in the body seems to be the amount of exposure to antigen. Also, because lymphocytes are capable of blast transformation and mitosis, they can serve as their own stem cell compartment in terms of replacement when needed.

LYMPHOCYTE FUNCTION

The primary function of lymphocytes is in the generation of immunity, of which two types have been defined: (1) synthesis of antibodies (immunoglobulin) primarily by the B lymphocytes and (2) establish-ment of cellular immunity by the T lymphocyte.

T LYMPHOCYTES

The T lymphocytes have none to very few immunoglobulin receptors on their surface membrane. They can and do recognize and respond to antigenic stimulation. Their primary responsibility concerns cellular immune responses or cell-mediated immunity and includes graft rejection and delayed hypersensitivity reactions. When the T lymphocytes are activated, they produce substances, called *lymphokines,* which play a role in the cellular immune response. Some of the more common lymphokines are described here. (1) *Lymphotoxin* (LT) may be produced by lymphocytes upon stimulation by antigens. These lymphotoxins are capable of destroying target cells and are important in cellular immunity reactions, where foreign cells are destroyed. Certain drugs, such as cortisone, are able to inhibit the release of lymphotoxin. (2) *Transfer factor* (TF) is nonantigenic and stimulates uncommitted lymphocytes to respond to specific antigens. Transfer factor is antigen-specific in that a specific antigen will stimulate transfer factor to act for that antigen only. (3) *Migration inhibitory factor* (MIF) is produced as a result of stimulation by any one of a number of antigens to inhibit migration of macrophages. (4) *Lymphocyte transforming factor* (LTF) will cause transformation of lymphocytes to blast cells. (5) *Interferon* is a group of various proteins, any of which can confer a resistance to viruses onto cells that otherwise would have been susceptible to the virus. The T lymphocytes are a major source of interferon. Other lymphokines mediate the interaction between T and B lymphocytes and macrophages. Growth inhibiting lymphokines, stimulatory or blastogenic lymphokines, and chemotactic, cytotoxin, maturation, and skin-reactive lymphokines have also been described.

In addition, T lymphocytes may act as helper cells (aid in antibody production by B lymphocytes), suppressor cells (inhibit antibody production by B lymphocytes), memory cells, and effector cells (act in delayed hypersensitivity and graft-vs.-host reactions).

In cellular immunity, the T lymphocytes and macrophages predominate. Cellular immunity can be passed from one person to another by transferring sensitized lymphocytes but not by the transfer of antibody. As a general rule, in cellular immunity, the cells undergo blast transformation followed by proliferation. These cells will then produce various substances (lymphokines) that interact with the antigen substance. There are several types of cellular immunity: (1) Delayed hypersensitivity reaction may be produced by bacterial, viral, parasitic, and contact antigens. The small lymphocytes become sensitized through receptor sites on their surface or from the transfer of information from macrophages. These lymphocytes then proliferate and release various soluble substances (lymphokines). (2) Transplantation reactions involve the HLA system, where the antibody response is directed against these HLA antigens. Skin grafts, for example, will survive if the sensitized lymphocytes can be kept from proliferating or if the lymphocytes have no access to the skin graft. (3) The lymphocytes in autoimmune disease are thought to have a decreased amount of suppressor T-cell activity. (4) Antitumor immunity is thought to exist because the tumor cells are antigenically different from normal cells.

B LYMPHOCYTES

B lymphocytes are active in the immune response by transforming into plasma cells and producing immunoglobulins, which are defined as a whole group of antibody proteins, including proteins found in pathologic states. All immunoglobulins consists of the basic subunit of four poly-

peptide chains connected by disulfide bonds. Of the four chains, two are classified as light chains and two are heavy chains. There are five classes of immunoglobulins: IgG, IgA, IgM, IgD, and IgE. These classes are further subdivided according to their antigenic characteristics. Usually, only one class of immunoglobulin is produced by a group (clone) of lymphocytes or plasma cells. This mechanism depends on the macrophage phagocytizing the antigen. The processed antigen is bound to RNA, and the antigen-RNA complex is transferred to the lymphocyte or plasma cell from the macrophage. The lymphocyte, upon accepting the antigen, becomes immunologically active, producing immunoglobulins specific for that antigen. At the same time, memory cells in the area remain which retain the capacity to respond to the same antigen in the future. There are also substances present that limit the intensity of the lymphocyte (immune) response. The concentration of immunoglobulins is directly proportional to the number of lymphocytes producing it. The half-lives of the various immunoglobulins are 6 days for IgA, 5 days for IgM, and 23 days for IgG.

MORPHOLOGY OF LYMPHOCYTES IN DISEASE

Lymphocytes will undergo transformations when they are stimulated. In the laboratory, under certain in vitro conditions, the lymphocyte can be made to transform into an immature cell that has the appearance of a blast cell. These cells have increased ribosomes, a well-developed Golgi apparatus, and some endoplasmic reticulum development, in addition to actively synthesizing RNA, DNA, immunoglobulins, complement components, and so on. This is similar to the reactions that occur in the body in response to various disease states such as drug reactions, viral infections, and so forth and the resultant finding of what are collectively termed *atypical lymphocytes* present in the Wright-stained blood smear. Various terms have been used to describe these morphologic changes in the lymphocyte in addition to the broad description of atypical lymphocyte: *virocytes, leukocytoid lymphocytes, reticular lymphocytes, reactive lymphocytes,* and *Türk cells.* Two additional terms used frequently are the *plasmacytoid lymphocyte* and *lymphocytoid plasma cell,* which more correctly describes the intermediate forms of the lymphocyte/plasma cell (the B lymphocyte in the process of developing into a plasma cell). When the lymphocyte is stimulated, the morphologic characteristics of the cell are transformed, and various changes take place. The cell first increases in size, and the nucleus becomes less dense and may show one or more nucleoli. Generally, the cytoplasm becomes basophilic and shows a greater increase in amount than the nucleus. A B lymphocyte transforming into a plasma cell also increases in size. The cytoplasm becomes basophilic and may show a lighter-staining area near the nucleus. The nuclear chromatin becomes more coarse and clumped and shows increased areas of parachromatin. Other characteristics exhibited by a stimulated lymphocyte are foamy (holes) or vacuolated cytoplasm, an irregularly shaped nucleus, increased numbers of azurophilic granules in the cytoplasm (normally, approximately one third of the lymphocytes contain these granules), radial and/or peripheral basophilia of the cytoplasm, sharper separation of the nuclear chromatin and parachromatin, and more abundant basophilic cytoplasm than is normally present in the cell. These cells have been separated into three groups by Dr. Hal Downey:

Downey type I: The nucleus may be irregularly shaped. The cytoplasm is relatively basophilic and may at times be foamy.

Downey type II: There is an increased amount of cytoplasm that also contains radial or peripheral basophilia. The nuclear chromatin is generally more coarse and clumped.

Downey type III: This group of cells increases in size and shows basophilic cytoplasm. The nucleus usually has visible nucleoli.

CELLS OF ACUTE AND SUBACUTE LYMPHATIC LEUKEMIA

The lymphocytic cells present in acute lymphatic leukemia show several morphologic variations from the normal lymphocyte. The leukemic lymphoblast is slightly larger than the lymphocyte of the circulating blood. It has a thin rim of clear, light blue cytoplasm. The chromatin pattern of the nucleus is delicate and fine but somewhat more coarse than that of the myeloblast. There are usually one or two well-defined nucleoli present. The immature lymphocyte or leukemic prolymphocyte is approximately the same size as the leukemic lymphoblast. It has only a small amount of cytoplasm. The nucleus shows more clumping of the chromatin. Nucleoli are usually visible.

Plasma Cells

Plasmablast

Size: 18 to 25 μm diameter.

Cytoplasm: Basophilic cytoplasm. Abundant. Nongranular.

Nucleus: Nuclear chromatin is more clumped than in the reticular lymphocyte.
Eccentric. (The nucleus is off center, located at one side of the cell.)

Round or oval in shape.
Multiple nucleoli that
may or may not be vis-
ible.

Proplasmacyte

Size: 15 to 25 μm in diameter.

Cytoplasm: Basophilic; usually bluer
than in the blast stage.
Nongranular.
Abundant, but slightly
less than in blast stage.
A lighter-staining area in
the middle of the cell
(in the cytoplasm, next
to the nucleus) may
become visible. This is
termed a *hof.*

Nucleus: Round or oval in shape.
Eccentric.
Chromatin is coarser and
more clumped than in
the plasmablast stage.
One or two nucleoli that
may or may not be vis-
ible.

Plasmacyte (plasma cell) (Fig. 120.)

Size: 8 to 20 μm in diameter.

Cytoplasm: Moderately abundant, but
less than in the pre-
vious stage.
Deeply basophilic.

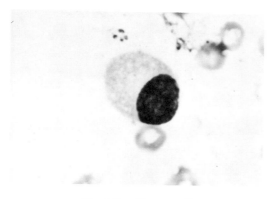

Fig. 120. Plasma cell.

Hof next to nucleus.
Nongranular, usually.

Nucleus: Chromatin is condensed
and coarse.
Round or oval in shape.
Eccentric.
No nucleoli are visible.

PLASMA CELLS

Most investigators believe that the plasma cell is derived from the B lympho-cyte. When the mature B lymphocyte is antigenically stimulated, it undergoes transformation first to a blast stage and then develops into a plasma cell. The ma-ture plasma cell contains a Golgi appara-tus located in the hof (clear zone or light-staining area near the nucleus). The cy-toplasm contains a well-developed rough endoplasmic reticulum and a few mito-chondria.

In certain pathologic states and when manufacturing immunoglobulins, the plasms cells may produce striking altera-tions in their appearance. Some of the changes possible are:

1. Red staining of the cytoplasm *(flame cell).*
2. Red-staining, crystalline, rod-shaped bodies present in the cytoplasm.
3. Red-staining globules in the cyto-plasm *(Russell bodies).*
4. Globular bodies present in the cyto-plasm *(grape, berry,* or *morula cell).*

The globules present in the cytoplasm are usually perfectly round, and the color may vary from pink, red, blue, or green to col-orless. These globules may become so tightly packed as to give a honeycombed appearance. At times, the protein material in the cytoplasm may crystallize, thus giv-ing rise to elongated and pointed struc-tures. Following the secretion of products from the plasma cell, the cytoplasm may have an uneven, tattered appearance to it.

For more details on the plasma cell and immunoglobulins, the reader is referred to the previous section describing B lymphocytes.

Monocytes

The monocyte is produced mainly in the bone marrow.

Promonocyte (immature monocyte) (Fig. 121.)

Size:	14 to 18 μm in diameter.
Cytoplasm:	Blue-gray. Contains fine dustlike azurophilic granules. Ground-glass appearance. Moderate amount.
Nucleus:	Oval or indented. One to five nucleoli. Fine chromatin pattern.

Monocyte (Fig. 122.)

Size:	14 to 20 μm in diameter.
Cytoplasm:	Abundant. Blue-gray. Many fine azurophilic granules, giving a ground-glass appearance. Vacuoles may sometimes be present.
Nucleus:	Round, kidney-shaped, or may show slight lobulation. It may be folded over on top of itself, thus showing brainlike convolutions. No nucleoli are visible. Chromatin is fine, arranged in skeinlike strands.

With the present staining techniques, it is often impossible to differentiate the various types of blast cells. Many times, the cell is merely termed a "blast." Otherwise, the cell is identified by the company it keeps, that is, by placing it in the same family of cells as the identifiable ones in the area surrounding the blast cell.

PHYSIOLOGY AND BIOLOGY OF THE MONOCYTE

Unlike the other white blood cells in the peripheral blood, the monocyte is considered to be an immature cell. When it leaves the blood, it travels to the tissues, where this cell line spends most of its time, maturing further into a macrophage. The immature monocyte, or promonocyte, is less phagocytic and less motile than the monocyte. The mature monocyte in the peripheral blood has a well-developed Golgi apparatus, rough endoplasmic reticulum, numerous mitochondria, and variable amounts of ribosomes and polyribosomes. There are nucleoli present in the nucleus in about 50% of the monocytes, as seen by

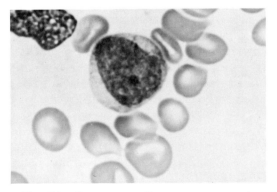

Fig. 121. Promonocyte (immature monocyte).

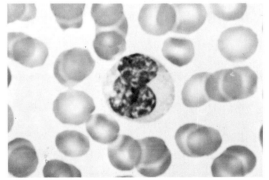

Fig. 122. Monocyte

(The above photographs have been enlarged in an attempt to show more nuclear and cytoplasmic detail)

electron microscopy. The granules in the cytoplasm of the monocyte are packaged by the Golgi apparatus and represent primary lysosomes. There are two types of granules present in the cytoplasm; one type contains peroxidase, and the second type does not contain this enzyme. Other enzymes present in both the monocyte and macrophage are sodium fluoride-resistant esterase, β-glucuronidase, lysozyme, galactosidases, and naphthylaminidase. The monocyte and macrophage are actively motile cells, capable of chemotaxis, capable of moving through blood vessel walls and migrating to areas of inflammation, and capable of extending multiple pseudopods. They respond to such substances as MIF (migration inhibitory factor), which is produced by the T lymphocytes to immobilize the macrophage, and to chemotactic inhibitors. The monocyte and macrophage are capable of phagocytosis and pinocytosis.

LIFE SPAN OF THE MONOCYTE

The bone marrow contains the developing monocyte precursors and supplies the monocytes to the peripheral blood. The proliferation of monocytes in the bone marrow takes about 54 hours. The mature monocytes, however, do not leave the bone marrow in any specific order. Some appear to enter the blood right after production, whereas other monocytes may spend several days in the bone marrow before going to the peripheral blood. The marginal pool of monocytes in the blood is about 3.5 times the size of the circulating pool. The mature monocyte spends about 12 hours in the peripheral blood before going to the tissues.

DEVELOPMENT OF THE MONOCYTE INTO THE MACROPHAGE

The monocyte moves via diapedesis through the blood vessels walls into the various tissues and transforms into the macrophage, at the same time becoming actively phagocytic. It is also thought that some macrophages are produced by cell division of existing macrophages. As the macrophage develops from the monocyte, the cell increases in size. One or more nucleoli develop and there is an increase in the hydrolytic enzymes. In addition, the Golgi apparatus and the number of mitochondria increase. There is also an increased number of secondary lysosomes as a result of increased phagocytosis. Overall, the macrophage is more active than the monocyte and has a much richer supply of acid hydrolases.

THE MACROPHAGE

The macrophage is a large cell, ranging in size from 15 to 80 μm in diameter. It has an eccentric nucleus that may be egg-shaped, indented, or elongated. The chromatin appears spongy, and there are generally one to two nucleoli. The cell has very abundant sky-blue cytoplasm that contains many coarse azure granules and is usually vacuolated. There is a large variation in the appearance of the macrophage, depending on the site from which the cell has been derived. Some macrophages may develop epithelioid characteristics and may then fuse to form giant multinucleated cells. Osteoclasts are thought to be formed from blood monocytes and histiocytes. Macrophages have been divided into two categories: fixed macrophages and unfixed, or wandering, macrophages. When stimulated, some of the fixed macrophages may become the actively motile, wandering macrophage. The unfixed, wandering macrophage has also been termed a *histiocyte*. Macrophages are found scattered throughout the body. There are macrophages lining the sinusoids of the spleen and bone marrow, the alveolar macrophages of the lungs, the Kupffer cells of the liver, and freely migrating macrophages of the pleural and peritoneal cavities. These cells are also found at sites of inflammation and in peritoneal, pleural, and synovial fluids. The macrophage lives much longer in the tissues than does the neutrophil. It is capable of cell division and can be stimulated to synthesize a number of enzymes and other substances, depending on the body's present needs.

PROPERTIES AND FUNCTIONS OF THE MONOCYTE AND MACROPHAGE

Both the monocyte and macrophage show active chemotaxis and *necrotaxis* (attraction to dead or dying cells). Pinocytosis and micropinocytosis increase as the cell matures toward the macrophage. Phagocytosis of antigens by the monocyte and macrophage requires that certain antigens be coated with an antibody *(opsonization)*. The monocytes and macrophages are also capable of *necrophagocytosis* (ingestion of dying cells and cellular debris) that, along with pinocytosis, does not require antibody coating of the material being ingested. The primary functions of the monocyte and macrophage are:

1. *Defense mechanism against intracellular parasites, including certain bacteria, fungi, and protozoa.* They primarily control such microbial infections of mycobacteria, brucella, listeria, and salmonella. When an antibody-coated antigen is present, the monocyte or macrophage travels to the site by the use of chemotaxis. It then attaches to the antigen and extends pseudopods around the material, forming a phagosome. Primary lysosomes in the cytoplasm of the monocyte or macrophage then fuse with the phagosome, emptying their acid hydrolases into the area to digest or degrade the antigen and become secondary lysosomes. The material may then be released from the cell *(exocytosis)*. It has been suggested that the monocyte and macrophage contain receptor sites for immunoglobulins on their surface. This then facilitates the recognition and ingestion of the foreign particles. Also, ingestion of particles by these cells is enhanced by certain factors present in the plasma such as antibodies and complement. The macrophage is able to phagocytize more quickly and has a greater capacity for phagocytosis than either the neutrophil or the monocyte. The cell is also capable of anaerobic phagocytosis, functioning in the center of wounds where oxygen is decreased. Unlike the neutrophil, both the monocyte and macrophage are able to synthesize new enzymes and replace lysosomes. Macrophages also are capable of destroying a variety of cells. They may produce substances that destroy some tumor cells or may destroy cells coated with specific antibodies.

2. *Removal of damaged and old cells.* They play an important part in the removal of old and damaged red blood cells and also in wound debridement. In red blood cells, the iron remains in the macrophage, binding with apoferritin (in the macrophage) to form ferritin. The ferritin later leaves the macrophage, binds to transferrin, and again is used in red blood cell production.

3. *Processes antigen information for lymphocytes.* Macrophages serve an important role in the immune response. They interact with antigens by membrane attachment, ingestion, and by subsequent modification of the antigen. This processed antigen is then presented to the lymphocyte by some type of cytoplasmic connection with the lymphocyte. The lymphocyte may then undergo blast transformation and antibody production. The macrophage can interact with both B and T lymphocytes and is, therefore, also active in cell-mediated immunity.

4. *Production and secretion of various substances.* The monocytes and macrophages release lysosomal enzymes

into the surrounding area in response to antigen-antibody complexes and during phagocytosis. They are an important source of colony-stimulating factor, which is felt to represent an important ingredient for the control of leukopoiesis. The macrophage produces and secretes high levels of pyrogen upon stimulation, which is the principal physiologic factor in fever. Complement factors are also synthesized and secreted by the macrophages, as are interferon and transferrin.

MEGAKARYOCYTES

The megakaryoblast develops into the megakaryocyte, which then gives rise to the blood platelet.

Megakaryoblast (Fig. 123.)

Size:	20 to 50 μm in diameter.
Cytoplasm:	Varying shades of blue. Usually darker than the myeloblast. May have small, blunt pseudopods. Small to moderate amount. Usually a narrow band around the nucleus. As the cell matures, the amount of cytoplasm increases. Usually nongranular.

Nucleus:	Round, oval, or may be kidney-shaped. Fine chromatin pattern. Multiple nucleoli that generally stain blue.

Promegakaryocyte

Size:	20 to 50 μm in diameter.
Cytoplasm:	Usually abundant. Less basophilic than the blast stage. Granules begin to form.
Nucleus:	Chromatin becomes more coarse. Multiple nucleoli are visible. Irregular in shape; may even show slight lobulation.

Megakaryocyte (the largest cell found in the normal bone marrow) (Fig. 124.)

Size:	30 to 160 μm in diameter.
Cytoplasm:	Abundant. Pinkish-blue in color. Very granular. Usually has an irregular peripheral border. The granules begin to aggregate into little bundles that bud off from the cell to become platelets.

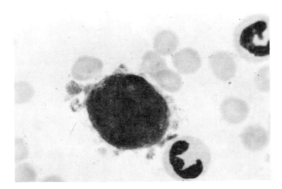

Fig. 123. Megakaryoblast. (Magnification ×1000)

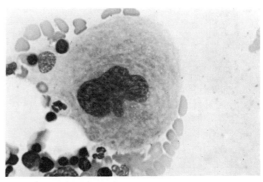

Fig. 124. Megakaryocyte. (Magnification ×500)

Nucleus: Small in comparison to
             cell size.
             Multiple nuclei may be
             visible or the nucleus
             may show multilobula-
             tion.
             Chromatin is coarser than
             in the previous stage.
             No nucleoli are visible.

Platelet (thrombocyte)

Size: 1 to 4 μm in diameter.

Cytoplasm: Light blue to purple.
             Very granular.
             Consists of two parts: (1)
             the chromomere,
             which is granular and
             located centrally, and
             (2) the hyalomere,
             which surrounds the
             chromomere and is
             nongranular and clear
             to light blue.

Nucleus: None present.

MATURATION OF THE MEGAKARYOCYTE

It is thought that the megakaryoblast originates (along with the granulocytes and erythrocytes) from the pluripotential stem cell. The maturation of the mega- karyoblast is unique. It is unable to undergo cell division, and, as it matures, the nucleus become lobulated, whereas the cytoplasm increases in amount and be- comes more granular. Nuclear and cyto- plasmic maturation do not occur together or on parallel levels. Initially, the nucleus contains a paired set of chromosomes (termed *diploid*). As the cell begins to ma- ture, DNA synthesis takes place, and the nuclear material duplicates itself, result- ing in a two-lobed nucleus in which each nuclear lobe contains a paired set of chro- mosomes (this process is termed *endo- mitosis*). The entire nucleus now contains two paired sets of chromosomes and may be termed 4 N, in which 4 represents the ploidy value of four single sets of chro-

mosomes and N stands for nuclear num- ber. The nuclear number generally under- goes further divisions, yielding four sets of paired chromosomes (four-lobed nu- cleus) and is termed 8 N. Further nuclear divisions give rise to eight sets of paired chromosomes (eight-lobed nucleus, or 16 N), then 16 sets of paired chromosomes (16-lobed nucleus, or 32 N), and so on. Another term used to describe the in- creased numbers of chromosomes over the diploid number is *polyploid*. The majority of mature megakaryocytes in the bone marrow are 16 N (eight nuclear lobes), whereas about 25% are 32 N and a few are 8 N. When the cell has acquired all of its nuclear lobes, the cytoplasm begins to ma- ture, becoming larger in size and more granular. During the entire process of nu- clear and cytoplasmic maturation, there is no division of the cytoplasm.

PHYSIOLOGY AND BIOLOGY OF THE MEGAKARYOCYTE

The maturing megakaryocyte contains a Golgi region around the nucleus where specific granules are packed to be distrib- uted throughout the cytoplasm, except at the peripheral borders of the cell, which remain free of granules until platelets begin to form. Polyribosomes and rough endoplasmic reticulum are present at the beginning of cytoplasmic maturation. It takes 4 to 5 days for the megakaryocyte to mature. Infrequently, megakaryocytes es- cape from the bone marrow and get into the peripheral blood. Megakaryocyte frag- ments may be seen in the blood in chronic myelogenous leukemia, various forms of cancer, myelofibrosis, polycythemia vera, Hodgkin's disease, leukocytosis due to in- fection, and following surgery.

PLATELET PRODUCTION

Platelets are produced directly from the megakaryocyte cytoplasm. As the mega- karyocyte matures, a network of tubules develops in the cytoplasm, many of which open to the outside of the cell. These tubules then fuse to form fissures, which ultimately form the margins and plasma membranes of individual platelets. The megakaryocyte extends these filaments of cytoplasm into the sinusoids, where they detach and fragment into individual platelets. The entire megakaryocyte cytoplasm is thus broken away, and the nucleus is left to degenerate eventually and be processed by reticuloendothelial cells. Each megakaryocyte generally produces between 2,000 to 4,000 platelets in this manner. Thus, the platelet is a portion of the megakaryocyte cytoplasm and, as such, contains no nucleus. As a general rule, the more nuclear lobes the megakaryocyte possesses, the larger the cytoplasmic mass, and, therefore, the more platelets that are produced. It is thought that platelet production is stimulated by *thrombopoietin* (as erythropoietin stimulates red blood cell production). When there is increased production of platelets, the number and size of the megakaryocytes in the bone marrow increases along with a decrease in the maturation time of the megakaryocyte. Major platelet production takes place in the bone marrow, where the megakaryocytes make up less than 1% of the nucleated cells of the marrow.

PLATELET LIFE SPAN

Once the platelet is released into the peripheral blood, it has a life span of 9 to 12 days. The young platelets are larger and less dense than older platelets. Also, they are metabolically more active and more effective in hemostasis. At any one time, approximately two thirds of the platelets are in the blood, whereas the remaining one-third are in the spleen. The platelets in the spleen are interchangeable with those in the blood. A high percentage of the platelets in the spleen are young platelets. Damaged and nonfunctioning platelets are generally removed from the blood, principally by the spleen. The platelet turnover rate is approximately 35,000 platelets (±4,300) per μl each day.

PLATELET STRUCTURE, COMPOSITION, AND METABOLISM

It has been suggested that the platelet membrane is derived from endoplasmic reticulum, but it is now thought that it most probably comes from the plasma membrane of the megakaryocyte. On the outside of the platelet membrane there is a fuzzy coating, termed the *surface coat.* This is an irregular layer that is primarily composed of proteins, glycoproteins, mucopolysaccharides, and sialic acids. Within the platelet, there is a system of canals *(canalicular system)* throughout the cytoplasm that communicates with the exterior of the platelet. Substances contained within the platelet are extruded to the outside of the platelet through this canal system, which is also involved in platelet phagocytosis. A microtubular system also exists that circles the periphery of the platelet beneath the platelet membrane (Fig. 125). These tubules are believed to contain the contractile protein, *thrombosthenin* (actomyosin), which helps to maintain platelet shape and may also be responsible for changes in platelet shape. (Actin and myosin molecules combine to form actomyosin.) The platelet cytoplasm contains a few mitochondria, granules, dense bodies, glycogen deposits, and many microfilaments. The granules, also termed *alpha granules,* are each enclosed in a membrane and contain acid hydrolases and phospholipids. The dense bodies are few in number and may be derived from undifferentiated granules. They contain serotonin, nucleotides, cal-

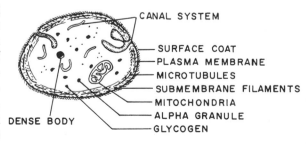

Fig. 125.   Normal platelet structure.

cium ions, catecholamines, and most probably, platelet factor 4. The platelet is composed of about 60% protein, 15% lipid, 8% carbohydrate, various minerals, water, and nucleotides. It contains over 90 different enzymes. Thrombosthenin comprises 15 to 20% of the platelet protein. Other proteins present include glycoproteins and coagulation factors. Fibrinogen, along with most of the other coagulation factors, has been demonstrated in association with the platelet. In addition, the platelet is able to synthesize amino acids, proteins, fatty acids, and phospholipids, and glycogen is the main carbohydrate present. The platelet has an active energy metabolism, using glucose as its main energy source.

PLATELET FUNCTION

Platelets function primarily in hemostasis (the stoppage of bleeding) and in maintaining capillary integrity. (This is discussed in greater detail in Chapter 5).

WHITE BLOOD CELL AND PLATELET MORPHOLOGY

In **toxic granulation** (Plate IVa), dark blue-black cytoplasmic granules are seen in the neutrophil. These are thought to be primary granules and show increased alkaline phosphatase activity. They are found in acute infections, drug poisoning, and burns.

Döhle bodies (Plate IVb) appear as a small, light blue-staining area in the cytoplasm of the neutrophil. The blue-staining area is a remnant of RNA and is found in infections, poisoning, burns, and following chemotherapy.

Hypersegmented neutrophils (Plate IVc) are neutrophils with a six- or more, lobed nucleus. This represents an abnormality in the maturation of the neutrophil. Normally, approximately 50 to 60% of the neutrophils contain three lobes, no more than 20% have four lobes, and there may be an occasional five-lobed neutrophil.

Any time there is an increased percentage of four- and/or five-lobed neutrophils present, hypersegmentation should be reported. In cases of pernicious anemia and folic acid deficiency, neutrophils with more than five lobes are commonly found. Hypersegmented neutrophils are also found in chronic infections.

The **Barr** (sex chromatin) **body** (Plate IVd) represents the second X chromatin in females and may be seen in 2 to 3% of the neutrophils in females. It is a small, well-defined, round projection of nuclear chromatin that is connected to the nucleus of the neutrophil by a single, fine strand of chromatin. The Barr body can be differentiated from small, nonspecific nodules of chromatin in that these projections are not attached to the nucleus with as fine a strand of chromatin. The number of Barr bodies in a cell is one less than the number of X chromosomes present in the cell. Another term used to describe the Barr body is a *drumstick*. These sex chromatins are not found in normal males.

Degenerated neutrophil and pyknotic nucleus (Plate IVe) results from condensation of nuclear chromatin to a solid, structureless mass with no pattern. These cells are not counted in a differential cell count.

A **vacuolated neutrophil** (Plate IIIr) results when the degenerating cytoplasm begins to acquire holes or as the result of active phagocytosis. This condition may be found in septicemia and severe infection.

Giant neutrophils may be seen occasionally in a normal peripheral blood smear. These cells are much larger than normal neutrophils and are generally hyperlobulated. They may be found normally in a frequency of about 1 in every 20,000 neutrophils but may increase somewhat in frequency in disease states.

Pelger-Huët anomaly (Plate Ve,f,g) is indicated by failure of the neutrophil nucleus to segment properly. All of the neutrophils have no more than a bi-lobed nucleus. The nuclear chromatin is coarsely clumped. This benign anomaly may be inherited or acquired, as in certain leukemias. A person heterozygous for this characteristic shows numerous bi-lobed (dumbbell-shaped) nuclei, whereas the homozygous person has round neutrophil nuclei. The neutrophils in this anomaly appear to function normally.

Chédiak-Higashi anomaly (Plate Va,b) is a rare, fatal disorder found in children. It is inherited as an autosomal recessive characteristic. The granulocytes usually contain several large, reddish-purple-staining masses in the cytoplasm, whereas they stain bluish purple in the lymphocytes and monocytes. These granules represent abnormal lysosomes. Neutropenia and thrombocytopenia generally develop, and patients with these conditions show increased susceptibility to infection.

Alder-Reilly anomaly (Plate IVf) shows heavy azurophilic granulation of the neutrophils, eosinophils, basophils, and sometimes, the lymphocytes and monocytes. This is an inherited condition and is commonly associated with Hurler's syndrome and Hunter's syndrome.

May-Hegglin anomaly is an inherited anomaly affecting the neutrophils and platelets. Döhle bodies are present in the neutrophils. Bizarre forms of the platelet are present, and the platelets may be decreased in number. Some patients are asymptomatic, whereas others may exhibit bleeding tendencies. Platelet function may be abnormal.

Auer rods (Plate Vh) are rodlike bodies that stain a reddish purple. They are found only in the cytoplasm of the blast cells in acute monocytic or acute myelogenous leukemia.

Smudge or basket cell (Plate IV,j,k) is the disintegrating nucleus of a ruptured white blood cell.

Atypical platelets (Plate III,o,p), abnormal in appearance, occur in some diseased states. In such cases, the platelet may have one or more of the following characteristics:
1. Large size.
2. Increased amount of hyalomere.
3. Granules decreased or absent.
4. Zoned appearance.

THE RETICULOENDOTHELIAL SYSTEM

The cells comprising the reticuloendothelial system are the reticulum cells of the lymph nodes and spleen, the Kupffer cells in the sinusoids of the liver, the blood monocytes (since they transform into tissue or fixed macrophages), and the sinusoid cells of the lymph nodes, bone marrow, adrenal gland, and pituitary gland. The reticuloendothelial system is of considerable size and is based on the ability of the cells to engulf particulate matter and damaged or dead cells. The phagocytosis may quickly kill and digest bacteria or red blood cells or may indefinitely store some particles. Phagocytosis is not always the primary function of these cells, however.

4

Special Hematology Procedures

EXAMINATION OF THE BONE MARROW

Examination of the bone marrow is a widely used method of diagnosing many hematologic diseases. It is a valuable procedure in conditions where diagnostic cells are present in the bone marrow but absent in the peripheral blood. Such conditions are found in Gaucher's disease, multiple myeloma, Niemann-Pick disease, some megaloblastic anemias, and when tumor cells are metastasizing (spreading) from other organs of the body. When pancytopenia exists, a bone marrow examination is helpful to rule out the diagnosis of leukemia and, where possible, to determine the cause of the pancytopenia. In addition to determining the presence of specific cells, the bone marrow procedure offers the opportunity for assessing the iron stores and cellularity of the marrow. Alterations in the normal distribution of cells may be noted, and the marrow cells may also be studied with special staining techniques.

Samples of bone marrow may be obtained from the sternum, the iliac crest, the spinous process of the lumbar vertebrae, and from the tibia in children under 4 years of age. The usual site of puncture in adults is the sternum, in the midline of the bone between the second and third ribs. The anterior or posterior iliac crest is also a common site for bone marrow biopsy. This area has an advantage in that there are no vital organs near the site of puncture. The patient is unable to see what is happening, which is helpful if he is apprehensive.

BONE MARROW BIOPSY

The bone marrow biopsy is carried out using sterile techniques, and sterile gloves are worn by the doctor performing the biopsy. If necessary, the skin at the puncture site may be shaved. A wide area around the puncture site is washed and cleaned with a suitable antiseptic solution, the same as for any minor surgical procedure. The area surrounding the puncture site is then draped with sterile towels. A solution of 1% procaine is injected into the skin and periosteum of the bone. After 1 or 2 minutes, a small one-eighth inch stab wound is made in the skin at the puncture site to avoid pushing the skin into the bone marrow. The area is now ready for the biopsy. A special needle is employed, of which there are several varieties available. The University of Illinois sternal needle (obtainable from V. Mueller and Company, Chicago, Illinois) consists of a heavy-duty, short, outer needle and a stylet that fits inside the needle. The outer needle has an adjustable guard to prevent it from entering too deeply into the bone. With the stylet in place, the needle is inserted until it impinges on the outer surface of the bone. The guard is then screwed down until it touches the skin. It is screwed back three

117

turns (each turn moves the guard a distance of 1 mm). The needle is inserted through the bone until the guard again comes in contact with the skin. In this way, the needle is inserted 3 mm deep into the bone. The stylet is removed from inside the needle, and a 10-ml syringe is attached to the needle. Firm, sharp pressure is applied to the plunger of the syringe to withdraw marrow. When this is done, the patient usually feels some pain. As soon as a few drops of marrow have entered the syringe, it is removed and passed to a technologist for the preparation of smears. If more marrow is desired, a second syringe may be attached to the needle and approximately 1 ml of marrow withdrawn. The syringe is then removed, and the blood is placed in a tube containing the proper amount of EDTA or heparin. The needle is removed from the bone, and a sterile dressing is applied.

PREPARATION OF THE BONE MARROW FOR STUDY

The exact procedures to be followed in preparing the bone marrow may vary according to the possible diagnosis of the patient. The most frequently used techniques are outlined below.

1. Using the first syringe containing only a few drops of marrow:
   A. Place the marrow on a slide in the form of a large drop.
   B. Using a spreader slide, immediately make five to eight thin smears. (Dip one end of the spreader slide into the pool of marrow. Transfer the marrow on the end of the slide to a clean glass slide and spread as for a routine blood smear.) It may also be desirable at this time to prepare several coverslip preparations. (The small clumps present in the blood are marrow particles.)
   C. When the pool of blood remaining on the original slide has clotted, transfer this to a small bottle of Zenker's fluid. This will be taken to the cytology department, where stained sections of the clot will be made.

2. Place the 1 ml of marrow obtained from the second syringe into a tube containing EDTA or heparin to prevent clotting, and return this specimen to the laboratory.

3. Using the fingerstick procedure, prepare several routine peripheral blood smears from the patient.

4. After adequate mixing of the anticoagulated bone marrow, place a large portion of the marrow onto a watch glass. Remove the fluid portion of the marrow from around the marrow particles, using this to fill a Wintrobe tube. Centrifuge at 2,500 RPM for 10 minutes. Four layers should then be seen (fat, plasma, nucleated cells, and red blood cells), and their relative volumes should be noted. Normally, there is 1 to 3% fat and 5 to 8% nucleated cells. Marrow that has been diluted with peripheral blood contains a smaller proportion of fat and nucleated cells. As the percent of nucleated cells increases, the amount of fat present decreases, and the marrow is termed *hypercellular*. If the fat layer increases, the percent of nucleated cells decreases, and the marrow is *hypocellular*. Remove the plasma and fat layers from the Wintrobe tube. Using a clean, disposable dropper, withdraw the nucleated cell layer and make several smears of this material. These are called *concentrate*, or *buffy coat*, smears.

5. To prepare particle smears, place several of the marrow particles, which remain on the watch glass, onto several slides or coverslips using the broken end of an applicator stick. Gently crush these marrow particles with a glass slide or coverslip.

6. The following smears are Wright-stained:

A. Thin direct smears (2).

B. Concentrate smear (1).

C. Particle smear (1).

(When Wright-staining bone marrow smears, it is advisable to double the staining times, especially when there is increased marrow cellularity.)

7. It is often advisable to routinely stain a concentrate smear with the Prussian-blue stain for iron. Other stains in widespread use for bone marrow smears are the peroxidase, Sudan black B, and the periodic acid-Schiff. Whether these stains are requested depends on the possible diagnosis of the patient.

8. The sections of clot prepared by the cytology department are generally stained with the hematoxylin and eosin stain unless further special stains are indicated.

EXAMINATION OF MARROW SLIDES

The bone marrow slides are studied and reported by the attending pathologist, with or without the aid of a technologist experienced in this area of hematology. A general outline of this procedure follows:

1. Examine the marrow section to determine the relative cellularity of the marrow. At this time, with experience, it is possible to detect certain abnormal cells if they are present. A differentiation between myeloid and erythroid cells is also possible.

2. A systematic examination of the direct marrow slide is made. The Wright-stained smear is examined first, using low power ($10 \times$). In scanning, megakaryocytes, abnormal cells of large size, and groups of abnormal cells may be detected. Using the oil immersion objective ($100 \times$), a differential cell count is made, based on a count of 200 to 500 nucleated cells. This will determine any abnormalities present in the distribution of cells, including any al-

teration in the myeloid:erythroid ratio. At the same time, the cells are also examined for morphologic abnormalities. (If the direct smear is very hypocellular, the concentrate smear may be examined.) The normal range for a differential count on bone marrow is shown in Table 3.

3. The Prussian-blue-stained concentrate smear is examined, and an estimate is made of the sideroblasts and particulate iron present.

4. Any marrow smears that had special stains are examined, evaluated, and reported.

LEUKOCYTE ALKALINE PHOSPHATASE STAIN

The granulocytic white blood cells contain alkaline phosphatase in the cytoplasm. The amount of alkaline phosphatase present varies in different diseases. Increased values for this test are found during pregnancy (last trimester), in infections accompanied by neutrophilia, in polycythemia vera, mongolism, Hodgkin's disease, and aplastic anemia. Low values occur in chronic myelogenous leukemia and paroxysmal nocturnal hemoglobinu-

TABLE 3. NORMAL VALUES FOR THE BONE MARROW

CELL	PERCENT
Myeloblasts	0.3– 5.0
Promyelocytes	1.0– 8.0
Myelocytes	
Neutrophil	5.0–19.0
Eosinophil	0.5– 3.0
Basophil	0.0– 0.5
Metamyelocytes	13.0–32.0
Neutrophils	7.0–30.0
Eosinophils	0.5– 4.0
Basophils	0.0– 0.7
Lymphocytes	3.0–17.0
Monocytes	0.5– 5.0
Megakaryocytes	0.1– 3.0
Plasma cells	0.1– 2.0
Reticulum cells	0.1– 2.0
Pronormoblast	1.0– 8.0
Basophilic normoblast	
Polychromatophilic normoblast	7.0–32.0
Orthochromic normoblast	
Mitotic cells	0.0– 2.0
Myeloid:erythroid ratio	2.1– 5.1

ria. Normal to high values are found in lymphocytic leukemia.

REFERENCE

Ackerman, G.A.: Substituted naphthol AS phosphate derivatives for the localization of leukocyte alkaline phosphatase activity, Lab. Invest., 11, 563, 1962.

REAGENTS AND EQUIPMENT

1. Formalin-methanol fixative.
   Formaldehyde, 40%   10 ml
   Methanol   90 ml
   Store in freezer.
2. Naphthol AS-MX phosphate, obtainable from Nutritional Biochemical Corporation, Cleveland, Ohio, in 1-g bottles.
3. N,N, dimethylformamide. Available from Eastman Organic Chemicals, Rochester, New York. Wash this reagent by shaking with activated charcoal and filter through a Seitz filter. (Note: This reagent is very toxic.)
4. Fast blue RR (4-benzoyl,2,5,-methoxyaniline dye), available from Dajac Laboratories, Division of Borden Company, Philadelphia, Pa., in 1-g bottles.
5. Neutral red, 1% (w/v), available from Coleman and Bell Company, Norwood, Ohio.
   Neutral red   1.0 g
   Distilled water   100 ml
   Filter immediately before use.
6. Stock solution.
   Naphthol AS-MX   12.5 mg
     phosphate
   N,N, dimethylformamide   5 ml
     (washed)
   Distilled water   20 ml
   To the preceding solution, add sufficient 1 M sodium carbonate (about one drop) to adjust the pH to 8.0.
   Distilled water   130 ml
   Tris (hydroxy) amino   95 ml
     methane (Tris) buffer,
     0.1 M, pH 8.3

Refrigerate and mix thoroughly prior to use.

7. Incubating solution.
   Fast blue RR   50 mg
   Stock solution   50 ml
   Prepare immediately before use. Filter. The solution is unstable and must be discarded immediately after use.
8. Coplin jar.

SPECIMEN

Collect five or six well-made fingerstick blood smears from the patient, from a positive control (pregnant woman in her last trimester), and from a normal control.

PRINCIPLE

The blood smears are fixed in cold formalin-methanol. When the smears are placed in the incubating solution, the alkaline phosphatase present in the white blood cells liberates naphthol, which couples with fast blue RR to form an insoluble brown-black compound. The smears are then counterstained. The degree of reactivity is determined by scoring each neutrophil according to the amount of precipitated dye present.

PROCEDURE

1. Immediately after collection, place the air-dried blood smears in a coplin jar containing cold formalin-methanol fixative for 30 seconds.
2. Rinse the smears in running tap water for 10 to 20 seconds.
3. Place the smears in a coplin jar containing freshly made incubating solution for 45 minutes at room temperature.
4. At the end of 45 minutes, wash the smears in running water.
5. Counterstain with 1% neutral red for 30 seconds. Allow the smears to airdry.
6. Examine the smears microscopically, using the oil immersion objective (100×). Count 100 consecutive neu-

trophils and grade each one from 0 to 4 on the basis of the appearance of the precipitated dye in the cytoplasm.

0 = Colorless.

1 = Diffuse pale brown cytoplasm.

2 = Cytoplasm is brown in color with or without an occasional clump of brownish-black precipitate.

3 = Brownish-black cytoplasm with clumps of precipitate.

4 = Deep brown-black precipitate uniformly throughout the cytoplasm.

7. The total of the ratings for 100 neutrophils is the score reported. The normal score for this test is 42 to 146.

DISCUSSION

1. Blood anticoagulated with EDTA may be used for this test, but the results will be inferior.
2. The preceding smears should be read within 1 to 2 hours of being stained because the stain tends to fade on standing.
3. In place of reporting the test score in numerical values, the result may be reported as below normal, normal, or above normal.
4. The blood smears must be fixed within 1 hour of collection. Once the smears are fixed, the specimen is stable for 24 hours.
5. An easy-to-use, prepared kit for the leukocyte alkaline phosphatase stain may be obtained from Sigma Chemical Company, St. Louis, Missouri.

PEROXIDASE STAIN

The peroxidase stain indicates the presence of peroxidases, which are normally present in the granulocytic white blood cells and, to a lesser degree, in the monocytes. The early myeloblast gives a negative reaction, whereas the immature and mature granulocytes give a positive stain.

Promonocytes and monocytes contain a few positively stained granules. Cells in the lymphocytic series yield negative staining, as do basophils. This stain is used to help differentiate leukemias.

REFERENCES

Graham, R.C., Lundholm, U., and Karnovsky, M.J.: Cytochemical demonstration of peroxidase activity with 3-amino-9-ethylcarbazole, J. Histochem. Cytochem., 13, 150, 1965.

Kaplow, L.S.: Substitute for benzidine in myeloperoxidase stains, Am. J. Clin. Path., 63, 451, 1975.

REAGENTS AND EQUIPMENT

1. Buffered formalin acetone fixative, pH 6.6 to 6.8.

Dibasic sodium phosphate (Na_2HPO_4)	0.2 g
Monobasic potassium phosphate (KH_2PO_4)	1.0 g

Dissolve the above in 300 ml of distilled water.

Acetone	450 ml
Formaldehyde, 40%	250 ml

Store in the refrigerator.

2. Acetic acid, 0.02 M.

Glacial acetic acid	1.16 ml

Dilute to 1 liter with distilled water.

3. Sodium acetate, 0.02 M.

Sodium acetate ($CH_3COONa \cdot 3 H_2O$)	2.72 g

Dilute to 1 liter with distilled water.

4. Acetate buffer, 0.02 M, pH 5.0 to 5.2.

Acetic acid, 0.02 M	176 ml
Sodium acetate, 0.02 M	800 ml

Store in the refrigerator.

5. Hydrogen peroxide, 0.3%.

Hydrogen peroxide, 30%	0.1 ml
Distilled water	9.9 ml

6. Stain, pH 5.5.

3-Amino-9-ethyl-carbazole	10 mg

(obtainable from Sigma Chemical Company, St. Louis, Missouri)

Dimethyl sulfoxide	6.0 ml
Acetate buffer, 0.02 M, pH 5.0 to 5.2	50 ml
Hydrogen peroxide, 0.3%	0.4 ml

Filter before use.

7. Mayer's hematoxylin.

Sodium iodate	0.5 g
Hematoxylin	5.0 g
Aluminum ammonium sulfate (ammonium alum)	50 g
Distilled water	700 ml
Acetic acid	20 ml
Glycerol	300 ml

Stable for several months.

8. Glycerol gelatin (obtainable commercially or may be prepared as outlined below).

Gelatin	20 g
Distilled water	105 ml
Glycerin	125 ml

Heat the above while mixing to dissolve the gelatin. Store in a jar. Refrigerate. Prior to use, remove a small portion and heat until liquified.

9. Coplin jars, three.
10. Coverslips.

SPECIMEN

Fresh blood smears made from capillary blood are recommended.

PROCEDURE

1. Prepare thin blood or bone marrow smears and allow to air-dry.
2. Place the smears in a coplin jar containing buffered formalin acetone for 15 seconds at room temperature.
3. Wash the smears under gently running tap water.
4. Place the smears in a coplin jar containing the stain mixture for 2½ minutes.
5. Wash the smears under gently running tap water.
6. Counterstain the smears in a coplin jar containing Mayer's hematoxylin for 8 minutes.
7. Wash the smears under gently running tap water.
8. Allow the smears to air-dry and immediately mount and coverslip in glycerol gelatin to prevent the stain from fading.
9. Examine the smears microscopically, using the oil immersion objective ($100 \times$). The presence of peroxidases is indicated by reddish-brown deposits present in the cytoplasm of the granulocytes and monocytes. The cytoplasm of the neutrophils is packed with these red-brown granules. The monocytes show a small to moderate number of the granules. The eosinophil exhibits darkly stained granules, whereas the basophil and lymphocyte remain unstained.

PERIODIC ACID-SCHIFF (PAS) REACTION

The periodic acid-Schiff stain indicates the presence of polysaccharides, mucopolysaccharides, mucoprotein, and glucoprotein. Granulocytes show a positive reaction in all stages of development, the mature neutrophils reacting the most strongly. Myelocytes and myeloblasts contain fewer positively stained granules. Eosinophil granules do not take up the stain, but the background cytoplasm stains positively. Lymphocytes contain a few fine or coarse, positively stained granules. Monocyte granules exhibit a small amount of positive staining, and nucleated red blood cells generally show no positively stained granules. In chronic lymphocytic leukemia, lymphosarcoma, and Hodgkin's disease, the lymphocytes contain an increased number of positively stained granules. In erythroleukemia (Di Guglielmo's disease) and thalassemia, the nucleated red blood cells may show a positive reaction. Some positive staining of the nucleated red blood cells has also been found in iron-deficiency anemia, some hemolytic anemias, pernicious anemia, aplastic anemia, and polycythemia.

REFERENCES

Dacie, J.V., and Lewis, S.M.: *Practical Hematology*, 5th ed., Churchill Livingstone, New York, 1975.

McManus, J.F.A.: Histological demonstration of mucin after periodic acid, Nature, *158*, 202, 1946.

REAGENTS AND EQUIPMENT

1. Periodic acid solution, 1% (w/v).
   Periodic acid ($HIO_4 \cdot 2H_2O$)   1.0 g
   Distilled water   100 ml
2. Schiff's leukobasic fuchsin.
   Basic fuchsin   1.0 g
   Boiling distilled water   400 ml
   Allow the preceding solution to cool to 50°C and filter. Add 1.0 g of thionyl chloride ($SOCl_2$) to it. Allow the mixture to stand in the dark for 12 hours. Add 2.0 g of activated charcoal to the mixture, shake for 1 minute, filter, and store in the dark at 0–4°C.
3. Methanol.
4. Aqueous hematoxylin.
   Hematoxylin   2.0 g
   Distilled water   100 ml
5. Coplin jars.

SPECIMEN

Air-dried blood or bone marrow smears.

PROCEDURE

1. Fix the blood or bone marrow smears with methanol for 10 minutes.
2. Wash the smears in running tap water for 15 minutes.
3. Place the slides in a coplin jar containing 1% periodic acid for 10 minutes.
4. At the end of 10 minutes, place the smears in a coplin jar containing Schiff's leukobasic fuchsin for 30 minutes.
5. Rinse the slides in tap water and then wash in distilled water for 5 minutes.
6. Place the smears in a coplin jar containing hematoxylin for 15 minutes.
7. Rinse the slides with tap water and allow to air-dry.
8. Examine the smears microscopically, using the oil immersion objective (100×). The polysaccharides, mucopolysaccharides, mucoproteins, and glucoproteins present in the cells will stain positively, taking on a reddish-purple color.

DISCUSSION

1. Blood or bone marrow smears that have been Wright-stained may be successfully stained according to the preceding procedure.
2. Smears several years old, whether Wright-stained or not, may also be stained by the periodic acid-Schiff stain.

SUDAN BLACK B STAIN

Sudan black B stains various lipids, among which are sterols, phospholipids, and neutral fats. As a stain, it is most often employed to distinguish the different types of acute leukemia. Myeloblasts stain faintly positive, whereas the lymphocytic cells show negative staining, and the monocytic cells show positive staining of the finely scattered granules.

REFERENCE

Sheehan, H.L., and Storey, G.W.: An improved method of staining leukocyte granules with Sudan black B, J. Path. Bact., *59*, 336, 1947.

REAGENTS AND EQUIPMENT

1. Stock buffer solution.
   Crystalline phenol   16 g
   Ethanol   30 ml
   Add the preceding two reagents to 100 ml of distilled water containing 0.3 g of disodium phosphate ($Na_2HPO_4 \cdot 12H_2O$).

2. Stock Sudan solution.

Sudan black B	0.3 g
Ethanol	100 ml

Prepare this solution several days prior to use. Allow it to sit at room temperature and shake frequently to ensure that all of the dye is dissolved.

3. Sudan black B staining solution.

Stock buffer solution	20 ml
Stock Sudan solution	30 ml

Stable for 2 to 3 months.

4. Formaldehyde, 40%.

5. Acetate buffer, 0.1 N, pH 5.0.

Sodium acetate (CH$_3$COONa·3 H$_2$O)	4.797 g
Acetic acid, 1 N	14.75 ml

(6 ml of glacial acetic acid diluted to 1 liter with distilled water)

Dissolve the sodium acetate in the 1 N acetic acid and dilute to 1 liter with distilled water. Refrigerate.

6. Buffered 1% neutral red solution.

Neutral red	1.0 g
Acetate buffer, 0.1 N, pH 5.0 (warm)	100 ml

Mix and filter when cool.

7. Ethyl alcohol, 70% (v/v).

8. Coplin jars.

SPECIMEN

Air-dried blood or bone marrow smears.

PROCEDURE

1. Place torn up filter paper in the bottom of a coplin jar and moisten with 40% formaldehyde (formalin).

2. Place the air-dried smears in the coplin jar and cover. Allow the smears to fix in the formalin vapor for 10 minutes. Wash in tap water and allow excess water to drain from smear.

3. Place the smears in a coplin jar containing Sudan black B staining solution for 30 minutes. (The time is variable, between 10 and 60 minutes.)

4. Rinse each slide with 70% ethyl alcohol just long enough to remove the excess stain.

5. Wash the smears in running tap water for 2 minutes.

6. Place the smears in a coplin jar containing 1% neutral red and counterstain for 10 minutes.

7. Wash the slides in tap water and coverslip with a synthetic mounting medium.

8. Examine the smears microscopically, using the oil immersion objective (100×). The neutrophils are packed with fine granules, taking up the black stain. The eosinophils have a similar appearance, whereas the monocytes have a moderate number of black-staining granules distributed evenly throughout the cell. The lymphocyte granules remain unstained.

DISCUSSION

1. Bone marrow or blood smears need not be fresh to obtain good results with the Sudan black B stain.

2. As the Sudan black B stain ages, it may be necessary to increase the staining time.

3. The granules are not readily decolorized by the 70% ethyl alcohol.

SIDEROCYTE (PRUSSIAN-BLUE) STAIN

Siderocytes are red blood cells that have one or more iron-containing granules. When these granules are found in nucleated red blood cells, the cell is termed a *sideroblast*. These iron-containing granules stain positively with the Prussian-blue stain but do not stain with Wright's stain. In contrast, *Pappenheimer bodies* (iron deposits in the mitochondria) stain positively with both the Prussian-blue and the Wright stains. *Basophilic stippling* (clusters of ribosomes) gives a positive reaction with Wright's stain but does not stain with Prussian-blue. It is thought that siderotic granules represent iron that has not yet been incorporated into hemoglobin. Normally, these granules are found in 20 to 60% of the nucleated red blood cells in the bone marrow. These granules are also found in some marrow reticulocytes but are not normally present in the mature red blood cell of the peripheral blood. In certain diseases in which the synthesis of hemoglobin is disturbed, an increased number of siderocyte granules are found. Also, the granules are generally larger in size. In sideroblastic anemias, the granules may be arranged in a ring around the nucleus of the nucleated red blood cell (ringed sideroblast). The iron stores of the body and the serum iron level are related to the percentage of the sideroblasts in the bone marrow. In iron-deficiency anemia, in which the iron stores are markedly decreased, the number of marrow sideroblasts is also reduced. Siderocytes are usually present in the peripheral blood following splenectomy because the spleen, as one of its functions, removes the red blood cell from the circulation until the heme synthesis is completed. The spleen may also remove these granules from the red blood cell.

REFERENCE

Lillie, R.D., and Fullmer, H.M.: *Histopathologic Technic and Practical Histochemistry,* McGraw-Hill Book Company, New York, 1976.

REAGENTS AND EQUIPMENT

1. Methyl alcohol, Mallinckrodt (absolute anhydrous, acetone-free).
2. Prussian-blue reagent.
   Potassium ferrocyanide   2.0 g
   Distilled water   36 ml
   Hydrochloric acid,   4 ml
      concentrated
   Use immediately after preparation.
3. Acetate buffer, 0.1 N, pH 5.0. (For preparation, see the following section entitled Reagents and Equipment under Acid Phosphatase.)
4. Buffered neutral red, 1%, pH 5.0.
   Neutral red   1.0 g
   Acetate buffer, 0.1 N,   100 ml
      pH 5.0
   Warm the solution and mix until the neutral red is in solution. Filter and store at room temperature.
5. Coplin jars, two.
6. Coverslips.

SPECIMEN

Air-dried blood or bone marrow slides.

PRINCIPLE

Prussian-blue reagent stains nonheme iron a vivid blue or green color. Nuclei and red cells are stained red or pink by the neutral red.

PROCEDURE

1. Fix blood or bone marrow smears by flooding the slide with methanol for 30 seconds. Allow to air-dry.
2. Place the smears in a coplin jar containing Prussian-blue reagent for 30 minutes.
3. Rinse the smears in distilled water.
4. Place the smears in a coplin jar containing neutral red and counterstain for 5 minutes.
5. Wash under running tap water.
6. Allow to air-dry and coverslip.

DISCUSSION

1. A positive control smear should be run each time this test is performed.
2. Wright-stained smears several years old may be effectively stained with the Prussian-blue reagent.

ACID PHOSPHATASE
(With Tartrate Resistance)

Acid phosphatase is present in myelogenous cells, lymphocytes, plasma cells, monocytes, and platelets. In this test, the acid phosphatase in the cytoplasm of the cells stains a red color. L(+) tartaric acid inhibits acid phosphatase activity, and, when added to the incubation mixture, the preceding cells exhibit no acid phosphatase activity (stain negatively). The acid phosphatase present in the "hairy" cells of leukemic reticuloendotheliosis, however, is resistant to L(+) tartaric acid and stains strongly positive even when this chemical has been added to the incubation mixture. The atypical lymphocyte of infectious mononucleosis and, rarely, the lymphocytes in chronic lymphocytic leukemia and lymphosarcoma may show less than complete resistance to L(+) tartaric acid. (They may stain faintly positive.)

REFERENCE

Katayama, I., and Yang, J.P.S.: Reassessment of a cytochemical test for differential diagnosis of leukemic reticuloendotheliosis, Am. J. Clin. Path., 68, 268, 1977.

REAGENTS AND EQUIPMENT

1. Buffered formalin acetone fixative, pH 6.6 to 6.8.

   Dibasic sodium phosphate   0.2 g
   (Na_2HPO_4)
   Monobasic potassium phosphate (KH_2PO_4) 1.0 g
   Dissolve the preceding compounds in 300 ml of distilled water.
   Acetone   450 ml
   Formaldehyde, 40%   250 ml
   Store in the refrigerator.

2. Sodium nitrite, 4% (w/v).

   Sodium nitrite   4.0 g
   Dilute to 100 ml with distilled water.

3. Pararosanilin solution.

   Pararosanilin hydrochloride 1.0 g
   (Obtainable from Sigma Chemical Company, St. Louis, Missouri.)
   Distilled water   20 ml
   Hydrochloric acid,   5.0 ml
      concentrated
   Gently warm the above while mixing to dissolve as much pararosanilin as possible. Allow the mixture to cool and filter and store it in a brown bottle at room temperature.

4. Acetic acid, 1 N.

   Glacial acetic acid   6.0 ml
   Dilute to 1 liter with distilled water.

5. Acetate buffer, 0.1 N, pH 5.0.

   Sodium acetate   4.797 g
   $(CH_3COONa \cdot 3 H_2O)$
   Acetic acid, 1 N   14.75 ml
   Dilute to 1 liter with distilled water. Store in the refrigerator.

6. Solution A.

   Sodium nitrite, 4%   2.4 ml
   Pararosanilin solution   2.4 ml
   Mix immediately before use in a 250-ml beaker.

7. Solution B.

   Naphthol AS-BI   40 mg
     phosphoric acid (obtainable from Sigma Chemical Company, St. Louis, Missouri.)
   N,N-dimethyl formamide   4.0 ml
   Acetate buffer, 0.1 N,   71.2 ml
     pH 5.0
   Mix immediately before use.

8. Incubation mixture I.

   Add solution B to solution A. Mix and place 40 ml in a separate beaker. Adjust the pH of mixture I to pH 5.1 with saturated sodium hydroxide. Filter into a coplin jar and use immediately.

9. Incubation mixture II.

   L(+) tartaric acid   300 mg
   Incubation mixture I   40 ml
   Mix and adjust pH to 5.1 with saturated sodium hydroxide. Filter into a coplin jar and use immediately.

10. Methyl green, 1%.

    Methyl green   1.0 g
    Acetate buffer, 0.1 N,   100 ml
      pH 5.0
    Adjust the pH of this solution to 4.2 to 4.5 with sodium hydroxide, 1 N, or hydrochloric acid, 1 N.

11. PVP mounting medium.

   Polyvinylpyrrolidone   8.0 g
   (PVP-40) (obtainable from Sigma
   Chemical Company, St. Louis,
   Missouri.)

   Distilled water   10 ml
   The PVP-40 takes 12 to 16 hours to
   dissolve. If it becomes too thick,
   add distilled water to obtain the
   proper consistency.
12. Incubator, 37°C.
13. Coplin jars, seven.
14. Coverslips.

SPECIMEN

Air-dried blood or bone marrow smears.

PROCEDURE

1. Prepare thin blood or bone marrow
   smears and allow to air-dry. At least
   two smears should be prepared for
   each patient and two normal control
   smears. Label one smear from each
   patient and normal control, I, and the
   second smear, II.
2. Place the slides in a coplin jar containing buffered formalin acetone at
   4 to 10°C for 30 seconds.
3. Wash the smears in three changes of
   distilled water.
4. Place the appropriately labeled slide
   for each patient and normal control
   in a coplin jar containing incubation
   mixture I and also in a coplin jar containing incubation mixture II. Incubate the smears at 37°C for 60 minutes.
5. Wash the smears in two changes of
   distilled water.
6. Place the smears in a coplin jar containing 1% methyl green for 2 minutes.
7. Wash the smears quickly in running
   tap water.
8. Allow the smears to air-dry, mount,
   and coverslip in PVP mounting medium.
9. Examine the smears microscopically
   using the oil immersion objective

(100×). Those smears from incubation mixture I should show acid
phosphatase activity in the cytoplasm of the white blood cells and
the platelets (varying degrees of reddish staining). The smears from incubation mixture II should show no
acid phosphatase activity or only a
minute amount of red staining. The
"hairy" cells of leukemic reticuloendotheliosis exhibit positive red staining from both incubation mixtures I
and II.

NONSPECIFIC ESTERASE STAIN
(With Flouride Inhibition)

White blood cells contain esterases, a
group of enzymes that are associated with
the azurophilic or nonspecific granules. In
this nonspecific esterase stain, the substrate employed is more specific for monocytic esterase, and there is positive staining in the monocytes, histiocytes, and
megakaryocytes. In the presence of fluoride, however, these cells show no positive staining. The nonspecific esterase
stain is negative in acute lymphocytic leukemia. In acute monocytic leukemia, the
cells show positive staining, which is inhibited by fluoride. In myelomonocytic
leukemia, the blasts are negative to weakly
positive, whereas the mature cells stain
positively, and the stain is not inhibited
by fluoride. Auer rods are esterase-posi-
tive, and in erythroleukemia, the abnormal erythroid cells show positive staining.
The nonspecific esterase stain is helpful
in differentiating lymphoid cells and in
diagnosing acute monocytic leukemia
using fluoride inhibition.

REFERENCE

Yam, L.T., Li, C.Y., and Crosby, W.H.:
Cytochemical identification of monocytes
and granulocytes, Am. J. Clin. Path., 55,
283, 1971.

REAGENTS AND EQUIPMENT

1. Cold, phosphate-buffered formalin
   acetone, pH 6.6.

Dibasic sodium phosphate   0.2 g
(Na$_2$HPO$_4$)
Monobasic potassium   1.0 g
phosphate (KH$_2$PO$_4$)
Dissolve the above reagents in 300 ml of distilled water and add:

Acetone   450 ml
Formaldehyde, 40%   250 ml
Store in the refrigerator.

2. Pararosanilin, 4% w/v, in 20% hydro-chloric acid, v/v.

Pararosanilin hydrochloride 1.0 g
Distilled water   20 ml
Hydrochloric acid,   5 ml
concentrated
Gently warm the above while mixing to dissolve as much pararosanilin as possible. Allow the mixture to cool and filter and store it in a brown bottle at room temperature.

3. Sodium nitrite, 4% w/v. Make fresh, just prior to use.

Sodium nitrite   0.4 g
Distilled water   10.0 ml

4. Phosphate buffer, M/15, pH 6.3. This reagent must be at room temperature when used.

Dibasic sodium phos-   1.183 g
phate (Na$_2$HPO$_4$)
Monobasic potassium   3.399 g
phosphate (KH$_2$PO$_4$)
Dilute to 500 ml with distilled water.
Store in the refrigerator.

5. Sodium hydroxide, 1 N.
6. Hydrochloric acid, 1 N.
7. Sodium fluoride, 0.1 M.

Sodium fluoride   0.42 g
Dilute to 100 ml with distilled water. Store at room temperature.

8. α-Naphthyl acetate in ethylene glycol monomethyl ether. Prepare just prior to use.

α-Naphthyl acetate   0.2 g
Ethylene glycol   10.0 ml
monomethyl ether.

9. Incubation mixture (A) without fluoride. Prepare just prior to use.

Pararosanilin (4% w/v   3.0 ml

in 20% hydrochloric
acid, v/v)
Sodium nitrite, 4% v/v   3.0 ml
Mix in a 200-ml beaker. Allow to sit for 1 minute and add:

Phosphate buffer M/15,   89.0 ml
pH 6.3
α-Naphthyl acetate in   5.0 ml
ethylene glycol
monomethyl ether
Mix. Remove 50 ml of this solution and place in a 100-ml beaker. This will be used to prepare the incubation mixture (B) with fluoride. Adjust the pH of incubation mixture A to approximately 6.1 (5.8 to 6.5), using 1 N sodium hydroxide. Filter directly into a coplin jar and use immediately.

10. Incubation mixture (B) with fluoride. Add 0.5 ml of the 0.1 M sodium fluoride to the 50 ml of the incubation mixture (A) that was set aside. Adjust the pH to 6.1 (5.8 to 6.5) using 1 N sodium hydroxide. Filter directly into a coplin jar and use immediately.

11. Acetic acid, 1 N.

Glacial acetic acid   6 ml
Dilute to 1 liter with distilled water.

12. Acetate buffer, 0.1 N, pH 5.0.

Sodium acetate   2.399 g
(CH$_3$COONa·3 H$_2$O)
Acetic acid, 1 N   7.38 ml
Dilute to 500 ml with distilled water.

13. Buffered methyl green, 1% w/v.

Methyl green   1.0 g
Acetate buffer, 0.1 N,   100 ml
pH 5.0
Adjust the pH to 4.2 to 4.5 with 1 N sodium hydroxide or 1 N hydrochloric acid. Filter. Store at room temperature.

14. Permount mounting medium.
15. Coplin jars.
16. Coverslips.

SPECIMEN

Air-dried blood or bone marrow smears.

PROCEDURE

1. Prepare thin blood or bone-marrow smears and allow to air-dry. At least two smears should be prepared for each patient and two normal control smears. Label one smear from each patient and normal control, A, and the second smear from each, B.

2. Fix the above smears in a coplin jar containing cold, phosphate-buffered formalin acetone for 30 to 60 seconds.

3. Wash the smears in three changes of distilled water.

4. Allow the smears to air-dry for 10 to 30 minutes while making up the incubation mixtures.

5. Place the appropriately labeled slide for each patient and normal control in a coplin jar containing incubation mixture A and in a second coplin jar containing incubation mixture B. Incubate the smears at room temperature for 60 minutes.

6. Wash the smears in three changes of distilled water.

7. Counterstain by placing the smears in a coplin jar containing 1% methyl green for 1 to 2 minutes.

8. Wash the smears in running tap water.

9. Allow the smears to air-dry and coverslip using Permount.

10. Examine the smears microscopically using the oil immersion objective (100 ×). Esterase activity is indicated by the presence of dark red-staining granules in the cytoplasm of the cell. Those smears from incubation mixture A without fluoride will show strong esterase activity in the cytoplasm of the monocytes, histiocytes, and megakaryocytes. The granulocytes and lymphocytes may show very weak to no nonspecific esterase activity. The smears from incubation mixture B, with fluoride, will show inhibition of the staining for nonspecific esterase, and, therefore, there will be no positive staining in the monocytes, histiocytes, or megakaryocytes.

DISCUSSION

1. Unfixed smears up to 2 weeks old that have been stored at room temperature may be successfully stained by this procedure. There appears to be no loss of enzyme activity during this time.

CHLOROACETATE ESTERASE STAIN

The chloroacetate stain is specific for esterases found in the granulocytic cells and is frequently performed in combination with the nonspecific esterase stain to differentiate monocytic from granulocytic cells.

REFERENCE

Yam, L.T., Li, C.Y., and Crosby, W.H.: Cytochemical identification of monocytes and granulocytes, Am. J. Clin. Path., 55, 283, 1971.

REAGENTS AND EQUIPMENT

1. Cold, phosphate-buffered formalin acetone, pH 6.6. Prepare as outlined in the previous section entitled Nonspecific Esterase Stain.

2. Acetic acid, 1 N. (See the section entitled Nonspecific Esterase Stain.)

3. Acetate buffer, 0.1 N, pH 5.0. (See the section entitled Nonspecific Esterase Stain.)

4. Buffered methyl green, 1% w/v. (See the section entitled Nonspecific Esterase Stain.)

5. Phosphate buffer, M/15, pH 7.4.
   Dibasic sodium phosphate (Na_2HPO_4) .... 3.786 g
   Monobasic potassium phosphate (KH_2PO_4) .... 0.907 g
   Dilute to 500 ml with distilled water.
   Adjust the pH to 7.4.

6. Naphthol AS-D chloroacetate (0.2% w/v in N,N-dimethylformamide)

Naphthol AS-D   0.01 g
  chloroacetate
N,N-dimethylformamide   5.0 ml
Prepare immediately before use.

7. Incubate the mixture. Prepare immediately before use.

Phosphate buffer (M/15,   47.5 ml
  pH 7.4)
Naphthol AS-D   2.5 ml
  chloroacetate
  (0.2% w/v in N,N-dimethylformamide)
Fast blue BB   30 mg
Mix and filter directly into a coplin jar.

8. Permount mounting medium.
9. Coplin jars.
10. Coverslips.

SPECIMEN

Air-dried blood or bone marrow smears.

PROCEDURE

1. Prepare thin blood or bone marrow smears on the patient and the normal control and allow to air-dry.
2. Fix the smears in a coplin jar containing cold, phosphate-buffered formalin acetone for 30 to 60 seconds.
3. Wash the smears in three changes of distilled water.
4. Allow the smears to air-dry for 10 to 30 minutes while preparing the incubation mixture.
5. Place the smears in a coplin jar containing the incubation mixture for 20 minutes.
6. Wash the smears in three changes of distilled water.
7. Counterstain by placing the smears in a coplin jar containing 1% methyl green for 1 to 2 minutes.
8. Wash the smears in running tap water.
9. Allow the smears to air-dry and coverslip using Permount.
10. Examine the smears microscopically using the high oil immersion objective (100×). Chloroacetate esterase activity will show up as blue-staining granules in the granulocytic cells. Basophils show little to no chloroacetate esterase activity. Granulocytes, including promyelocytes, will show very strong activity, as do many, but not all, myeloblasts. Monocytes show little to no activity. Lymphocytes, eosinophils, plasma cells, megakaryocytes, and erythroblasts show no chloroacetate esterase activity.

DISCUSSION

1. Unfixed smears up to 2 weeks old that were stored at room temperature may be successfully stained by this procedure. There appears to be no loss of enzyme activity during this time.
2. The nonspecific esterase stain and the chloroacetate esterase stain may be combined and performed on the same patient and control slides. To do the combined nonspecific esterase stain and chloroacetate esterase stain, perform steps 1 through 6 as outlined for the nonspecific esterase stain (see the previous section). Continue the procedure by performing steps 5 through 9 as described above for the chloroacetate esterase stain. The staining results for the combined stain are very similar to the individual stain results. Nonspecific esterase activity is indicated by dark red granules in the monocytes, histiocytes, and megakaryocytes. Blue-staining granules in the cytoplasm of the granulocytes indicates chloroacetate esterase activity.

NITROBLUE-TETRAZOLIUM TEST

The nitroblue-tetrazolium test (NBT) is helpful in diagnosing chronic granulomatous disease. In this disorder, markedly decreased values for the NBT test are obtained. In normal individuals, less than 10% of the neutrophils are NBT-positive, whereas in patients with bacterial infections, greater than 10% of the neutrophils are NBT-positive.

REFERENCES

Cocchi, P., Mori, S., and Becattini, A.: N.B.T. tests in premature infants, Lancet, 2, 1426, 1969.

Park, B.H., Fikrig, S.M., and Smithwick, E.M.: Infection and nitroblue-tetrazolium reduction by neutrophils, Lancet, 2, 532, 1968.

Silverman, E.M., and Ryden, S.E.: The nitroblue-tetrazolium (N.B.T.) test: A simple, reliable method and a review of its significance, Am. J. Med. Tech., 40–4, 151, 1974.

REAGENTS AND EQUIPMENT

1. Phosphate buffered sodium chloride, pH 7.2.

    Dibasic sodium phosphate (Na_2HPO_4) 7.6 g

    Monobasic potassium phosphate (KH_2PO_4) 2.48 g

    Dilute to 500 ml with 0.85% sodium chloride and adjust pH to 7.2.

2. Nitroblue-tetrazolium solution.

    Dissolve 100 mg nitroblue-tetrazolium in 50 ml of 0.85% sodium chloride. Mix at room temperature for 1 to 2 hours. Filter. Prepare the working nitroblue-tetrazolium solution just prior to use by mixing equal parts of the phosphate-buffered sodium chloride (pH 7.2) with the nitroblue-tetrazolium sodium chloride solution.

3. Plastic syringe, 5 ml.
4. Test tubes, plastic.
5. Heparin.
6. Water bath, 37°C.
7. Coverslips.
8. Wright's stain and buffer.

SPECIMEN

Heparinized whole blood, 2 ml. Collect blood for a normal control at the same time the patient's blood is drawn.

PRINCIPLE

Increased enzyme activity normally present in neutrophils during a bacterial infection is capable of reducing nitroblue-tetrazolium to formazan, which forms a black precipitate. In fatal granulomatous disease, the neutrophils do not have a normal ability to kill certain organisms and are also unable to reduce nitroblue-tetrazolium. In this procedure, blood is mixed with nitroblue-tetrazolium, allowed to incubate, and smears made and counterstained with Wright's stain. The smears are examined microscopically for neutrophils containing formazan. In healthy adults, 3 to 10% of the neutrophils contain formazan. In the presence of a bacterial infection, 12 to 70% of the neutrophils normally reduce the nitroblue-tetrazolium.

PROCEDURE

1. Collect 2 ml of blood using a plastic syringe.
2. Immediately place the blood in a plastic tube containing 150 to 200 units of heparin (75 to 100 units of heparin per 1 ml of whole blood).
3. Mix well by gentle shaking.
4. Place six drops of well-mixed heparinized blood into a second plastic test tube.
5. Add six drops of nitroblue-tetrazolium solution. Gently mix.
6. Incubate this mixture at 37°C for 30 minutes.
7. At the end of 30 minutes, gently mix the solution and carefully make coverslip smears. (Avoid damaging the white blood cells.)
8. When the smears are dry, counterstain with Wright's stain.
9. Using the oil immersion objective $(100 \times)$, count 100 neutrophils, enumerating those neutrophils that contain the reduced nitroblue-tetrazolium. The formazan appears as large black deposits in the neutrophils. Report results as the percent-

age of neutrophils containing reduced nitroblue-tetrazolium (percentage of NBT-positive neutrophils).

DISCUSSION

1. Control blood from a normal person should be tested along with the patient's blood.
2. The absolute number of NBT-positive neutrophils may be determined by performing a white count on the test blood. In the absence of infection, there are normally 145 to 725 NBT-positive neutrophils per µl of blood. When a bacterial infection is present, this number increases to a range of 1,115 to more than 13,000 NBT-positive neutrophils per µl of blood.
3. In chronic granulomatous disease, there is a negligible to zero reduction of the nitroblue-tetrazolium.
4. An increased concentration of heparin may give false-positive results.

LUPUS ERYTHEMATOSUS PREPARATION (L.E. PREP)

In patients suffering from systemic lupus erythematosus, a specific characteristic cell, termed the *L.E. cell,* is found in the bone marrow and peripheral blood when the smears are prepared according to a specific procedure. This L.E. cell phenomenon is caused by an immunoglobulin present in the patient's plasma, called the *L.E. factor.*

REFERENCES

Cartwright, G.E.: *Diagnostic Laboratory Hematology,* Grune & Stratton, Inc., New York, 1963.

Dacie, J.V., and Lewis, S.M.: *Practical Hematology,* 5th ed., Churchill Livingstone, New York, 1975.

Magath, T.B., and Winkle, V.: Technic for demonstrating "L.E." (lupus erythematosus) cells in blood, Am. J. Clin. Path., 22, 586, 1952.

REAGENTS AND EQUIPMENT

1. Wire sieve and pestle.
2. Petri dish.
3. Wintrobe erythrocyte sedimentation rate tubes, three or four.
4. Clean glass slides.
5. Wright's stain and buffer.
6. Disposable droppers with a long narrow tip. These should be long enough to reach the bottom of a Wintrobe tube.

SPECIMEN

Clotted whole blood, 10 ml.

PRINCIPLE

Clotted blood is allowed to sit at room temperature for 2 hours. The clot is then macerated by forcing it through a sieve. The trauma produced when the blood is forced through the strainer causes extrusion of nuclei from the polymorphonuclear cells. The L.E. factor present in the blood lyses the nuclear material, which is then phagocytized by other neutrophils. This forms the L.E. cell.

PROCEDURE

1. Place 10 ml of whole blood in a plain test tube and allow the blood to clot.
2. Incubate the tube of clotted blood at room temperature for 2 hours.
3. Using an applicator stick to hold the clot in the test tube, pour off the serum and discard it.
4. Place the sieve over a Petri dish.
5. Place the clot in the sieve.
6. Mash the clot through the sieve, using the pestle.
7. Transfer the blood from the Petri dish to three or four Wintrobe erythrocyte sedimentation rate tubes, using disposable droppers of the proper length.
8. Centrifuge the filled Wintrobe tubes at 2,500 RPM for 20 minutes.
9. Remove the serum from each of the tubes, using a disposable dropper. Be

careful not to remove any of the buffy coat (layer of white blood cells).

10. Using a clean disposable dropper, remove the buffy coat and transfer a small drop to each of three or four slides and make smears.

11. Wright-stain the smears and examine for the presence of L.E. cells (Figs. 126 and 127). Report as positive or negative. The characteristic L.E. cell appears as a neutrophil containing a large spherical body in its cytoplasm. Ordinarily, the nucleus of the neutrophil is pushed to one side of the cell and may appear to wrap itself around the ingested material. The L.E. cell shows no nuclear structure and stains as a pale purple homogeneous mass. It has a velvety appearance. In rare instances, the ingesting cell may be a monocyte or eosinophil. The L.E. phenomenon also includes rosettes, which consist of a free L.E. cell surrounded by neutrophils. These are readily seen using low-power (10×) magnification. The *tart cell*, which may be confused with the L.E. cell, is usually a monocyte that has ingested another cell or the nucleus of another cell. In this case, the ingested material usually resembles a lymphocyte nucleus or phagocytized material with a definite nuclear pattern. Another form of ingested material found in the tart cell is an intensely stained body termed a *pyknotic nucleus*. The significance of these cells is not known. Their presence in an L.E. preparation does not signify a positive test for systemic lupus erythematosus.

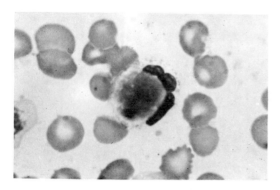

Fig. 126. L.E. cell. (Magnification 1000×.)

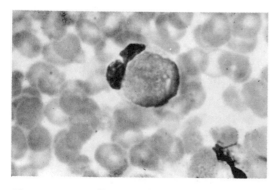

Fig. 127. L.E. cell. (Magnification 1000×.)

DISCUSSION

1. An alternative method to the preceding procedure employs the use of 5 ml of whole blood mixed with 0.5 ml of dilute heparin. Five glass beads (4 to 5 mm in diameter) are added to the tube. After incubating the blood at room temperature for 30 minutes, the blood is mixed on a rotator for 30 minutes and reincubated at room temperature for 1 hour. The blood is then placed in Wintrobe sedimentation tubes, centrifuged, and blood smears are made from the buffy coat, as previously described. This method is considered to be more sensitive than the procedure employing clotted blood. The concentration of heparin, however, is important because high concentrations of anticoagulants are thought to inhibit L.E. cell formation.

2. When examining the blood smear, each of three slides should be studied for approximately 10 minutes before a report is made. The smear should be examined, using the high-dry objective (40×) or on low power (10×)

when enough experience has been gained. All suspicious cells should be examined under the oil immersion objective (100×).

3. The presence of one L.E. cell is not a substantial basis for reporting a positive result. Several typical L.E. cells should be seen before a positive report is made.

4. If a patient has severe leukopenia, a false-negative result may be obtained due to the decrease in neutrophils present. Therefore, because the L.E. factor is present in the serum, add 5 ml of patient's serum to 5 ml of washed red blood cells (type O blood) obtained from a normal individual. Carry out the test as previously described.

5. Occasionally, false-positive results are obtained in patients having disorders such as drug sensitivity caused by rheumatoid arthritis and hepatitis.

6. Patients with systemic lupus erythematosus who are on adrenocorticosteroid therapy may have false-negative L.E. tests. Also, L.E. cells are not demonstrated in some people who have the active clinical disease.

7. The L.E. factor is also termed an *antinuclear factor* because it reacts against cell nuclei. Two other methods employed to detect the presence of this factor are (1) an immunofluorescent method and (2) a serologic method that tests the ability of the serum to agglutinate latex particles.

8. The 2-hour incubation of whole blood at room temperature does not have to be critically timed. It should incubate a minimum of 2 hours, but no longer than 7 hours.

OSMOTIC FRAGILITY TEST

The osmotic fragility test is employed to help diagnose different types of anemias, in which the physical properties of the red blood cell are altered. The main factor affecting the osmotic fragility test is the shape of the red blood cell, which, in turn, is dependent on the volume, surface area, and functional state of the red blood cell membrane. An increased osmotic fragility is found in hemolytic anemias, hereditary spherocytosis, and whenever spherocytes are found. Decreased osmotic fragility occurs following splenectomy, in liver disease, sickle cell anemia, iron-deficiency anemia, thalassemia, polycythemia vera, and in conditions in which target cells are present.

REFERENCES

Dacie, J.V., and Lewis, S.M.: *Practical Hematology*, 5th ed., Churchill Livingstone, New York, 1975.

Parpart, A.K., Lorenz, P.B., Parpart, E.R., Gregg, J.R., and Chase, A.M.: The osmotic resistance (fragility) of human red cells, J. Clin. Invest., *26*, 636, 1947.

REAGENTS AND EQUIPMENT

1. Buffered sodium chloride stock solution.

   Sodium chloride 180 g
   (dry for 24 hours in a desiccator with calcium chloride prior to weighing out)
   Dibasic sodium 27.31 g
   phosphate (Na_2HPO_4)
   Monobasic sodium 4.86 g
   phosphate ($NaH_2PO_4 \cdot 2\ H_2O$)
   Dilute to 2,000 ml with distilled water. This solution is stable for several months at room temperature if it is kept well stoppered.

2. Buffered sodium chloride solution, 1% (w/v).

   Buffered sodium chloride 20 ml
   stock solution, 10%
   Distilled water 180 ml

3. Distilled water.

4. Erlenmeyer flask, 250 ml.

5. Glass beads, 3 to 4 mm in diameter.
6. Test tubes, 13 × 100 mm.

SPECIMEN

Heparinized venous blood or, preferably, defibrinated whole blood, 15 to 20 ml. A normal control blood should be collected at the same time the patient's blood is drawn.

PRINCIPLE

If red blood cells are placed in an isotonic solution, 0.85% sodium chloride, water will neither enter nor leave the red blood cell. If red blood cells are placed in a 0.25% solution of sodium chloride, however, water enters the red blood cell, the cell swells up, and eventually hemolyzes or ruptures. A spherocyte, which is almost round, swells up in 0.25% sodium chloride and ruptures much more quickly than a normal red blood cell or more quickly than cells that have a large surface area per volume, such as target cells or sickle cells. The fragility of the red blood cell is said to be increased when the rate of hemolysis is increased. When the rate of hemolysis is decreased, the fragility of the red blood cells is considered to be decreased. In the osmotic fragility test, whole blood is added to varying concentrations of buffered sodium chloride solution and allowed to incubate at room temperature. The amount of hemolysis is then determined by reading the supernatants on a spectrophotometer. A normal control blood is run at the same time the patient's blood is being tested.

PROCEDURE

1. Prepare dilutions of buffered sodium chloride and place in the appropriately labeled test tube. See Table 4.
2. Mix the preceding dilutions well, using Parafilm to cover each test tube while mixing.
3. Transfer 5 ml of each dilution to a second set of test tubes, labeled No. 1 through No. 14. This set of dilu-

tions will be used for the normal control blood.

4. If defibrinated blood is to be used, proceed as follows:
   A. Place 15 to 20 ml of whole blood into an Erlenmeyer flask containing 15 glass beads.
   B. Gently rotate the flask until the hum or noise of the beads on the glass can no longer be heard (about 10 minutes).
   C. Repeat steps 4A and 4B for the normal control blood.
5. Add 0.05 ml of the patient's heparinized or defibrinated blood to each of the 14 test tubes. Repeat, adding the normal control blood to the set of 14 control test tubes.
6. Mix each test tube immediately by gentle inversion.
7. Allow the test tubes to stand at room temperature for 30 minutes.
8. Remix the test tubes gently and centrifuge at 2,000 RPM for 5 minutes.
9. Carefully transfer the supernatants to cuvettes and read on a spectrophotometer at a wavelength of 550 nm. Set the optical density at 0, using the supernatant in test tube No. 1, which represents the blank, or 0% hemolysis. Test tube No. 14 represents 100% hemolysis.
10. Calculate the percent hemolysis for each supernatant as follows:

$$\text{Percent hemolysis} = \frac{\text{Optical density of supernatant}}{\text{Optical density of supernatant in test tube No. 14}} \times 100$$

11. The results of the test should then be graphed, with the percent hemolysis plotted on the ordinate, or vertical, axis and the sodium chloride concentration on the abscissa, or horizontal, axis, as shown in Figure 128.
12. Normal results are shown in Table 5.

DISCUSSION

1. Instead of determining the amount of hemolysis on the spectrophotometer,

TABLE 4.   DILUTIONS FOR THE OSMOTIC FRAGILITY TEST

TEST TUBE NO.	ml of 1% (w/v) BUFFERED SODIUM CHLORIDE	ml of DISTILLED WATER	CONCENTRATION OF BUFFERED SODIUM CHLORIDE (%)
1	10.0	0.0	1.00
2	8.5	1.5	0.85
3	7.5	2.5	0.75
4	6.5	3.5	0.65
5	6.0	4.0	0.60
6	5.5	4.5	0.55
7	5.0	5.0	0.50
8	4.5	5.5	0.45
9	4.0	6.0	0.40
10	3.5	6.5	0.35
11	3.0	7.0	0.30
12	2.0	8.0	0.20
13	1.0	9.0	0.10
14	0.0	10.0	0.00

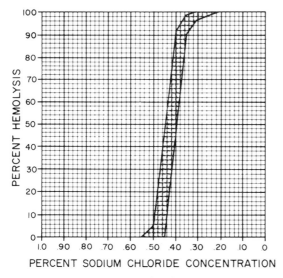

Fig. 128.   Normal osmotic fragility curve.

TABLE 5.   NORMAL RANGES FOR THE OSMOTIC FRAGILITY TEST

TEST TUBE NO.	CONCENTRATION OF SODIUM CHLORIDE (%)	HEMOLYSIS (%)
1	1.00	0
2	0.85	0
3	0.75	0
4	0.65	0
5	0.60	0
6	0.55	0
7	0.50	0–5
8	0.45	0–45
9	0.40	50–90
10	0.35	90–99
11	0.30	97–100
12	0.20	100
13	0.10	100
14	0.00	100

the test may be read visually. In this method, the first test tube (the highest concentration of sodium chloride) showing a trace of hemolysis in the supernatant determines the beginning of hemolysis. The first test tube, having the highest concentration of sodium chloride in which hemolysis is complete, determines complete hemolysis. Hemolysis should be complete in 0.3% sodium chloride. Beginning hemolysis should not occur in a concentration over 0.45% sodium chloride.

2. The pH of the blood-saline mixture is important and should be 7.4.

3. There are many possible sources of technical error in this procedure. It is, therefore, important to report the control results and interpret the patient's test in light of the normal control values.

4. Oxalated blood is not recommended for use in this test. The salts present in the anticoagulant may alter the pH of the blood-saline mixture.

OSMOTIC FRAGILITY TEST WITH INCUBATION

The incubated osmotic fragility test shows a greater increase of hemolysis in hereditary spherocytosis and in at least one nonspherocytic hemolytic anemia, pyruvate kinase deficiency. The test is helpful in detecting mild cases of spherocytosis.

REFERENCE

Dacie, J.V., and Lewis, S.M.: *Practical Hematology,* 5th ed., Churchill Livingstone, New York, 1975.

REAGENTS AND EQUIPMENT

1. Water bath, 37°C.
2. Glass beads, 3 to 4 mm in diameter.
3. Buffered sodium chloride stock solution.

> Sodium chloride   180 g
> (dry for 24 hours in a desiccator with calcium chloride prior to weighing out)
> Dibasic sodium   27.31 g
> phosphate (Na_2HPO_4)
> Monobasic sodium   4.86 g
> phosphate ($NaH_2PO_4 \cdot 2\ H_2O$)
> Dilute to 2,000 ml with distilled water. This solution is stable for several months at room temperature if it is kept well stoppered.

4. Buffered sodium chloride solution, 1% (v/v).

> Buffered sodium chloride   20 ml
> stock solution
> Distilled water   180 ml

5. Distilled water.
6. Erlenmeyer flask, 250 ml (sterile).
7. Sterile screw-cap vials, 10 ml.
8. Test tubes, 13 × 100 mm.

SPECIMEN

Collect 20 ml of whole blood and defibrinate. A normal control blood must be collected at the same time the patient's blood is obtained.

PRINCIPLE

Whole blood is allowed to incubate at 37°C for 24 hours. It is then added to varying concentrations of buffered sodium chloride, and the amount of hemolysis is determined by reading the supernatants on a spectrophotometer. A normal control blood is run at the same time the patient's blood is being tested.

PROCEDURE

1. Defibrinate the patient and control bloods, according to the following procedure:
   A. Place 15 to 20 ml of whole blood into a sterile Erlenmeyer flask containing 15 glass beads.
   B. Gently rotate the flask until the hum or noise of the beads on the glass can no longer be heard (about 10 minutes).
2. Place 5 ml of the patient's defibrinated blood into each of two sterile screw-cap vials. Repeat, using the control blood.
3. Incubate the preceding four test tubes of blood at 37°C for 24 hours.
4. In each of two test tube racks, number a set of 17 test tubes.
5. Prepare dilutions (see Table 6) of buffered sodium chloride and place in the appropriately labeled test tube.
6. Mix the preceding dilutions well, using Parafilm to cover each test tube while mixing.
7. Transfer 5 ml of each dilution to the second set of labeled test tubes. This is to be used for the normal control blood.
8. Gently mix the incubated blood samples. Pool the contents of the two patient test tubes together and combine the contents of the two control test tubes. The blood should not be grossly hemolyzed.
9. Add 0.05 ml of the patient's incubated blood to each of the 17 test tubes. Repeat, adding the normal incubated control blood to the set of 17 control test tubes.
10. Mix each test tube immediately by gentle inversion.
11. Allow the test tubes to stand at room temperature for 30 minutes.

TABLE 6.   DILUTIONS FOR THE INCUBATED OSMOTIC FRAGILITY TEST

TEST TUBE NO.	ml of 1% (w/v) BUFFERED SODIUM CHLORIDE	ml of DISTILLED WATER	CONCENTRATION OF BUFFERED SODIUM CHLORIDE (%)
1	10.0	0.0	1.00
2	9.0	1.0	0.90
3	8.5	1.5	0.85
4	8.0	2.0	0.80
5	7.5	2.5	0.75
6	7.0	3.0	0.70
7	6.5	3.5	0.65
8	6.0	4.0	0.60
9	5.5	4.5	0.55
10	5.0	5.0	0.50
11	4.5	5.5	0.45
12	4.0	6.0	0.40
13	3.5	6.5	0.35
14	3.0	7.0	0.30
15	2.5	7.5	0.25
16	2.0	8.0	0.20
17	1.0	9.0	0.10

12. Remix the test tubes gently and centrifuge at 2,000 RPM for 5 minutes.

13. Carefully transfer the supernatants to cuvettes and read on a spectrophotometer at a wavelength of 550 nm. Set 0 optical density using the supernatant in test tube No. 1, which represents the blank, or 0% hemolysis. Test tube No. 17 represents 100% hemolysis.

14. Calculate the percent hemolysis for each supernatant:

$$\text{Percent hemolysis} = \frac{\text{Optical density of supernatant}}{\text{Optical density of supernatant in test tube No. 17}} \times 100$$

15. The results of the test should be graphed with the percent hemolysis plotted on the ordinate, or vertical, axis and the sodium chloride concentration on the abscissa, or horizontal, axis, as shown in Figure 129.

16. Normal results are shown in Table 7.

DISCUSSION

It is important to maintain the sterility of the blood during incubation at 37°C. Bacterial contamination may produce hemolysis and inaccurate test results.

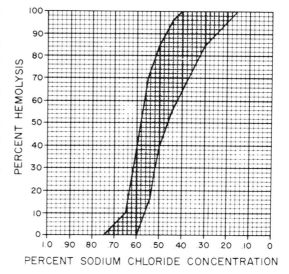

Fig. 129. Normal curve for the incubated osmotic fragility test.

AUTOHEMOLYSIS TEST

Autohemolysis of the red blood cell is increased in many types of hemolytic anemia and spherocytosis. The real value of the procedure, however, lies in its ability to differentiate between several types of congenital nonspherocytic hemolytic anemias, namely type I (Dacie) congenital nonspherocytic hemolytic anemia (paroxysmal nocturnal hemoglobinuria, glucose-6-phosphodehydrogenase deficiency), and type II (Dacie) congenital nonspher-

TABLE 7. NORMAL RANGES FOR THE INCUBATED OSMOTIC FRAGILITY TEST

TEST TUBE NO.	CONCENTRATION OF BUFFERED SODIUM CHLORIDE (%)	HEMOLYSIS (%)
1	1.00	0
2	0.90	0
3	0.85	0
4	0.80	0
5	0.75	0
6	0.70	0–5
7	0.65	0–10
8	0.60	0–40
9	0.55	15–70
10	0.50	40–85
11	0.45	55–95
12	0.40	65–100
13	0.35	75–100
14	0.30	85–100
15	0.25	90–100
16	0.20	95–100
17	0.10	100

ocytic hemolytic anemia (pyruvate kinase deficiency).

REFERENCES

Cartwright, G.E.: *Diagnostic Laboratory Hematology,* Grune & Stratton, Inc., New York, 1963.

Dacie, J.V., and Lewis, S.M.: *Practical Hematology,* 5th ed., Churchill Livingstone, New York, 1975.

REAGENTS AND EQUIPMENT

1. Water bath, 37°C.
2. Glass beads, 3 to 4 mm in diameter.
3. Drabkin's reagent. (See the section entitled Cyanmethemoglobin Method [Reagents and Equipment] in Chapter 2.)
4. Glucose solution, 10% (w/v).
   Glucose   10.0 g
   Sodium chloride,   100 ml
      0.85% (w/v)
   This solution must be sterile. Autoclave or sterilize by Seitz filtration.
5. Sterile, screw-cap vials.
6. Sterile Erlenmeyer flask, 125 ml

SPECIMEN

Whole defibrinated blood (15 to 20 ml) from the patient and a normal control.

PRINCIPLE

Sterile, defibrinated blood is incubated for 48 hours at 37°C. A second sample of defibrinated blood is incubated with a specific amount of glucose. The percent hemolysis in each specimen is determined spectrophotometrically. Normally and in certain disorders, glucose inhibits or reduces the amount of autohemolysis. In other pathologic states, the presence of added glucose does not effectively decrease the autohemolysis.

PROCEDURE

1. The entire test procedure must be run under sterile conditions.
2. Defibrinate the patient and control bloods according to the following procedure:
   A. Place 15 to 20 ml of whole blood in a 125-ml, sterile Erlenmeyer flask containing 15 glass beads.
   B. Gently rotate the flask until the hum or noise of the beads on the glass can no longer be heard (about 10 minutes).
3. Label eight sterile screw-cap vials, No. 1 through No. 8.
4. Place 2 ml of the patient's defibrinated blood in test tube Nos. 1, 2, 3, and 4. Place the remainder of the patient's defibrinated blood in an empty sterile screw-cap vial and centrifuge at 2,500 RPM for 10 minutes. Remove the serum and place in a sterile screw-cap tube in the refrigerator.
5. Place 2 ml of the normal control's defibrinated blood in test tubes Nos. 5, 6, 7, and 8. Place the remainder of the normal defibrinated blood into an empty sterile screw-cap vial and centrifuge at 2,500 RPM for 10 minutes. Remove the serum and place in a sterile screw-cap tube in the refrigerator.
6. Add 0.1 ml of 10% glucose solution to test tubes Nos. 3, 4, 7, and 8. Mix the tubes gently.

7. Incubate the preceding eight test tubes at 37°C for 24 hours.
8. At the end of 24 hours, gently mix the eight test tubes by inverting them carefully 5 to 10 times. Incubate the tubes for an additional 24 hours.
9. At the end of 48 hours, inspect each test tube for contamination (a greenish discoloration or bad odor).
10. If there is no contamination, pool test tubes No. 1 and No. 2 together, tubes No. 3 and No. 4 together, tubes No. 5 and No. 6 together, and tubes No. 7 and No. 8 together.
11. Perform a duplicate hematocrit on each of the four preceding test tubes. Average the duplicate readings and record the results.
12. Pipet 0.02 ml of blood from each test tube to four separate tubes containing 5.0 ml of Drabkin's reagent. (This is a 1:251 dilution.)
13. Centrifuge the four test tubes of pooled blood at 2,500 RPM for 10 minutes.
14. Remove the supernatant serums and pipet 0.5 ml of each serum into appropriately labeled test tubes containing 5.0 ml of Drabkin's reagent. (This is a 1:11 dilution.)
15. Pipet 0.5 ml of the nonincubated (refrigerated) patient's serum into an appropriately labeled test tube containing 5.0 ml of Drabkin's reagent. Repeat, pipetting 0.5 ml of the nonincubated (refrigerated) control serum into a second test tube containing 5.0 ml of Drabkin's reagent.
16. Record the optical density of the following solutions diluted with Drabkin's reagent, using a spectrophotometer set at a wavelength of 550 nm and using Drabkin's reagent as the solution blank (0 optical density):
    A. Patient's incubated whole blood.
    B. Patient's incubated serum without glucose.
    C. Patient's incubated serum with glucose.
    D. Patient's nonincubated serum.
    E. Control's incubated whole blood.
    F. Control's incubated serum without glucose.
    G. Control's incubated serum with glucose.
    H. Control's nonincubated serum.
17. Calculate the percent hemolysis for the control and patient bloods incubated with and without glucose according to the following formula:

$$\text{Percent hemolysis} = (D_2 - D_3) \times \frac{\text{Dilution factor of serum}}{}$$

$$\times \frac{100 - \text{hematocrit}}{D_1 \times \text{dilution factor of blood}}$$

D_1 = The optical density of diluted whole blood.
D_2 = The optical density of the diluted serum after incubation.
D_3 = The optical density of the diluted nonincubated serum.
Dilution factor of serum = 11.
Dilution factor of whole blood = 251.

18. The normal values for this test and the results found in types I and II congenital nonspherocytic hemolytic anemia are shown in Table 8.

DISCUSSION

1. There may be considerable methemoglobin formation in the preceding procedure. Therefore, the cyanmethemoglobin method must be employed for measuring the amount of hemoglobin in the serum.
2. Hemolysis may be increased by bacterial contamination.
3. In addition to glucose being used as an additive, adenosine triphosphate (ATP) may be incubated with the blood.

GLUCOSE-6-PHOSPHATE DEHYDROGENASE TEST

When red blood cells are exposed to an oxidant drug, the activity of the hexose monophosphate shunt increases. If one of

TABLE 8. INTERPRETATION OF THE AUTOHEMOLYSIS TEST

WHOLE BLOOD PLUS	NORMAL HEMOLYSIS (%)	TYPE I HEMOLYSIS (%)	TYPE II HEMOLYSIS (%)
No additive	0.4 to 4.5	0.7 to 5.9	8.0 to 44.0
Glucose	0.3 to 0.7	0.5 to 4.1	3.5 to 48.0

the enzymes in this pathway is decreased or absent, reduced glutathione cannot be produced and oxidation of the hemoglobin takes place.

REFERENCES

Beutler, E.: A series of new screening procedures for pyruvate kinase deficiency, glucose-6-phosphate dehydrogenase deficiency, and glutathione reductase deficiency, Blood, *28*, 553, 1966.

Sigma Chemical Company: *A Qualitative Screening Procedure for the Determination of Glucose-6-Phosphate Dehydrogenase in Blood*, Sigma Technical Bulletin No. 202, Sigma Chemical Company, St. Louis, Missouri, 1979.

REAGENTS AND EQUIPMENT

1. Phosphate buffer, 0.075 M (pH 7.4) (obtainable from Sigma Chemical Company, St. Louis, Missouri). Store in refrigerator.
2. Glucose-6-phosphate dehydrogenase test reagent, containing glucose-6-phosphate and nicotinamide-adenine dinucleotide phosphate (NADP). Reconstitute with 2.0 ml of phosphate buffer, 0.075 M, pH 7.4 (item No. 1 above). Allow to stand for 2 minutes. Mix carefully. Use as quickly as possible. (When reconstituted, this reaction mixture is stable for approximately 2 weeks when it is stored at 0°C.) (Available from Sigma Chemical Company, St. Louis, Missouri.)
3. Test tubes, 12 × 75 mm.
4. Microhematocrit tubes.
5. Pipets, 2 ml, 0.2 ml, and 10 μl.
6. Filter paper, 32.0 cm, No. 1.
7. Long-wave ultraviolet lamp. (This is available from various laboratory suppliers for about $50.)
8. Normal control blood.

SPECIMEN

Whole blood, 1 ml, using EDTA, heparin, or ACD (acid citrate dextrose) as the anticoagulant.

PRINCIPLE

When red blood cells containing glucose-6-phosphate dehydrogenase (G-6-PD) are mixed with the test reagent (containing glucose-6-phosphate and NADP), the following reaction occurs:

$$\text{Glucose-6-phosphate}$$

$$+ \text{ NADP} \xrightarrow{\text{G-6-PD}} \text{NADPH}$$

$$+ \text{ 6-phosphogluconate}$$

The resultant NADPH fluoresces under long-wave ultraviolet light. NADP does not fluoresce.

PROCEDURE

1. Reconstitute one vial of the G-6-PD test reagent as described previously.
2. Label one 12 × 75-mm test tube for each patient and control to be tested. Label one tube as a blank.
3. Pipet 0.2 ml of G-6-PD test reagent into each of the preceding test tubes.
4. Fold a piece of 32.0 cm filter paper in half and label as shown in Figure 130.
5. Pipet 10 μl of whole, well-mixed blood from the first specimen and add to the appropriately labeled test tube containing the G-6-PD test reagent. Rinse the pipet several times. Mix the contents of the test tube and, using a microhematocrit tube,

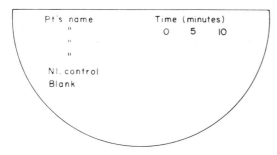

Fig. 130. Folded filter paper for G-6-PD procedure.

quickly place a drop of the mixture on the filter paper under the 0 column (0 time) across from the appropriate name. Place the test tube in a test tube rack at room temperature and immediately set a clock for 5 minutes.

6. Repeat step 5 for each specimen and the normal control. Add 10 μl of 0.85% sodium chloride to the blank.

7. At the end of the first 5-minute incubation period, place one small drop of the mixture in the appropriate line in the 5-minute column on the filter paper. Reset the clock for a second 5-minute incubation period. At the completion of the incubation period, place a small drop of the mixtures in the appropriate place on the filter paper.

8. Allow 10 to 15 minutes for the sample application to dry. In a dark room, place the filter paper under a long-wave ultraviolet light and observe for fluorescence. Record the results, using + for the presence of fluorescence, − for lack of fluorescence, and ± for weak fluorescence (outer rim fluoresces, whereas the center of the spot does not).

9. Interpretation of results. There should be little or no fluorescence at 0 time. Normal G-6-PD activity is indicated by maximum fluorescence at 10 minutes. Little or no fluorescence is seen in the 10-minute column on patients with a gross G-6-PD defi-

ciency. The normal control should show strong fluorescence at 10 minutes, whereas the blank should show no fluorescence. Patients with a mild deficiency (about 50%) generally show about half the fluorescence that is seen with the normal control.

DISCUSSION

1. Whole blood samples can be stored for several days at 4°C without loss of G-6-PD activity.

2. If it is preferred, this procedure may be performed at 37°C. In this case, greater fluorescence will be noted than when the test is performed at 25°C.

3. The 32-cm filter paper should be folded in half (not torn in half). The drops placed on the filter paper generally seep through one layer of the filter paper and, unless they are protected, may pick up contamination from the counter top (from the previous drop).

4. Hemoglobin has a quenching effect on fluorescence.

5. Once the drop of mixture has been placed on the filter paper, the reaction will continue until the drop completely dries.

6. No fluorescence or decreased fluorescence will be present as long as the drop is moist.

7. In this procedure, the rate of formation of fluorescence generally parallels the concentration of G-6-PD in the blood sample. For example, a blood sample with a G-6-PD concentration that is 50% of normal will take twice as long to form a strong fluorescence as a normal blood sample.

8. Quantitative assays should be performed when abnormal results are obtained by this procedure.

9. This test procedure may be used to differentiate normal and grossly deficient levels of G-6-PD.

PYRUVATE KINASE TEST

Pyruvate kinase is an enzyme in the Embden-Meyerhof pathway. A deficiency in this enzyme causes congenital non-spherocytic hemolytic anemia and is probably the most common cause of this type of anemia. Crenated red blood cells and irregularly contracted red blood cells may also be found in this deficiency.

REFERENCES

Beutler, E.: A series of new screening procedures for pyruvate kinase deficiency, glucose-6-phosphate dehydrogenase deficiency, and glutathione reductase deficiency, Blood, *28*, 553, 1966.

Sigma Chemical Company: *A Qualitative Screening Procedure for the Detection of Pyruvate Kinase Deficiency in Red Blood Cells*, Sigma Technical Bulletin No. 205, Sigma Chemical Company, St. Louis, Missouri, 1981.

REAGENTS AND EQUIPMENT

1. Pyruvate kinase reaction mixture. Reconstitute with 2.0 ml of distilled water. Allow to stand for 2 minutes. Mix gently. Reconstituted reaction mixture can be stored at 0°C for approximately 5 days. (Available from Sigma Chemical Company, St. Louis, Missouri.)
2. Test tubes, 12 × 75 mm.
3. Microhematocrit tubes.
4. Pipets, 2.0 ml, 0.2 ml, 0.1 ml, and 20 μl.
5. Conical centrifuge tubes, 15 ml.
6. Sodium chloride, 0.85% (w/v).
7. Filter paper, 32.0 cm, No. 1.
8. Long-wave, ultraviolet lamp.
9. Water bath, 37°C.

PRINCIPLE

The pyruvate kinase reaction mixture contains phosphoenolpyruvic acid, adenosine diphosphate (ADP), and reduced nicotinamide-adenine dinucleotide (NADH). When red blood cells containing pyruvate kinase and lactate dehydrogenase (LDH) are added to the test reagent, the following reactions occur:

Phosphoenolpyruvic acid

$$+ \text{ ADP } \xrightarrow{\frac{\text{Pyruvate}}{\text{Kinase}}} \text{ATP } + \text{ Pyruvic acid}$$

Pyruvic acid

$$+ \text{ NADH } \xrightarrow{\text{LDH}} \text{Lactic Acid } + \text{ NAD}$$

Under long-wave ultraviolet light, NADH fluoresces, whereas NAD does not fluoresce. Normally, all fluorescence should disappear within 30 minutes after the patient's red blood cells have been mixed with the pyruvate kinase reaction mixture.

SPECIMEN

Whole blood, 2 ml, using EDTA, heparin, or ACD as the anticoagulant. For a fingerstick specimen, obtain a minimum of 1 ml of whole blood, using heparinized microbilirubin tubes. As soon as each tube is collected, allow the blood to flow back and forth six or seven times to ensure complete anticoagulation of blood.

PROCEDURE

1. Place approximately 2 ml of patient's whole blood into an appropriately labeled conical centrifuge tube. Repeat using a normal control blood. Fill both tubes with 0.85% sodium chloride. Centrifuge at 2,500 RPM for 5 to 10 minutes. Remove supernatant sodium chloride and plasma, being careful not to disturb the packed red blood cells.
2. Place 0.4 ml of 0.85% sodium chloride into 12 × 75-mm test tubes appropriately labeled for each of the preceding specimens.
3. Without disturbing the packed red blood cell layer, carefully place a disposable pipet into the very bottom of the packed red blood cells. Carefully pipet 0.1 ml of red blood cells. Wipe off the outside of the pipet and trans-

fer the cells to the appropriate test tube containing 0.4 ml of sodium chloride. Rinse the pipet several times with the now diluted red blood cells.

4. Reconstitute the pyruvate kinase reaction mixture.

5. Pipet 0.2 ml of pyruvate kinase reaction mixture into the appropriately labeled 12 × 75-mm test tubes (one tube for negative control, one tube for the blank, and one tube for each patient).

6. Fold a piece of 32-cm filter paper in half and label with patients' names as shown in Figure 130 for the glucose-6-phosphate dehydrogenase test procedure. Insert reading times of 0, 10, 20, and 30 minutes.

7. Pipet 20 µl of the diluted red blood cell suspension into the appropriately labeled test tube containing 0.2 ml of reaction mixture. Rinse the pipet several times. Mix the test tube and, using a microhematocrit tube, quickly place a drop of the mixture on the filter paper under the 0 column (0 time). Place the test tube in a 37°C incubator. Set the clock for 30 minutes.

8. Repeat step 7 for each specimen and control, working as quickly as possible. (Use only one clock.) Add 20 µl of 0.85% sodium chloride to the blank in place of the red blood cell suspension.

9. When 10 minutes have elapsed on the clock, place one drop of the mixture in the 10-minute column. Repeat at 20 and 30 minutes.

10. Allow 10 to 15 minutes for the sample application to dry. In a dark room, place the filter paper under a long-wave ultraviolet light and observe for fluorescence. Record the results, using + for the presence of fluorescence, − for lack of fluorescence, and ± for weak fluorescence (outer rim fluoresces, whereas the center of the spot does not).

11. Interpretation of results. There should be strong fluorescence at 0 time. With normal pyruvate kinase activity, all NADH should have been oxidized to NAD and there should be no fluorescence at 30 minutes. Any fluorescence present at 30 minutes or after indicates decreased pyruvate kinase activity. The normal control blood should show no fluorescence at 30 minutes, whereas the blank mixture shows fluorescence throughout the 30 minutes.

DISCUSSION

1. Pyruvate kinase is present in the plasma and in the white blood cells. Since this procedure is used to test for the pyruvate kinase activity of the red blood cells, it is important that no plasma or white blood cells contaminate the red blood cell suspension.

2. The 32-cm filter paper should be folded in half (not torn in half). The drops placed on the filter paper generally seep through one layer of the filter paper and, unless they are protected, may pick up contamination from the counter top (from the previous drop).

3. Once the drop of mixture has been placed on the filter paper, the reaction will continue until the drop completely dries.

4. Hemoglobin has a quenching effect on fluorescence.

5. No fluorescence or decreased fluorescence will be present as long as the drop is moist.

6. Pyruvate kinase activity of the red blood cells is stable for 2 to 3 weeks when the blood is stored at refrigerator temperature.

7. Quantitative assays should be performed when abnormal results are obtained by this procedure.

8. This test procedure may be utilized to differentiate normal and grossly deficient levels of pyruvate kinase.

GLUTATHIONE REDUCTASE TEST

Glutathione reductase is a red blood cell enzyme. It functions in the hexose monophosphate shunt to catalyze the reaction of the transfer of electrons from NADPH to glutathione in forming reduced glutathione.

A severe hemolytic anemia, frequently drug-induced, is caused by a deficiency in glutathione reductase.

REFERENCES

Beutler, E.: A series of new screening procedures for pyruvate kinase deficiency, glucose-6-phosphate dehydrogenase deficiency, and glutathione reductase deficiency, Blood, 28, 553, 1966.

Sigma Chemical Company: A Qualitative Screening Procedure for the Determination of Glutathione Reductase Deficiency in Blood, Sigma Technical Bulletin No. 190, Sigma Chemical Company, St. Louis, Missouri, 1981.

REAGENTS AND EQUIPMENT

1. Glutathione reductase reaction mixture. Reconstitute with 2.0 ml of distilled water. Allow to stand for 2 minutes. Mix gently. Reconstituted reaction mixture can be stored at 0°C for 3 days without losing activity. (Available from Sigma Chemical Company, St. Louis, Missouri.)
2. Test tubes, 12 × 75 mm.
3. Microhematocrit tubes.
4. Pipets, 2.0 ml, 0.2 ml, and 20 μl.
5. Filter paper, 32.0 cm, No. 1.
6. Long-wave ultraviolet lamp.
7. Sodium chloride, 0.85% (w/v).
8. Water bath, 37°C.

SPECIMEN

Whole blood (2 ml), using EDTA, heparin, or ACD as the anticoagulant. For fingerstick specimen, obtain six or seven heparinized microhematocrit tubes (about three-fourths full). As soon as each tube is collected, allow the blood to flow back and forth six or seven times to ensure complete anticoagulation of the blood.

PRINCIPLE

The glutathione reductase reaction mixture contains oxidized glutathione (GSSG) and reduced nicotinamide-adenine dinucleotide phosphate (NADPH). When red blood cells containing glutathione reductase (GSSG-R) are added to the reaction mixture, the following reactions occur:

$$GSSG + NADPH \xrightarrow{\text{GSSG-R}} \begin{matrix} \text{Reduced} \\ \text{glutathione} \end{matrix} + NADP$$

Under long-wave ultraviolet light, NADPH shows fluorescence, whereas NADP does not. Generally, in normal patients, fluorescence begins to disappear within 30 minutes after the patient's red blood cells have been mixed with the glutathione reductase reaction mixture. In blood samples from patients with decreased activity of glutathione reductase, fluorescence may continue for 1 hour or longer.

PROCEDURE

1. Reconstitute the glutathione reductase reaction mixture with 2.0 ml of distilled water. Mix gently until in solution.
2. Pipet 0.2 ml of glutathione reductase reaction mixture into the appropriately labeled 12 × 75 mm test tubes (one tube for negative control, one tube for blank, and one tube for each patient).
3. Fold a piece of 32-cm filter paper in half and label with patients' names as shown in Figure 130 for the glucose-6-phosphate dehydrogenase test procedure. Insert reading times of 0, 20, 40, and 60 minutes.
4. Pipet 20 μl of whole, well-mixed

blood from the first specimen into the appropriately labeled test tube containing 0.2 ml of reaction mixture. Rinse the pipet several times. Mix the test tube and, using a microhematocrit tube, quickly place a drop of the mixture on the filter paper under the 0 column (0 time). Place the test tube in a test tube rack and incubate at 37°C. Set the clock for 60 minutes.

5. Repeat step 4 for each specimen, working as quickly as possible. (Use only one clock.) Add 20 µl of 0.85% sodium chloride to the blank in place of the whole blood.

6. When 20 minutes have elapsed on the clock, place one small drop of the mixtures in the 20-minute column. Repeat at 40 and 60 minutes.

7. Allow 10 to 15 minutes for the sample application to dry. In a dark room, place the filter paper under a long-wave ultraviolet light and observe for fluorescence. Record the results, using + for the presence of fluorescence, − for lack of fluorescence, and ± for weak fluorescence (outer rim fluoresces, whereas the center of the spot does not).

8. Interpretation of results. There should be strong fluorescence at 0 time. With normal glutathione reductase activity, all NADPH should have been oxidized to NADP and there should be no fluorescence at 20 to 30 minutes. Fluorescence at 60 minutes is abnormal. The normal control blood should show no fluorescence at 60 minutes, whereas the blank mixture does show fluorescence.

DISCUSSION

1. Blood samples may be stored at refrigerator temperature for 3 weeks without a loss of glutathione reductase activity.

2. The 32-cm filter paper should be folded in half (not torn in half). The drops placed on the filter paper generally seep through one layer of the filter paper and, unless they are protected, may pick up contamination from the counter top (from the previous drop).

3. Hemoglobin has a quenching effect on fluorescence.

4. Once the drop of mixture has been placed on the filter paper, the reaction continues until the drop completely dries.

5. No fluorescence or decreased fluorescence is present as long as the drop is moist.

6. Quantitative assays should be performed when abnormal results are obtained by this procedure.

7. This test procedure may be used to differentiate normal and grossly deficient levels of glutathione reductase.

ASCORBATE-CYANIDE SCREENING TEST

The ascorbate-cyanide screening test is used to detect deficiencies in glucose-6-phosphate dehydrogenase and certain other enzymes present in the red blood cell. It is also capable of detecting defective glutathione synthesis. It should be noted, however, that this procedure is only a screening test and cannot differentiate the specific enzyme deficiency. It indicates only that a defect or an enzyme deficiency exists in the hexose monophosphate shunt.

Jacob and Jandl Method

REFERENCES

Dacie, J.V., and Lewis, S.M.: *Practical Hematology*, 5th ed., Churchill Livingstone, New York, 1975.

Jacob, H.S., and Jandl, J.H.: A simple visual screening test for glucose-6-phosphate dehydrogenase deficiency employing ascorbate and cyanide, N. Eng. J. Med., 274, 1162, 1966.

REAGENTS AND EQUIPMENT

1. Ascorbate.

Sodium ascorbate	10.0 mg
Glucose	5.0 mg

   Place the preceding chemicals in each of several 13 × 100-mm test tubes. (One test tube is used for each test and one test tube for each control.) These tubes may be stoppered and stored at −20°C indefinitely.

2. Iso-osmotic phosphate buffer, pH 7.4.

   Solution 1

Monobasic sodium phosphate (NaH$_2$PO$_4$·2 H$_2$O)	23.4 g

   Dilute to 1,000 ml with distilled water.

   Solution 2

Dibasic sodium phosphate (Na$_2$HPO$_4$)	21.3 g

   Dilute to 1,000 ml with distilled water.

   For iso-osmotic phosphate buffer, pH 7.4, mix together:

Solution 1	18 ml
Solution 2	82 ml

3. Sodium cyanide.

Sodium cyanide	50 mg
Distilled water	50 ml
Iso-osmotic phosphate buffer	20 ml

   Neutralize the preceding solution to a pH of 7.0 using hydrochloric acid. Dilute to 100 ml with distilled water. This solution is stable at room temperature indefinitely.

4. Test tubes, 13 × 100 mm.
5. Water bath, 37°C.

SPECIMEN

Collect 3 ml of whole blood, using heparin or EDTA as the anticoagulant. A normal control blood should be collected at the same time the patient's blood is obtained.

PRINCIPLE

In the red blood cell, catalase normally inhibits, or decomposes, hydrogen peroxide. Sodium cyanide, however, added to the blood inhibits catalase and allows hydrogen peroxide to be generated. If the enzymes in the hexose-monophosphate shunt are not able to utilize the added glucose, the red blood cells are oxidized by the hydrogen peroxide and change to a brown color (methemoglobin).

PROCEDURE

1. Aerate both patient and control bloods to a bright red color by gently swirling the blood under air.
2. Add 2 ml of the patient's whole blood to a test tube containing sodium ascorbate and glucose. Place 2 ml of control blood into a second test tube containing sodium ascorbate and glucose.
3. Mix both tubes well.
4. Add two drops of sodium cyanide solution to each of the preceding test tubes.
5. Gently mix the tubes well by blowing into the solutions with a disposable pipet. Leave the pipet in the test tubes, and place in a 37°C water bath for 2 hours.
6. During the 2 hours of incubation, remix each solution several times, using the pipet to blow into the mixtures.
7. At the end of 2 hours' incubation, mix the test tubes and note the color of each solution. The normal control solution should be a red color. If the patient's mixture is red, the test result is normal. If, however, the patient's solution has turned a brown color, the test is positive, and there is probably an enzyme deficiency in the hexose-monophosphate shunt,

most often a glucose-6-phosphate dehydrogenase deficiency.

DISCUSSION

1. If the blood specimen has a hematocrit below 20%, the volume of blood added to the ascorbate tube should be adjusted so that the amount of red blood cells added is equivalent to a hematocrit of 30 to 40%. For example, if the hematocrit is 20%, add 3 to 4 ml of whole blood to the ascorbate tube. As an alternative method, an appropriate amount of plasma may be removed from the whole blood until a hematocrit reading of 30 to 40% is attained.
2. Ammonium-potassium oxalate cannot be used as an anticoagulant for this procedure.

HEINZ BODY PREPARATION

Heinz bodies represent precipitated hemoglobin and appear as single or multiple, round, oval, or serrated, refractile granules in the red blood cell. They are present in a number of hemolytic disorders. Heinz bodies are formed when the glycolytic enzymes in the red blood cell are unable to prevent the oxidation of hemoglobin. As a result, the hemoglobin is eventually denatured and precipitated to form Heinz bodies. Because the normal aging of a red blood cell is accompanied by a decrease in the red blood cell enzyme systems, occasional Heinz bodies will be seen normally. Increased numbers of Heinz bodies occur in hemolytic anemias secondary to the action of certain oxidant drugs (glucose-6-phosphate dehydrogenase deficiency and glutathione deficiency) and in the presence of unstable hemoglobins such as hemoglobin Zurich and hemoglobin H.

REFERENCES

Cartwright, G.E.: *Diagnostic Laboratory Hematology,* Grune & Stratton, Inc., New York, 1963.

Dacie, J.V., and Lewis, S.M.: *Practical Hematology,* 5th ed., Churchill Livingstone, New York, 1975.

Fertman, M.H., and Fertman, M.B.: Toxic anemia and Heinz bodies, Medicine, *34,* 131, 1955.

REAGENTS AND EQUIPMENT

1. Sodium chloride, 0.85% (w/v).
2. Crystal violet, 1% (w/v).
   Crystal violet 2.0 g
   (Color Index number 42555)
   Sodium chloride, 100 ml
   0.85% (w/v)
   Shake the preceding mixture for 15 minutes and filter. Dilute the filtered stain with an equal volume of 0.85% sodium chloride. This stain is stable at room temperature for several months.
3. Test tubes, 13 × 100 mm.

SPECIMEN

Whole blood, using heparin, EDTA, or ammonium-potassium oxalate as the anticoagulant.

PRINCIPLE

Whole blood is mixed with crystal violet stain and allowed to incubate. Moist preparations are made of the blood and stain mixture, and the red blood cells are examined for the presence of Heinz bodies.

PROCEDURE

1. Place 0.5 ml (1 volume) of well-mixed whole blood into a 13 × 100-mm test tube.
2. Add 1.0 ml (2 volumes) of the 1% saline solution of crystal violet.
3. Mix well and allow to incubate at room temperature for 15 minutes.
4. At the end of 15 minutes, remix the blood and stain solution. Place a small drop of the mixture on a glass slide and cover with a cover glass.
5. Examine the red blood cells microscopically, using the oil immersion objective (100×). The Heinz bodies

appear as purple, irregularly shaped bodies of varying sizes, up to 2 μm in diameter. There may be more than one Heinz body present in a red blood cell, and they generally lie close to the cell membrane (Color Plate IV, H).

DISCUSSION

1. Heinz bodies are detectable in wet preparations and by using supravital stains such as methyl violet, new methylene blue N, and brilliant cresyl blue, in addition to the aforementioned crystal violet. They are not seen when Wright's stain is used.
2. Red blood cells with a suspectibility to Heinz body formation may also be detected with acetylphenylhydrazine. This chemical, an oxidant, is incubated for 4 hours with the patient's blood. The red blood cells are then stained with crystal violet. In those patients whose red blood cells have defective reducing systems, 45 to 92% of the red blood cells contain five or more Heinz bodies. In this method, the amount of acetylphenylhydrazine added to the red cells is critical. A normal control blood must be run at the same time the patient's blood is tested and must show a low percentage of Heinz bodies.

HEAT PRECIPITATION TEST

The heat precipitation test demonstrates unstable hemoglobins, which are present in the various types of hereditary Heinz body anemias. Normally, less than 1% of the hemoglobin precipitates out when the test is performed by the following procedure.

REFERENCE

Dacie, J.V., and Lewis, S.M.: *Practical Hematology*, 5th ed., Churchill Livingstone, New York, 1975.

REAGENTS AND EQUIPMENT

1. Phosphate buffer, pH 7.4.
   Solution 1
   Monobasic sodium phosphate (NaH₂PO₄·2 H₂O) — 23.4 g
   Distilled water — 1,000 ml
   Solution 2
   Dibasic sodium phosphate (Na₂HPO₄) — 21.3 g
   Distilled water — 1,000 ml
   For phosphate buffer, pH 7.4, mix together:
   Solution 1 — 18 ml
   Solution 2 — 82 ml
2. Cyanmethemoglobin reagent. (See the section entitled Cyanmethemoglobin Method [Reagents and Equipment] in Chapter 2.)
3. Sodium chloride, 0.85% (w/v).
4. Test tubes, 13 × 100 mm.
5. Water bath, 50°C.

SPECIMEN

Whole blood, using EDTA, ammonium-potassium oxalate, or heparin as the anticoagulant. A normal control blood must be collected at the same time the patient's blood is obtained.

PRINCIPLE

Washed red blood cells are hemolyzed with water, a phosphate buffer is added, and the resultant mixture is allowed to incubate at 50°C for 3 hours. The percentage of unstable hemoglobin precipitated during incubation is then calculated from the amount of hemoglobin in the unheated and heated samples.

PROCEDURE

1. Pipet 1 ml of patient's fresh whole blood into a 13 × 100-mm test tube. Place 1 ml of normal control blood into a second test tube.
2. Fill both test tubes with 0.85% sodium chloride to wash the red blood cells. Centrifuge at 2,500 RPM for 5 minutes. Remove the supernatant.

3. Wash the red blood cells a second time by repeating step 2.
4. Add 5 ml of distilled water to both test tubes to lyse the red blood cells. Mix the test tubes gently to dislodge all the red blood cells from the bottom of the tube.
5. Add 5 ml of phosphate buffer to each test tube. Mix gently.
6. Centrifuge the tubes at 2,500 RPM for 10 minutes.
7. Remove 4 ml of the supernatant from each of the preceding test tubes.
8. Place 2 ml of the patient's hemolysate into each of two 13 × 100-mm test tubes. Place one of these tubes in the 50°C water bath and leave the second test tube at room temperature.
9. Repeat step 8 for the normal control blood.
10. Incubate both test tubes at 50°C for 3 hours.
11. At the end of 3 hours, centrifuge the preceding two incubated tubes at 2,500 RPM for 10 minutes.
12. Using cyanmethemoglobin reagent, determine the hemoglobin content of the supernatant in each of the four test tubes as follows:
    A. Add 0.5 ml of the hemolysate (supernatant) to 9.5 ml of cyanmethemoglobin reagent.
    B. Mix well and allow to sit at least 10 minutes.
    C. Transfer to a cuvette and read in a spectrophotometer at a wavelength of 540 nm (or with a yellow-green filter), using the cyanmethemoglobin reagent to blank the machine (set optical density at 0).
    D. Record the optical density for each of the four hemolysates.
13. Calculate the results for the patient and for the normal control as shown at the top of the next column.

$$\text{Percent of unstable hemoglobin} = \frac{\begin{array}{c}\text{Optical} \\ \text{density of} \\ \text{unheated} \\ \text{sample}\end{array} - \begin{array}{c}\text{Optical} \\ \text{density of} \\ \text{heated} \\ \text{sample}\end{array}}{\begin{array}{c}\text{Optical density of} \\ \text{unheated sample}\end{array}} \times 100$$

DISCUSSION

Normally, the hemolysate remains clear after incubation for 1 hour at 50°C. At the end of 3 hours, only trace amounts of precipitate are found (less than 1%).

ISOPROPANOL PRECIPITATION TEST

The isopropanol precipitation test detects unstable hemoglobins. According to the following procedure, normal hemoglobins will begin to show precipitation in a 17% isopropanol solution after about 40 minutes, whereas unstable hemoglobins will begin to precipitate after 5 minutes and show heavier flocculation at 20 minutes.

REFERENCE

Carrell, R.W.,. and Kay, R.: A simple method for the detection of unstable haemoglobins, Br. J. Haematol., 23, 615, 1972.

REAGENTS AND EQUIPMENT

1. Isopropanol-tris buffer, pH 7.4.
   Tris (hydroxymethyl)   12.11 g
   aminomethane
   Isopropyl alcohol, 100%   170 ml
   Dilute to 1 liter with distilled water. Adjust to pH 7.4 using concentrated hydrochloric acid. Store in the refrigerator. This solution may be used for several weeks.
2. Water bath, 37°C.
3. Test tubes, 10 × 75 mm, with caps.
4. Centrifuge tubes, polypropylene or glass, 15 ml.
5. Sodium chloride, 0.85%, w/v.
6. Distilled water.
7. Toluene.
8. Pasteur pipets.
9. Pipets, 0.2 ml and 2.0 ml.
10. Vortex mixer (optional).

11. Parafilm.
12. Timer.

SPECIMEN

Whole anticoagulated blood. The type of anticoagulant used is not critical. A normal control blood should be collected at the same time the patient's blood is obtained.

PRINCIPLE

Washed red blood cells are hemolyzed and mixed with a 17% solution of isopropanol and incubated at 37°C. The specimens are then examined at 5 minutes and 20 minutes for precipitation of hemoglobin. The isopropanol solution weakens the internal bonding of hemoglobin, causing a faster rate of precipitation of unstable hemoglobins than that of normal hemoglobin.

PROCEDURE

1. Preparation of hemolysate.
   A. Place 2 to 3 ml of patient's whole blood into a graduated, polypropylene centrifuge tube. Place 2 to 3 ml of normal control blood into a second tube.
   B. Fill both tubes with 0.85% sodium chloride to wash the red blood cells. Centrifuge at 2,000 RPM for 5 minutes. Remove the supernatant.
   C. Wash the red blood cells two more times by repeating step B above.
   D. Remove 1 ml of washed red blood cells from each tube and place in a clean, labeled, polypropylene or glass centrifuge tube. Add 1 ml of distilled water to each tube. Mix. Add 0.5 ml of toluene to each tube. Stopper each tube.
   E. Vortex each tube for 2 to 3 minutes or shake tubes manually for 5 minutes.
   F. Centrifuge the tubes at 3,000 RPM

for 10 minutes. Carefully remove the tubes from the centrifuge.
   G. Remove the middle hemolysate layer from each tube. Be very careful performing this step: hold the tube against a well-lit background so that you are able to see well and avoid mixing the toluene or red blood cell stroma in with the hemolysate. Contamination with the red blood cell stroma may cause false-positive test results. Place the hemolysate in a separate, labeled test tube, making certain the hemolysate is crystal clear.

2. For each patient and control to be tested, place 2.0 ml of the isopropanol-tris buffer solution into a 10 × 75 mm test tube. Stopper each tube and place in the 37°C water bath for 10 minutes. Be certain the liquid in the tubes is completely immersed in the water of the incubator. (To save time, place the test tubes in the water bath just prior to the last centrifugation in the preparation of the hemolysate.)

3. Add 0.2 ml of each hemolysate to the appropriately labeled test tubes of buffer in the water bath. Stopper each tube and gently invert two times to mix.

4. Check each test tube at 5, 20, and 45 minutes for evidence of precipitation or flocculation. When reading the test tubes, extreme care must be taken not to mix the solution too much. (The precipitate will quickly break up if the solution is physically mixed.) Carefully remove the test tube from the water bath, tilt the tube horizontally, and examine the solution for precipitation against a light source.

5. Interpretation of results.
   A. Negative for unstable hemoglobin: No precipitation or flocculation at 5 minutes or 20 minutes.

Precipitation should begin to appear at 45 minutes.

B. Positive for unstable hemoglobin: Precipitation present at the 5-minute reading, with definite flocculation at 20 minutes.

C. The normal control should be negative for hemoglobin precipitation at 5 and 20 minutes. To ensure that the buffer solution is effective, precipitation should begin appearing at 45 minutes. If these results are not obtained for the normal control, fresh buffer reagent should be prepared and the entire test repeated.

DISCUSSION

1. Blood that is several days old may be used for this test. The hemolysate, however, must be prepared immediately prior to the performance of the test.
2. The concentration of isopropanol (17%) in the buffer solution is very critical.
3. The pH of the buffer solution is not critical but must be at least 7.2.
4. The temperature of the water bath is very important and must be at 37°C.
5. Increased amounts of methemoglobin may give false-positive results because it is less stable than oxyhemoglobin.

HEMOGLOBIN ELECTROPHORESIS BY CELLULOSE ACETATE

The hemoglobin molecule is made up of globin and heme. There are numerous types of hemoglobins, based on the structure of the globin chains. These polypeptide chains differ in the number, type, and sequence of amino acids, depending on the type of hemoglobin involved. Hemoglobin electrophoresis is a procedure used to detect the types of hemoglobin present in a patient's red blood cells.

There are several electrophoretic methods in use today for differentiating the various types of hemoglobin. To date, the most widely used technique employs the use of cellulose acetate. Other media in use are starch block, agar gel, and paper. The technical details of the procedure vary between different laboratories and according to the apparatus used.

REFERENCES

Helena Laboratories: *Sickle Cell Hemoglobinopathies*, Helena Laboratories, Beaumont, Texas, 1979.

Schmidt, R.M., and Brosious, E.M.: *Basic Laboratory Methods of Hemoglobinopathy Detection*, HEW Pub. No. (CDC) 74-8266, U.S. Department of Health, Education, and Welfare, Public Health Service, Center for Disease Control, Atlanta, 1974.

REAGENTS AND EQUIPMENT

1. Supre-Heme Buffer, obtainable from Helena Laboratories, Beaumont, Texas. Dissolve one packet of the buffer in 980 ml of distilled water.
2. Hemolysate reagent.
   Stock saponin solution, 1% (w/v)

   Saponin, certified grade   1.0 g
   Add approximately 50 ml of distilled water and mix. When the saponin is completely in solution, dilute to 100 ml.
   Hemolysate reagent

   Stock saponin solution   10 ml
   Dilute to 100 ml with distilled water. Add 2.0 ml of 3% (w/v) potassium cyanide. Store at 4°C.
3. Ponceau stain.
   Ponceau S   0.5 g
   Dilute to 100 ml with 5% (w/v) trichloroacetic acid.
4. Disposable wicks.
5. New Titan III H cellulose acetate strips with Mylar backing.
6. Sample applicator (Fig. 131).
7. Sample plate (contains hemolysate samples to be tested) (Fig. 131).
8. Aligning base (holds cellulose ace-

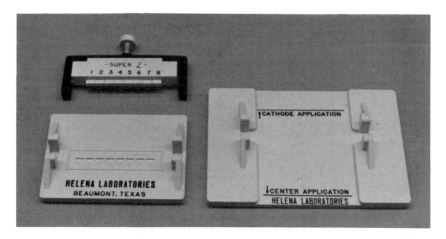

Fig. 131. Equipment used in hemoglobin electrophoresis by cellulose acetate. Sample applicator (top left), sample plate (left), and aligning base (right).

tate strip while inoculating with patient samples) (Fig. 131).

9. Electrophoresis chamber (Fig. 132). (Note: All preceding items, No. 1 through 9, are obtainable from Helena Laboratories, P.O. Box 752, Beaumont, Texas, 77704.)
10. Blotting paper, grade 470, size $5\frac{7}{8} \times 8\frac{7}{8}$, 100 per package. Obtainable from Schleicher and Schuell, Keene, New Hampshire. (Routine laboratory filter paper may be used in place of the blotting paper.)
11. Test tubes, 12 × 75 mm.
12. Disposable pipet droppers.
13. Squeeze bottle of distilled water to rinse the applicator and sample plate.
14. Small, shallow pans, five. (Used for buffer, stain, and acetic acid rinse solutions.)
15. Hemostats, two.
16. Acetic acid, 5% (v/v).
17. A DC-regulated power supply (Fig. 133).
18. Sodium chloride, 0.85% (w/v).
19. Microhematocrit tubes.
20. Glass slides, 1 × 3 inches.
21. Known control samples. These may be liquid, lyophilized, or frozen red blood cells and may be prepared from blood with known abnormal hemoglobins or purchased from any one of several commercial companies.

SPECIMEN

Whole blood, using EDTA, heparin, or ammonium-potassium oxalate as the an-

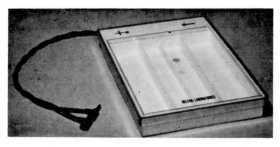

Fig. 132. Electrophoresis chamber. (Courtesy of Helena Laboratories, Beaumont, Texas.)

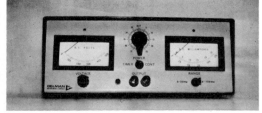

Fig. 133. Power supply. (Courtesy of Gelman Instrument Company, Ann Arbor, Michigan.)

ticoagulant. Capillary blood may also be used. When using whole blood, at least 0.5 ml of blood should be obtained. When utilizing capillary blood, three to four hematocrit tubes three-fourths filled should be collected.

PRINCIPLE

The hemoglobin molecule contains globin chains made up of amino acids. The sequence of these amino acids influences the properties of the globin chain and, therefore, the hemoglobin molecule. Basically, an amino group consists of a carboxyl group (COOH), an amino group (NH$_3$), and an R group attached to a carbon atom, as shown in the following diagram.

$$\begin{array}{c} NH_3 \\ | \\ H-C-COOH \\ | \\ R \end{array}$$

The carboxyl and amino groups are able to carry a charge, and the amino acid has a positive or negative charge, depending on the pH of the solution it is in. For example, in an alkaline solution, the amino acid shows a negative charge as indicated in the following diagram.

$$\begin{array}{c} NH_2 \\ | \\ H-C-COOH \\ | \\ R \end{array} \xrightarrow[\text{(OH$-$)}]{\text{Alkaline Solution}} H_2O + \begin{array}{c} NH_2 \\ | \\ H-C-COO^- \\ | \\ R \end{array}$$

In an acid solution, in which there is an excess of hydrogen ions, the amino acid has a positive charge. In hemoglobin electrophoresis, the hemoglobin is placed in an alkaline buffer solution (pH approximately 8.0–8.6). The net negative charge of the various hemoglobins depends on the amino acids (and their R groups) making up the hemoglobin molecule.

$$\begin{array}{c} NH_2 \\ | \\ H-C-COOH \\ | \\ R \end{array} \xrightarrow[\text{Solution (H$+$)}]{\text{Acid}} \begin{array}{c} NH^+_3 \\ | \\ H-C-COOH \\ | \\ R \end{array}$$

The first step in hemoglobin electro-phoresis is the preparation of a hemolysate to destroy the red blood cell membranes and free the hemoglobin. A small quantity of hemolysate is then placed on a cellulose acetate membrane and positioned in an electrophoresis tray with the inoculated hemolysate near the cathode (negative). One end of the cellulose acetate strip is immersed in the buffer (pH 8.4) on the cathode side and the other end is placed in the buffer on the anode side. An electric current of specific voltage and milliamps is allowed to run for a specified time. During this period, the hemoglobin molecules migrate toward the anode (positive) because of their negative charge. Because of variations in the amino acid content of different hemoglobins, the net negative charge of various types of hemoglobin at a specific pH differs from that of other hemoglobin types. This difference in the net charge of the hemoglobin molecule determines its mobility in an electric field and manifests itself by the speed with which it migrates to the positive pole. The cellulose acetate membrane is then placed in stain that colors the proteins (hemoglobins) red. By noting the distance each hemoglobin has migrated and comparing this distance with the migration distance of known controls, the different types of hemoglobins present can be identified.

PROCEDURE

1. Preparation of hemolysate from whole blood.
   A. Label one 12 × 75-mm test tube for each patient's blood to be tested.
   B. Place one drop of patient's whole blood into the preceding appropriately labeled tube.
   C. Fill the test tube with 0.85% sodium chloride and centrifuge at 2,500 RPM for 5 minutes to wash the red blood cells and remove the plasma.
   D. Decant the supernatant and drain the test tube against gauze to re-

move all the sodium chloride-plasma possible.

E. Add three drops of hemolysate reagent to each test tube. Mix well and stopper each test tube.

F. Place each test tube in the freezer for approximately 10 minutes or longer.

G. Upon thawing, the red blood cells should be completely hemolyzed (crystal-clear solution). If the hemolysate is slightly cloudy, refreeze and thaw the specimen to obtain complete hemolysis.

H. If the patient's hemoglobin is low (less than 9 g per dl), add two to three drops of whole blood to the tube for the hemolysate.

2. Preparation of hemolysate from hematocrit tubes.

A. Centrifuge two hematocrit tubes from each patient to be tested for approximately 3 minutes.

B. Using a small file, place a small nick in the hematocrit tube a small distance below the buffy coat and plasma layers. Break the hematocrit tube at the cut and discard the plasma and buffy coat portions.

C. In the same manner as in step B, remove the sealed end at the bottom of the hematocrit tube so that only the packed red blood cell layer remains.

D. Using the small file, cut the packed red blood cell layer into three or four small pieces and place in an appropriately labeled 12 × 75-mm test tube.

E. Repeat the preceding procedure for the second hematocrit tube, placing it in the same labeled tube with the first hematocrit.

F. Add six drops of hemolysate reagent to the tube. Mix vigorously to shake the red blood cells out of the hematocrit tubes. Stopper the test tube. If the hemoglobin elec-trophoresis is to be performed at this time, the hemolysate need not be frozen. Allow 10 minutes after adding the hemolysate reagent for the red blood cells to hemolyze completely.

3. Fill a small pan with approximately 40 ml of buffer solution.

4. Using a clean, dry hemostat, slowly and uniformly immerse a cellulose acetate strip into the buffer solution. This should take 10 to 15 seconds. If the membrane is immersed too quickly, white areas appear on the cellulose acetate and it must be discarded. Allow the strip to soak in the buffer a minimum of 20 minutes prior to use. (Do not touch the cellulose acetate portion of the membrane with your fingers at any time prior to or after electrophoresing. After the strip has been stained and the stain removed, it is permissible to touch the cellulose acetate side of the strip.)

5. Pour 50 ml of buffer into each of the outer compartments of the electrophoresis chamber. Moisten two disposable paper wicks in the buffer and drape one over each of the middle support bridges, ensuring that it makes buffer contact and that there are no air bubbles underneath the wicks.

6. Using microhematocrit tubes, two-thirds fill each well in the sample well plate (one patient sample per well). It is a good idea to place the known control samples in well number 1 and/or number 2. Position the applicator directly over the sample well plate in the two lateral indentations.

7. Cover the sample well plate with a glass slide if the hemolysates are not inoculated within 5 minutes.

8. Remove the cellulose acetate strip from the buffer, being careful not to touch the cellulose acetate side of the

strip with your fingers. Carefully blot the strip between the two pieces of filter paper or blotters. The object is to remove only the shiny excess surface buffer. Do not blot the membrane too much.

9. With the Mylar (plastic) backing facing up and the long side of the strip on the horizontal, label the strip at the top right-hand corner with a black magic marker.

10. Quickly turn the strip over (cellulose acetate side up) and place it in the aligning base with the label in the bottom left corner (now on the back of the strip) with the long side now vertical. The back edge of the strip should be flush with the back of the aligning base to allow the samples to be inoculated approximately 1 inch from the front edge of the cellulose acetate strip.

11. Depress the applicator tips into the sample wells for 1 to 2 seconds.

12. Quickly transfer the applicator to the aligning base. Press the button down quickly, lowering the applicator tips to the cellulose acetate strip. Hold the button down for 1 to 2 seconds and release.

13. Quickly place the strip, cellulose side down and with the long side of the strip on the horizontal, in the chamber with the application site nearest the cathode (negative) side. The label should be at the top right corner. Place a glass slide on top of the strip to act as a weight. Carefully place the cover on top of the chamber.

14. Attach the electrode terminal pins to the power supply. Turn the power supply on and adjust the voltage to 350 V. Time for 25 minutes.

15. At the end of 25 minutes, turn the power supply off, carefully remove the strips from the chamber, and blot the side edges to remove the excess buffer.

16. Place the strips in a pan containing Ponceau S stain for approximately 3 minutes.

17. Remove the membrane from the stain and place it in a 5% acetic acid solution to rinse the excess stain off. Agitate the membrane gently.

18. Repeat step 17 two or three more times in clean 5% acetic acid until all of the excess stain is removed. The strip should return to its white color, with only the hemoglobin taking up the pink or red stain.

19. After the last acetic acid wash, remove the excess moisture with filter or blotting paper. Allow 5 to 10 minutes for air-drying.

20. Identify the hemoglobin types present in the patient samples by comparing the migration distances with the known controls. See Figure 134 for the mobilities of various hemoglobins.

DISCUSSION

1. A third method of hemolysate preparation is available employing a special type of filter paper (available from Rochester Paper Company, Rochester, Michigan, as ROPACO #1023, 0.038 inch). A drop of cap-

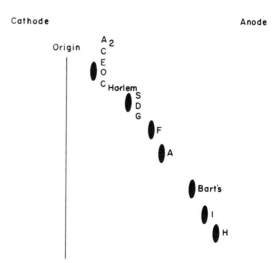

Fig. 134. Electrophoretic mobility of various hemoglobins at pH 8.4.

illary blood is placed on this filter paper to cover a circular area with a minimum 12-mm diameter. When the blood sample has dried, it is ready for use, or it may be stored in a plastic bag at refrigerator temperatures. To prepare the hemolysate, punch out a disk 1 cm in diameter (of the blood specimen) and place in a 12 × 75-mm test tube. Add two drops of hemolysate reagent, mix, and allow to elute for 30 minutes. Remove the filter paper. The hemolysate may be used immediately or placed in the freezer for future testing.

2. It is easy and economical for a laboratory to prepare its own hemoglobin electrophoresis controls. Using known blood samples, prepare any number of hemolysates as outlined in step 1 of the previous procedure. Stopper the test tubes tightly and place in the freezer. Each time hemoglobin electrophoresis is performed, remove one test tube of each known hemoglobin control from the freezer and thaw. Discard the remaining hemolysate after use. In the frozen state, these hemolysates will remain effective controls for several months.

3. If the Ponceau S is kept tightly covered, it may be used for approximately 1 month.

4. The buffer solution used for soaking the cellulose acetate strips may be used for 5 days if it is kept covered when not in use.

5. Fresh chamber buffer should be used daily.

6. The staining time is not critical.

7. On patients showing hemoglobin S, perform the sodium dithionite sickle cell test. (The results should be positive.) If the sickle cell test is negative and the patient shows hemoglobin S electrophoretically, this is possibly hemoglobin D. Agar gel electropho-

resis may then be performed for further diagnosis.

8. If desired, the sodium dithionite sickle cell test may also be performed on hemoglobin C patients. Hemoglobin C_{Harlem} is a sickling hemoglobin and shows a positive sodium dithionite tube test.

9. Three cellulose acetate strips may be run in the electrophoresis tray at one time.

10. Sometimes, when eight samples are inoculated on a strip, distortion may occur in the first and eighth samples. For consistently good results, use only the second through seventh slots in the sample well plate.

11. The hemoglobin electrophoresis may also be run at 450 V for 15 minutes.

12. If semiquantitative results are desired, the membrane may be placed in a densitometer and scanned. The Beckman R-110 Microzone Densitometer is obtainable from Beckman Instruments, Palo Alto, California. Models available from other companies are equally satisfactory. The instructions accompanying the equipment should be followed for the quantitation of the hemoglobins. Prior to quantitation, however, the cellulose acetate strip must be cleared (to develop a transparent background). This is accomplished by placing the strip in absolute methanol for 3 minutes after the acetic acid washes and then placing it in an acetic acid-methanol solution (one part acetic acid and four parts methanol) for 10 minutes. Dry in a 65°C oven for approximately 10 minutes.

13. This procedure shows particularly good separation of hemoglobins A and F. For accurate quantitation of hemoglobin F, however, the alkali denaturation procedure must be utilized.

14. When interpreting the hemoglobin electrophoresis results, the unknown

hemoglobins may only be identified by comparing their mobility (distance traveled) with the mobility of known hemoglobins run on the same membrane.

15. There may be a small amount of hemoglobin that distributes itself along the pathway of the migrating hemoglobin. This is called *trailing*. A small amount of this trailing is not unusual. Excessive amounts may be due to (1) denaturation of the hemoglobin because of excessive heat or samples that are too old, (2) too large a sample of blood used, or (3) a dirty membrane.

CITRATE AGAR GEL ELECTROPHORESIS

Many abnormal hemoglobins have similar electrophoretic ability on cellulose acetate. To further classify an unusual hemoglobin, agar gel electrophoresis may be employed. In this procedure, a different media (agar) and buffer pH (pH 6.0 to 6.3) are utilized.

It is suggested that the reader be familiar with the previous section, Hemoglobin Electrophoresis, before continuing with the following.

REFERENCES

Helena Laboratories: *Titan III Citrate Hemoglobin Procedure*, Helena Laboratories, Beaumont, Texas, 1973.

Schmidt, R.M., and Brosious, E.M.: *Basic Laboratory Methods of Hemoglobinopathy Detection.* HEW Pub. No. (CDC) 74-8266, U.S. Department of Health, Education, and Welfare, Public Health Service, Center for Disease Control, Atlanta, 1974.

REAGENTS AND EQUIPMENT

1. Stock citrate buffer, 0.5 M.
   Place 147 g of sodium citrate $(C_6H_5O_7Na_3 \cdot 2H_2O)$ in a 1-liter volumetric flask. Add 800 ml of distilled water. Mix until in solution. Adjust the pH to 6.0 with 30% citric acid. Dilute to 1 liter with distilled water. If stored in the refrigerator, this solution should keep for approximately 1 month.

2. Working buffer.
   Just prior to use, dilute 30 ml of the stock buffer to 300 ml with distilled water. The pH of this solution should be 6.0 to 6.3. (Note: Pre-weighed packages of working buffer are available from Helena Laboratories, Beaumont, Texas. Order citrate buffer.)

3. Disposable double wicks.

4. Electrophoresis chamber (Fig. 132). (Note: Items 1 through 4 are obtainable from Helena Laboratories, P.O. Box 752, Beaumont, Texas, 77704.)

5. Bromphenol blue
   Bromphenol blue   0.1 g
   Dilute to 1 liter with distilled water and add 10 ml of glacial acetic acid.

6. Bacto-Agar (purified, Difco) 1% (w/v), in working citrate buffer.

7. Pipets, 0.02 ml, 5.0 ml, and 10 ml.

8. Beaker, 500 ml.

9. Polypropylene centrifuge tubes, 15 ml.

10. Sodium chloride, 0.85% (w/v).

11. Toluene.

12. Cotton-tipped applicators.

13. Disposable dropper pipets.

14. Test tubes, 12 × 75 mm.

15. Cyanmethemoglobin reagent.

16. Glass slides, 2 × 3 inches or 1 × 3 inches.

17. Hot plate or bunsen burner.

18. Parafilm.

19. Disposable blood lancets.

20. DC-regulated power supply.

21. Small shallow pan.

22. Acetic acid, 5% (v/v).

23. Hydrogen peroxide, 3%.

24. Sodium nitroferricyanide, 1% (w/v).

25. Blotting paper. (Obtainable from Schleicher and Schuell, Keene, New

Hampshire. Order grade 470, size 5⅞ × 8⅞, 100 per package.)

26. Plastic bags, one or two, of such size that, when three-fourths filled with ice, they cover the bottom area of the electrophoresis chamber.
27. Ice cubes.
28. Potassium cyanide, 5% (w/v).
29. Vacutainer tubes, 15 ml.

SPECIMEN

Whole blood, using EDTA, heparin, or ammonium-potassium oxalate as the anticoagulant. Capillary blood may also be used. When using whole blood, at least 2.0 ml should be obtained. When utilizing capillary blood, four to six hematocrit tubes three-fourths filled with whole blood should be collected.

PRINCIPLE

A red blood cell hemolysate is prepared to destroy the red blood cell membrane and free the hemoglobin. Toluene is employed in this procedure to remove the red blood cell stroma. A thin, uniform layer of agar is placed on a glass slide and inoculated with a small amount of the hemolysate. The agar slide is then placed face down across the support bridges of the electrophoresing tray. An electric current of specific voltage and milliamps is allowed to run for a specific period of time. At an acid pH, hemoglobin F has a positive charge and, therefore, migrates to the cathode (negative) side, whereas the negatively charged molecules of hemoglobins C and S move toward the anode. The media through which the hemoglobins travel and the difference in the net charge of the hemoglobin in an acid pH determine the mobility of each type of hemoglobin. The agar gel slide is then placed in a stain that colors the hemoglobin. By noting the distance each hemoglobin has migrated and comparing this distance with the migration distance of known controls, the different types of hemoglobins present can be identified. These results must be correlated with the results of the hemoglobin electrophoresis.

PROCEDURE

1. Preparation of the agar.
   A. Place 1 g of Bacto-Agar (purified Difco) in a large beaker.
   B. Add 100 ml of working citrate buffer (pH 6.0–6.3).
   C. Heat on a hot plate only until the agar has dissolved completely. (A magnetic stirrer helps prevent burning.)
   D. Allow to cool to approximately 50°C and add one drop of 5% potassium cyanide. Mix well.
   E. Place 12 to 15 ml of the agar into 15-ml disposable Vacutainer tubes. Replace the stoppers and refrigerate.
   F. Just prior to use, remove a tube of agar from the refrigerator (one tube contains sufficient agar for one run). Place the tube in a beaker of water and boil the water until the agar is completely melted. (Prior to boiling, remove the stopper from the agar and replace it with a gauze plug.)
   G. Allow the tube of agar to remain in the beaker of hot water until it is ready to use.
2. Preparation of the hemolysate.
   A. Place approximately 2 ml of whole blood into an appropriately labeled disposable polypropylene centrifuge tube. Fill the tube with 0.85% sodium chloride. Mix and centrifuge at 2,500 RPM for 10 minutes.
   B. Remove the supernatant sodium chloride and plasma.
   C. Remove all but 0.5 ml of the packed red blood cells from each tube and discard. Add 0.7 ml of distilled water and 0.2 ml of toluene to each tube. Stopper the tubes and shake for 5 minutes.

D. Centrifuge the tubes at 2,500 RPM for 10 minutes.

E. Remove the top layer of toluene from each tube with a cotton-tipped applicator.

F. Using a disposable dropper pipet, remove the hemolysate layer from underneath the red blood cell stroma layer and place in an appropriately labeled centrifuge tube.

G. Centrifuge at 2,500 RPM for 10 minutes.

H. Remove the supernatant hemolysate and place it in an appropriately labeled 12 × 75-mm test tube. Discard the sediment.

I. Perform a hemoglobin determination on the hemolysate, using the cyanmethemoglobin procedure. Dilute the hemolysate with distilled water until the hemoglobin reads approximately 3 g per dl. When the specimen is a cord blood or blood from an infant under 3 months of age, dilute the hemoglobin until it reads approximately 6 g per dl.

J. If the agar gel is not going to be run at this time, stopper the tube and place it in the freezer.

3. Preparation of the hemolysate from hematocrit tubes.

A. Centrifuge four microhematocrit tubes. Using a file, remove the plasma, buffy coat, and sealed end. Separate the red blood cell layer into smaller sections and place it in an appropriately labeled 12 × 75-mm test tube. Add six drops of hemolysate reagent and mix vigorously. Allow 15 to 30 minutes for complete hemolysis of the red blood cells or freeze and thaw the hemolysate until complete hemolysis is achieved.

B. Add two to three drops of toluene. Stopper and mix for 3 to 5 minutes.

C. Centrifuge at 2,500 RPM for 10 to 15 minutes.

D. Using a disposable dropper, carefully place the tip of the pipet in the very bottom of the test tube (underneath the toluene and red blood cell stroma layers). Remove as much of the hemolysate as possible (without contamination from the red blood cell stroma and toluene). Remove the pipet from the test tube and wipe the outside of the pipet tip with a piece of gauze. Place the hemolysate in a second, appropriately labeled 12 × 75-mm test tube.

E. Centrifuge the hemolysate for 10 minutes at 2,500 RPM.

F. Carefully remove the supernatant hemolysate with a disposable dropper pipet and place in an appropriately labeled 12 × 75-mm test tube. (The hemolysate should be crystal clear.)

G. Adjust the hemoglobin to read approximately 6 g per dl (if the patient is younger than 3 months) or 3 g per dl (if the patient is older than 3 months).

H. Stopper the tube. Place it in the freezer if the agar gel test is not to be performed that day.

4. Remove a tube of agar from the refrigerator. Replace the stopper with a gauze plug. Place the tube in a beaker of water and boil until the agar is completely dissolved. (Allow the tube of agar to remain in the beaker of hot water until it is ready to use.)

5. While the agar is being heated, fill two plastic bags with ice. Seal the bags and place them underneath the electrophoresis tray, ensuring that the tray remains level.

6. Remove the hemolysates from the freezer and allow them to thaw.

7. Fill the electrophoresis tray with citrate buffer, pH 6.0 to 6.3. Place 100 ml of buffer into each of the outer

compartments and 50 ml of buffer in each of the center compartments. Wet two disposable wicks in the chamber buffer and drape over each support bridge, ensuring that one side of the wick touches the bottom of the outer compartment and that the other side touches the bottom of the inner compartment.

8. Cut a piece of Parafilm and label for the hemolysates. Place one drop of each hemolysate behind the labeled area on the Parafilm.

9. Label as many 2 × 3 inch slides as needed on the back left corner with a magic marker.

10. With a pipet, place 3 ml of the hot melted agar on each 2 × 3 inch slide to be used. Place the agar on the slide quickly to ensure a uniform film of agar.

11. As soon as the agar hardens (approximately 2 to 5 minutes), inoculate with the hemolysate, using a disposable blood lancet. The inoculation should be in the center of the slide or slightly to the right of center (long side of the slide horizontal). The top inoculation on each slide should be the control. Six or seven samples may be inoculated on each slide (Fig. 135).

12. Immediately after the slide has been inoculated, turn the slide upside down so that the agar is now face down, and the inoculation is slightly left of center. (The number of the slide should be at the positive pole.)

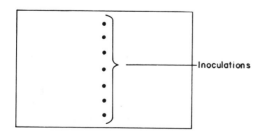

Fig. 135. Inoculated agar gel slide.

Place the slide in the chamber gently, being careful not to cut or tear the agar.

13. When all the slides have been inoculated and placed in the electrophoresis tray, carefully place the cover on top of the chamber.

14. Attach the electrode terminal pins to the power supply. Turn the power supply on and adjust the voltage so that there are 10 milliamps per slide. The voltage will be approximately 60 to 90 V. Electrophorese for 2 hours and 30 minutes. Periodically during this time, recheck the milliamps, adjusting the voltage so that the proper milliamp reading is maintained.

15. Before electrophoresing is complete, place the stain (75 to 100 ml) in a flat shallow pan.

16. Place two or three applicator sticks in the bottom of the stain pan.

17. At the end of the electrophoresing period, remove the chamber cover. Carefully remove the slides, turn them agar side up, and place them in the stain pan on top of the applicator sticks. Tilt the stain tray as needed to allow the stain to cover the agar. Keep the slides in the stain until all hemoglobin components are stained (about 20 minutes).

18. Place the slides in distilled water to rinse or carefully rinse them under running distilled water.

19. Remove the slides from the water and place the slides, agar side down, on blotter paper until the moisture is absorbed (5 to 10 minutes). (Slides may be carefully moved to a dry blotter to hasten drying.)

20. When a majority of the moisture has been removed, allow the slides to air-dry and read.

21. Identify the hemoglobin types present in the patient samples by comparing the migration distance with the known controls. See Figure 136 for the mobilities of various hemo-

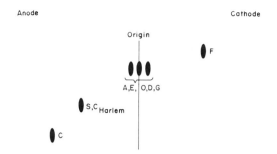

Fig. 136. Electrophoretic mobility of various hemoglobins on agar gel at pH 6.0 to 6.3.

globins. The interpretation of agar gel results must be correlated with the hemoglobin types found on the hemoglobin electrophoresis by cellulose acetate method.

DISCUSSION

1. The regular 1 × 3-inch slide may be used in place of the larger ones. In this case, only 1.5 ml of agar is placed on the slide and during electrophoresis the voltage should be adjusted to 5 milliamps per slide.
2. Once the agar has cooled and hardened on the slide, it should be inoculated as quickly as possible. There is only a thin film of agar on the slide and it will dry out quickly.
3. With agar gel, it is possible to detect very small amounts of a hemoglobin. This procedure is helpful, therefore, in diagnosing the hemoglobin types present in the newborn. At birth the major portion of hemoglobin is F. If the baby has inherited hemoglobins A and S from the parents, extremely small quantities of these two hemoglobins will be present at birth. Because of the low concentration, it is often impossible to detect their presence on cellulose acetate, but they can be seen on agar gel.
4. When the agar gel slide is stained, hemoglobin F has a round shape, whereas hemoglobins C and S are bullet-shaped.
5. The size of the inoculation and the hemoglobin concentration of the hemolysate are important factors in agar gel. Heavy inoculations appear to migrate faster than light inoculations. When first setting this test up in a laboratory, a moderate amount of practice is needed to master the sample inoculation. Of critical importance is the inoculation of specimens from a newborn. The hemoglobin concentration and size of the inoculation must be high enough so that very small quantities of a hemoglobin will be detected.
6. As seen in Figure 136, hemoglobins A, E, O, D, and G remain at the site of inoculation or migrate slightly to the right or left of the origin.
7. Agar gel results should be correlated with the hemoglobin electrophoresis results and should not supplant cellulose acetate hemoglobin electrophoresis. Agar gel electrophoresis should be performed when it is desirable to know the hemoglobin types of a newborn and to verify abnormal hemoglobin types. For example, a hemoglobin that migrates on cellulose acetate as hemoglobin C may in reality be hemoglobin E, O, or C_{Harlem}.

ACID ELUTION TEST

The acid elution test is employed to detect hemoglobin F present in the red blood cells. Approximately 80% of the total hemoglobin at birth is hemoglobin F. By the age of 4 months, there is approximately 10% hemoglobin F present, and at the end of infancy only trace amounts remain. Normal adult blood will contain less than 0.4%. Increased amounts of hemoglobin F are found in hereditary persistence of fetal hemoglobin, sickle cell anemia, acquired aplastic anemia, thalassemia, and other hemoglobinopathies.

Kleihauer and Betke Method
(Modified by Shepard,
Weatherall, and Conley)

REFERENCE

Shepard, M.K., Weatherall, D.J., and Conley, C.L.: Semiquantitative estimation of the distribution of fetal hemoglobin in red cell populations, Bull. J. Hopkins Hosp., *110*, 293, 1962.

REAGENTS AND EQUIPMENT

1. Ethyl alcohol, 80% (v/v).
2. Citric acid-phosphate buffer, pH 3.2 to 3.3.

    Dibasic sodium phosphate, 0.2 M

Dibasic sodium phosphate (Na_2HPO_4)	14.2 g

    Dilute to 500 ml with distilled water.

    Citric acid, 0.1 M

Citric acid ($C_6H_8O_7 \cdot H_2O$)	10.5 g

    Dilute to 500 ml with distilled water.

    Prior to use, prepare the citric acid-phosphate buffers as indicated below:

Dibasic sodium phosphate, 0.2 M	13.3 ml
Citric acid, 0.1 M	36.7 ml

    A pH of 3.2 to 3.3 is critical and must be checked on a pH meter prior to use. Store the stock solutions of dibasic sodium phosphate and citric acid in the refrigerator.

3. Erythrosin B, 0.1% (w/v), aqueous solution. Eosin yellowish, 1.25% (w/v), may be used as an alternative (0.5 g of eosin yellowish in 120 ml of absolute alcohol and 280 ml of distilled water). Add two to three drops of glacial acetic acid.
4. Mayer's hematoxylin.
5. Coplin jar.
6. Parafilm.

SPECIMEN

Obtain four blood smears from the fingertip (or earlobe, toe, or heel), or make blood smears from venous blood collected in EDTA anticoagulant. Obtain a similar blood specimen for a normal control at the same time the patient's blood is obtained.

PRINCIPLE

Blood smears are fixed with ethyl alcohol. A citric acid-phosphate buffer solution elutes (removes) hemoglobin other than hemoglobin F from the red blood cells. The fetal hemoglobin that remains may then be seen when it is stained with the appropriate blood stains.

PROCEDURE

1. Pour citric acid-phosphate buffer solution into a coplin jar and cover with Parafilm. Incubate at 37°C for 30 minutes.
2. Make four thin blood smears each of the patient and the normal control.
3. Allow the blood smears to air-dry for 10 to 60 minutes.
4. Fix the blood smears for 5 minutes in 80% ethyl alcohol.
5. Rinse the smears thoroughly with distilled water and allow to air-dry.
6. After the smears are completely dry, place the slides (both control and patient) in the prewarmed citric acid-phosphate buffer solution for 5 minutes. At the end of 1 minute, remove the slides from the coplin jar and replace immediately. Repeat again at 3 minutes. This provides gentle agitation of the blood smears.
7. After 5 minutes, remove the slides from the citric acid-phosphate buffer solution and rinse with distilled water. Air-dry.
8. After the smears are completely dry, stain with Mayer's hematoxylin for 3 minutes. Rinse with distilled water.
9. Counterstain the smears with erythrosin B for 4 minutes. Rinse with distilled water and allow to air-dry.
10. Examine the slides microscopically, using the oil immersion objective (100×), for the presence of hemoglo-

bin F. Those red blood cells containing hemoglobin F are deeply stained, depending on the concentration of hemoglobin F in the cell. Normal red blood cells (those not containing hemoglobin F) appear as scarcely visible ghost cells.

DISCUSSION

1. Reticulocytes may resist elution and would, therefore, give the appearance of cells containing hemoglobin F.
2. In hereditary persistence of fetal hemoglobin, the amount of hemoglobin F in each cell is constant and, therefore, all of the red blood cells are consistently stained.
3. In diseases such as sickle cell anemia, thalassemia, acquired aplastic anemia, and several other hemoglobinopathies, the amount of hemoglobin F present in the red blood cells varies. This shows up as an inconsistent staining of the red blood cells. Those cells containing small amounts of hemoglobin F will stain more lightly than cells having a higher concentration of hemoglobin F. (This indicates that a single red blood cell is capable of synthesizing more than one type of hemoglobin.)
4. Ethyl alcohol in concentrations of less than 80% do not give satisfactory results.
5. The pH of the citric acid-phosphate buffer is critical and must be within a pH range of 3.2 to 3.3.
6. After 10 minutes of incubation in the citric acid-phosphate buffer, there is some loss of hemoglobin F.
7. As soon as the blood smears have been made, the test must proceed as outlined.
8. The blood for the acid elution test may be stored in EDTA at refrigerator temperatures for no longer than 2 weeks before the smears are made.

ALKALI DENATURATION TEST

The alkali denaturation test measures the amount of fetal hemoglobin present in the blood. Normally, a result of less than 2% for this method is normal. Values between 0.8 and 2.0% are borderline, and results above 2.0% are considered abnormal. Increased amounts of fetal hemoglobin are found in newborns and in early infancy. Hemoglobin F is also increased in hereditary persistence of fetal hemoglobin, sickle cell anemia, acquired aplastic anemia, and in other hemoglobinopathies.

Singer, Chernoff, and Singer Method
(Modified by Betke, Marti, and Schlict)

REFERENCES

Betke, K., Marti, H.R., and Schlict, I.: Estimation of small percentages of foetal haemoglobin, Nature, *184*, 1877, 1959.

Singer, K., Chernoff, A.I., and Singer, L.: Studies on abnormal hemoglobin. 1. Their demonstration in sickle cell anemia and other hematologic disorders by means of alkali denaturation, Blood, *6*, 413, 1951.

REAGENTS AND EQUIPMENT

1. Cyanmethemoglobin reagent. (See the section entitled Cyanmethemoglobin Method [Reagents and Equipment] in Chapter 2.)
2. Saturated ammonium sulfate.
3. Sodium hydroxide, 1.2 N.
   Sodium hydroxide   48 g
   Dissolve the sodium hydroxide and dilute it to 1,000 ml with distilled water.
4. Sodium chloride, 0.85% (w/v).
5. Chloroform.
6. Whatman #42 filter paper.
7. Triton X-100 wetting agent or saponin.
8. Glycerin, USP.
9. Graduated centrifuge tube, 15 ml.
10. Normal hemolysate control.
11. Fetal hemolysate control.

12. Test tubes, 13 × 125 mm.
13. Water bath, 20°C.

SPECIMEN

Whole blood, using EDTA as the anticoagulant.

PRINCIPLE

A red blood cell hemolysate is prepared to lyse the red blood cells completely. This test utilizes the characteristic of fetal hemoglobin to resist denaturation in an alkaline solution. The hemolysate is added to the cyanmethemoglobin reagent and then exposed to an alkaline reagent, sodium hydroxide, for a specified period. During this time, normal hemoglobin is denatured or destroyed, but the fetal hemoglobin is intact. Ammonium sulfate is added to halt the denaturation process and to precipitate the denatured hemoglobin. The solution is filtered, measured spectrophotometrically, and compared with the spectrophotometric readings of the original cyanmethemoglobin solution.

PROCEDURE

1. Preparation of the red blood cell hemolysate.
   A. Transfer 3 to 5 ml of the patient's whole blood to a graduated centrifuge tube.
   B. Add approximately 6 to 7 ml of 0.85% sodium chloride to the preceding tube. Centrifuge at 2,500 RPM for 5 to 10 minutes. Remove the supernatant.
   C. Wash the red blood cells two more times by repeating step 1B.
   D. Note the volume of packed red blood cells. Add one to two drops of Triton-X or 1 mg of saponin. Mix and allow to sit for 15 minutes. Add an amount of chloroform estimated to be about one-half of the volume of the packed red blood cells.
   E. Stopper the tube and shake for 5 minutes. If hemolysis is not com-
   plete, the mixture should be frozen and rapidly thawed.
   F. Centrifuge the mixture at 2,500 RPM for 20 minutes.
   G. Carefully remove the hemolysate and place it in a test tube.
   H. Add an equal volume of glycerin to the hemolysate.
   I. Determine the hemoglobin content of the hemolysate by the cyanmethemoglobin method. Adjust the hemoglobin concentration to about 10 g per dl by the addition of distilled water. The hemolysate is now ready. It may be stored in the freezer at 0°C.

2. Pipet 0.5 ml of the patient's hemolysate, the normal control hemolysate, and the fetal control hemolysate into respective tubes containing 9.5 ml of cyanmethemoglobin reagent. This gives a cyanmethemoglobin solution of 0.5 g per dl.

3. Mix and transfer 2.8 ml of each of the preceding cyanmethemoglobin solutions into each of two test tubes. (Each test is performed in duplicate.) Place the test tubes in a 20°C water bath.

4. Add 0.2 ml of 1.2 N sodium hydroxide to each test tube and rapidly mix. Allow to incubate for exactly 2 minutes.

5. At the end of 2 minutes, add 2 ml of saturated ammonium sulfate to all test tubes and allow to stand for 5 to 10 minutes to coagulate the protein.

6. Filter each of the preceding solutions through Whatman #42 filter paper. If the filtrate is not absolutely clear, refilter the solution using the same filter paper.

7. Prepare the total hemoglobin specimen for the patient, normal control, and fetal control: add 0.4 ml of each of the original 0.5 g per dl solutions of cyanmethemoglobin, prepared in step 2, to 6.75 ml of distilled water.

8. Transfer the filtrate and total hemo-

globin solutions to cuvettes and read in a spectrophotometer at a wavelength of 540 nm (or with a yellow-green filter), using cyanmethemoglobin reagent to set the machine at 0 optical density. Record the optical density of all specimens. The optical density readings should fall within a range of 0.05 to 0.50 for maximum sensitivity. If the filtrate is too concentrated, dilute it, using distilled water.

9. Calculate the results as follows:

$$\text{Percent of alkali-resistant hemoglobin} = \frac{\text{Optical density of alkali-resistant hemoglobin}}{\text{Optical density of the total hemoglobin}} \times 10$$

The optical density of the total hemoglobin is multiplied by 10 because this solution is 10 times more dilute than the alkali-resistant solution.

DISCUSSION

1. It is unnecessary to prepare the hemolysate with an exact concentration of 10 g per dl. A concentration in the range of 9 to 11 g per dl does not alter the final results.
2. A temperature variation from 19 to 20°C does not appreciably alter the results of this test.

SERUM HAPTOGLOBIN TEST

The major breakdown, or hemolysis, of red blood cells takes place in the reticuloendothelial system. Approximately 10% of red blood cell destruction, however, occurs intravascularly. In this circumstance, free hemoglobin is released directly into the blood and undergoes dissociation into α, β dimers, which are then bound to a serum globulin called *haptoglobin*. The binding of the hemoglobin to the haptoglobin prevents renal excretion of the pigment. This complex is then removed from the plasma by the reticuloendothelial system. In normal plasma, the haptoglobin is present in amounts sufficient to bind 30 to 200 mg of hemoglobin per dl of plasma. Haptoglobin decreases and begins to disappear when hemolysis is increased to two times the normal. Increased amounts of haptoglobin are found in infections, malignancy, Hodgkin's disease, rheumatoid arthritis, and systemic lupus erythematosus.

REFERENCES

Colfs, B., and Verkeyden, J.: A rapid method for the determination of serum haptoglobin, Clin. Chem. Acta, *12*, 470, 1965.

Dacie, J.V., and Lewis, S.M.: *Practical Hematology*, 5th ed., Churchill Livingstone, New York, 1975.

Lathem, W., and Worley, W.E.: The distribution of extracorpuscular hemoglobin in circulating plasma, J. Clin. Invest., *38*, 474, 1959.

REAGENTS AND EQUIPMENT

1. Phosphate buffer, pH 7.0.
   Solution 1
   Dibasic sodium phosphate (Na_2HPO_4)   7.10 g
   Dilute to 1,000 ml with distilled water.
   Solution 2
   Monobasic sodium phosphate ($NaH_2PO_4 \cdot H_2O$)   3.45 g
   Dilute to 500 ml with distilled water.
   For a phosphate buffer, pH 7.0, mix:
   Solution 1   1,000 ml
   Solution 2   500 ml
   Refrigerate this solution.
2. O-dianisidine reagent. Prepare just prior to use.
   O-dianisidine   100 mg
   Ethanol   70 ml
3. Acetate buffer, pH 4.7. Prepare just prior to use.
   Sodium acetate   11.2 g
   Acetic acid, 96% (v/v)   4 ml
   Dilute to 100 ml with distilled water.

4. Hydrogen peroxide.
5. Staining reagent. Prepare 10 minutes before use.

O-dianisidine reagent	70 ml
Acetate buffer	10 ml
Distilled water	18 ml
Hydrogen peroxide	2 ml

6. Tweezers, one pair.
7. Equipment, which may also be used for electrophoresis by cellulose acetate.
   A. Microzone cell, model No. R-101, obtainable from Beckman Instruments, Palo Alto, California.
   B. Cellulose acetate membranes, obtainable from Beckman Instruments, Palo Alto, California.
   C. Sample applicator, part No. 324399, obtainable from Beckman Instruments. Palo Alto, California.
   D. DC-regulated power supply.
   E. Drying oven, capable of reaching 100 to 110°C temperatures.
   F. Glass drying plates (same size as the cellulose acetate membranes).
8. Rinsing solution, acetic acid, 5% (v/v).
9. Dehydrating solution. Ethanol or methanol may be used, whichever yields better results.
10. Clearing solution.

Methanol	87 ml
Glacial acetic acid	13 ml

Ethanol may be used in place of methanol. It may be necessary to vary the amounts of glacial acetic acid and methanol (ethanol) depending on the membranes used.
11. Triton-X wetting agent.
12. Sodium chloride, 0.85% (w/v).
13. Chloroform.
14. Glycerin.
15. Graduated centrifuge tubes, 15 ml.
16. Applicator sticks.
17. Parafilm.
18. Hemoglobin solutions of 0.25, 0.50, 1.0, and 2.0 g per dl.
    A. Preparation of the hemolysate.

1) Place 3 or 4 ml of normal, whole anticoagulated (EDTA) blood in a 15-ml graduated centrifuge tube.
2) Centrifuge the blood at 2,500 RPM for 5 minutes. Remove the plasma and discard.
3) Fill the tube to the 15-ml mark with 0.85% sodium chloride. Mix well.
4) Centrifuge at 2,500 RPM for 5 minutes. Remove the supernatant sodium chloride.
5) Wash the red blood cells two more times.
6) Note the volume of the packed red blood cells.
7) Add one drop of Triton-X wetting agent. Mix the tube and allow to stand approximately 15 minutes to ensure complete hemolysis of red blood cells.
8) Add a volume of chloroform equal to one-half the volume of the red blood cells. Stopper and shake the tube vigorously for 1 minute.
9) Centrifuge for 5 minutes at 2,500 RPM.
10) Carefully remove the upper layer of the hemolysate.
11) Add an equal volume of glycerin to the hemolysate. This should yield a hemoglobin concentration of approximately 10 g per dl. This hemolysate may be stoppered and placed in the freezer until ready for use.
B. Using the cyanmethemoglobin method, determine the exact hemoglobin concentration of the hemolysate. Using distilled water, adjust the hemoglobin concentration to 10 g per dl.
C. Prepare the following dilutions as indicated:
   1) Hemoglobin solution of 2.0 g per dl

Hemolysate   2.0 ml
  (10 g per dl)
Distilled water   8.0 ml

2) Hemoglobin solution of 1.0 g per dl

Hemoglobin   2.0 ml
  solution of 2.0 g per dl
Distilled water   2.0 ml

3) Hemoglobin solution of 0.5 g per dl

Hemoglobin   2.0 ml
  solution of 1.0 g per dl
Distilled water   2.0 ml

4) Hemoglobin solution of 0.25 g per dl

Hemoglobin   2.0 ml
  solution of 0.5 g per dl
Distilled water   2.0 ml

SPECIMEN

Clotted blood, 6 ml. Collect a blood specimen from a normal control at the same time the patient's blood is obtained.

PRINCIPLE

The patient and control serums are incubated with varying concentrations of hemoglobin solutions. During this time, the haptoglobin present in the serum binds the hemoglobin, depending on the amount of haptoglobin available. An electrophoretic pattern of the serum-hemoglobin samples is then obtained and stained, and the cellulose acetate strips are examined. The approximate amount of haptoglobin present in the serum can be ascertained by noting at what hemoglobin concentration a second band of free hemoglobin appears.

PROCEDURE

1. Collect 5 to 6 ml of whole blood from both the patient and the normal control. Place the blood into test tubes and incubate at 37°C for 2 hours.
2. At the end of 2 hours, remove the clot from both tubes, using applicator sticks.
3. Centrifuge the serum at 2,500 RPM

for 10 minutes. Remove the supernatant serum and place in clean test tubes. If the test will not be performed at this time, freeze the serum. (If either of the samples is hemolyzed, the blood must be re-collected.)

4. Number eight test tubes, No. 1 through No. 8, and set up the following serum hemolysate dilutions.
   A. 0.2 ml of normal control serum and 0.02 ml of hemoglobin solution of 0.25 g per dl (tube No. 1).
   B. 0.2 ml of normal control serum and 0.02 ml of hemoglobin solution of 0.5 g per dl (tube No. 2).
   C. 0.2 ml of normal control serum and 0.02 ml of hemoglobin solution of 1.0 g per dl (tube No. 3).
   D. 0.2 ml of normal control serum and 0.02 ml of hemoglobin solution of 2.0 g per dl (tube No. 4).
   E. Same as tube No. 1, using the patient's serum in place of the normal control serum (tube No. 5).
   F. Same as tube No. 2, using the patient's serum in place of the normal control serum (tube No. 6).
   G. Same as tube No. 3, using the patient's serum in place of the normal control serum (tube No. 7).
   H. Same as tube No. 4, using the patient's serum in place of the normal control serum (tube No. 8).
5. Incubate the preceding eight tubes at 37°C for 30 minutes.
6. Fill both sides of the microzone cell with phosphate buffer.
7. Fill a small tray (of a size to accommodate one cellulose-acetate membrane) with approximately 40 ml of buffer solution.
8. Using tweezers, place a cellulose-acetate membrane in the tray of buffer. The membrane should be allowed to float on the surface of the buffer to allow capillary action to draw the buffer up evenly through the membrane. As soon as the entire

membrane has become wet, immerse it completely in the buffer by carefully agitating the tray. Immediately remove the membrane from the buffer using the tweezers. Carefully blot the membrane between two pieces of filter paper or blotters by passing a hand lightly over the top blotter one time.

9. Immediately suspend and mount the wet membrane on the bridge, ensuring that the membrane lies evenly and that each end hangs freely in the opposite chambers containing the buffer.

10. Replace the upper lid of the microzone cell to guard against drying of the membrane.

11. Attach the connecting cables of the power supply to the electrode terminal pins. Do not turn on the power supply yet.

12. Allow the membrane to equilibrate for about 2 minutes before applying the blood samples. (The serum-hemolysates are inoculated on the cathode side.)

13. Place a small drop of each of the eight serum-hemolysate dilutions on a strip of Parafilm.

14. Using the applicator, depress the white button on the top to extend the applicator tip. Without breaking the surface tension of the serum-hemolysate drop, carefully and slowly move the applicator tip across the top surface. In this way, a 0.25-μl sample is picked up by the applicator tip. Retract the applicator tip by carefully depressing the red button.

15. Remove the lid of the microzone cell and place the applicator in the appropriate grooves. Remove your hand from the applicator. Touch the white button carefully. Allow the applicator tip to remain in contact with the membrane for 10 to 15 seconds. Press the red button carefully, causing the applicator tip to retract. Re-

move the applicator and replace the lid on the microzone cell.

16. Repeat steps 14 and 15 two more times, using the same serum-hemolysate dilution, and inoculating the cellulose-acetate membrane in the same place. This gives a 0.75-μl sample.

17. Rinse the applicator tip with a thin stream of distilled water and blot dry.

18. Repeat steps 14 through 17, applying each serum-hemolysate sample in one of the eight positions on the cellulose-acetate membrane.

19. As soon as all samples have been applied to the membrane, turn on the power supply to 150 V for 40 minutes.

20. At the end of 40 minutes, turn off the power supply and remove the plugs from the electrode terminal pins.

21. Carefully remove the membrane from the bridge without allowing any buffer to splash or run over the membrane.

22. Immediately immerse the membrane in a pan containing the freshly prepared stain for 5 minutes.

23. Remove the membrane from the stain and wash in a series of three pans of distilled water for approximately 5 minutes.

24. Place the membrane in a pan containing 5% acetic acid for approximately 10 minutes.

25. Allow the excess acetic acid to drain from the membrane and place it in methanol for 1 minute.

26. Drain the excess methanol from the membrane and place it in the clearing solution for exactly 1 minute. While the membrane is immersed in the clearing solution, place the glass drying plate directly over the membrane. As soon as 1 minute has elapsed, hold the membrane and glass together at one end. Lift this end from the clearing solution first, allowing the membrane to become

positioned on the glass plate. Make certain the membrane lies flat on the glass plate and contains no air bubbles.

27. Place the glass plate holding the membrane in the drying oven at 100 to 110°C for 10 to 15 minutes.

28. Carefully remove the glass plate and membrane from the oven and allow it to cool. The membrane should be completely transparent when removed from the oven.

29. When the glass plate has cooled sufficiently, loosen one corner of the membrane and carefully peel it from the glass, taking care that it does not tear.

30. The membrane may then be placed in a storage envelope (in between two pieces of plastic) to preserve it and avoid curling at the edges.

31. Interpretation: the free hemoglobin and hemoglobin bound to haptoglobin migrate as shown in Figure 137. The serum-hemolysate dilution containing the greatest amount of hemoglobin determines the amount of haptoglobin present in the serum. For example, if the serum-hemolysate mixture from tube No. 8 does show a free hemoglobin band, 100 to 200 mg per dl of haptoglobin is reported present in the serum.

DISCUSSION

If the freshly incubated serum sample is allowed to stand, methemalbumin is formed. In this situation, the methemalbumin will be present on the membrane as a band located on the right of the hemoglobin-haptoglobin band.

SUGAR-WATER TEST

The sugar-water test is a simple diagnostic procedure for paroxysmal nocturnal hemoglobinuria.

REFERENCE

Hartmann, R.C., and Jenkins, D.E.: The "sugar-water" test for paroxysmal nocturnal hemoglobinuria, New Eng. J. Med., 275, 155, 1966.

REAGENTS AND EQUIPMENT

Sugar-water solution: approximate pH of 7.4.

Sucrose (commercial granulated sugar)	9–10 g
Distilled water	100 ml

SPECIMEN

Whole oxalated blood: one part 0.1 M sodium oxalate to nine parts whole blood or one part sodium citrate to nine parts whole blood. One to 2 ml of defibrinated whole blood may also be used. Obtain a specimen of blood for the normal control at the same time the patient's blood is collected.

PRINCIPLE

Whole blood is mixed with a sugar-water solution and incubated at 37°C. The red blood cells from patients with paroxysmal nocturnal hemoglobinuria show hemolysis under these circumstances,

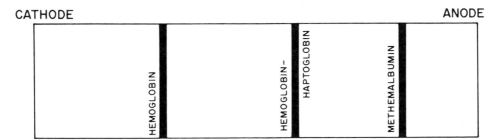

CATHODE   ANODE

HEMOGLOBIN   HEMOGLOBIN-HAPTOGLOBIN   METHEMALBUMIN

Fig. 137. Electrophoretic migration of free hemoglobin, hemoglobin-haptoglobin, and methemalbumin.

whereas blood from a normal person shows no hemolysis. The exact cause of the red blood cell breakdown is not known but may be related to an increased sensitivity of the paroxysmal nocturnal hemoglobinuria red blood cells to complement damage. The presence of hemolysis in this test, therefore, indicates a positive result for paroxysmal nocturnal hemoglobinuria.

PROCEDURE

1. Pipet 4.5 ml of sugar-water solution into each of two 13 × 100-mm test tubes, labeled patient and control.
2. Add 0.5 ml of well-mixed control and patient's whole blood to the respective test tubes.
3. Invert each test tube gently to mix.
4. Place both tubes in the 37°C water bath for 30 minutes.
5. At the end of 30 minutes, centrifuge the test tubes at 2,500 RPM for 5 minutes.
6. Observe the supernatants for the presence of hemolysis.
7. Hemolysis indicates a positive test for paroxysmal nocturnal hemoglobinuria.

DISCUSSION

1. It is not necessary to incubate the test tubes at 37°C. Allowing the test tubes to sit at room temperature for 30 minutes will yield valid results.
2. Prior to performing the test, it may be desirable to centrifuge a small portion of the patient and control bloods to ensure that no hemolysis is present in the plasma as a result of poor venipuncture techniques.

ACID-SERUM TEST

Paroxysmal nocturnal hemoglobinuria may also be reliably diagnosed by means of the acid-serum test.

Ham Method

REFERENCES

Cartwright, G.E.: *Diagnostic Laboratory Hematology*, Grune & Stratton, Inc., New York, 1963.

Dacie, J.V., and Lewis, S.M.: *Practical Hematology*, 5th ed., Churchill Livingstone, New York, 1975.

Ham, T.H.: Studies on destruction of red blood cells, Arch. Intern. Med., 64, 1271, 1939.

REAGENTS AND EQUIPMENT

1. Glass beads, 3 to 4 mm in diameter.
2. Sodium chloride, 0.85% (w/v).
3. Sterile test tubes.
4. Hydrochloric acid, 0.2 N.
5. Water bath, 37°C.
6. Water bath, 56°C.
7. Sterile flask.
8. Ammonium hydroxide, 0.04% (v/v).
9. Erlenmeyer flask, 125 ml.

SPECIMEN

Whole blood, 10 ml, to be defibrinated. Collect blood to use as a normal control and process in the same way as for the patient's blood. (The control blood must be of the same blood type as the patient's blood.)

PRINCIPLE

It is believed that complement present in serum is responsible for lysis of the red blood cells in patients with paroxysmal nocturnal hemoglobinuria due to a defect in the red blood cells. In this procedure, the patient's red blood cells are mixed with normal serum and also with the patient's own serum, acidified, incubated at 37°C, and examined for hemolysis. The serum in one test tube is inactivated to destroy the complement. Weak acid is added to each test tube to adjust the pH of the mixture so that the hemolytic activity will be at a maximum. Normally, there should be no lysis of the red blood cells in this test.

PROCEDURE

1. Defibrinate the patient and control blood in the following manner:
   A. Place 10 ml of whole blood in an Erlenmeyer flask containing 10 glass beads.
   B. Gently rotate the flask until the hum or noise of the beads on the glass can no longer be heard (about 10 minutes).
2. Decant the blood into a graduated centrifuge tube and centrifuge at 2,500 RPM for 5 minutes.
3. Remove the serum and save.
4. Add at least an equal volume of 0.85% sodium chloride to the red blood cells. Mix and centrifuge at 2,500 RPM for 5 minutes. Remove the sodium chloride.
5. Wash the red blood cells two more times by repeating step 4. After the last wash, note the volume of the packed red blood cells.
6. Add an equal volume of 0.85% sodium chloride to the packed red blood cells. Mix. This gives a 50% suspension of red blood cells.
7. Place seven sterile test tubes in the 37°C water bath and number accordingly.
8. Pipet 0.5 ml of patient's serum into tubes Nos. 1, 2, 6, and 7.
9. Pipet 0.5 ml of normal serum into test tubes Nos. 3, 4, and 5.
10. Place test tube No. 3 in a 56°C water bath for 30 minutes. This inactivates the serum, destroying the complement. At the end of 30 minutes, return the test tube to the 37°C water bath.
11. Pipet 0.05 ml of 0.2 N hydrochloric acid into test tubes Nos. 2, 3, 5, and 7.
12. Add 0.05 ml of the 50% suspension of patient's red blood cells to test tubes Nos. 1, 2, 3, 4, and 5.
13. Add 0.05 ml of the 50% suspension of normal red blood cells to test tubes Nos. 6 and 7.
14. Incubate all test tubes at 37°C for 1 hour.
15. At the end of 1 hour, centrifuge the preceding seven test tubes at 1,000 RPM for 2 minutes.
16. Examine the supernatant for hemolysis.
17. The presence of hemolysis in test tubes Nos. 2 and 5 only indicates paroxysmal nocturnal hemoglobinuria. See Table 9.
18. The percent hemolysis present in each tube may be quantitated as follows:
    A. Add 0.05 ml of the cell suspension to 0.55 ml of 0.85% sodium chloride. This mixture represents 100% hemolysis.
    B. Add 5 ml of 0.04% ammonium hydroxide to nine test tubes and label accordingly.
    C. To test tubes No. 1 though No. 7 add 0.3 ml of the supernatants to the respectively numbered test tubes containing ammonium hydroxide.
    D. To test tube No. 8, add 0.3 ml of the cell suspension representing 100% hemolysis. (The mixture prepared in step 18A.)
    E. To tube No. 9, add 0.3 ml of the original preincubated serum. This represents 0% hemolysis.
    F. Read the above solutions in a spectrophotometer at a wavelength of 550 nm, using tube No. 9 to set the instrument at 0 optical density.
    G. Calculate the percent hemolysis as shown:

$$\text{Percent hemolysis} = \frac{\text{Optical density of test}}{\text{Optical density of test tube representing 100\% hemolysis}} \times 100$$

    H. A positive test usually shows 10 to 50% hemolysis in the "test" tubes. Ranges of from 5 to 80%,

TABLE 9.   ACID-SERUM TEST RESULTS INDICATING PAROXYSMAL NOCTURNAL HEMOGLOBINURIA

TUBE	0.05 ml OF RED BLOOD CELLS	0.5 ml OF SERUM	ml of 0.2 N HYDROCHLORIC ACID	HEMOLYSIS
1	P	P	0.00	0
2	P	P	0.05	+
3	P	N (heated)	0.05	0
4	P	N	0.00	0
5	P	N	0.05	+
6	N	P	0.00	0
7	N	P	0.05	0

P = Patient's serum or cells. N = Control serum or cells.

however, may be considered positive.

DISCUSSION

1. Test tube No. 1 serves as a control for tube No. 2, tube No. 4 is a control for tube No. 5, and tube No. 6 is the control for tube No. 7.
2. Hemolysis present in test tubes 1, 2, 6, and 7, but absent in test tube 5, indicates the presence of a warm hemolysin.
3. There may be a trace of hemolysis in test tubes 1, 3, and 4 when the test is positive for paroxysmal nocturnal hemoglobinuria.
4. Hemolysis in test tubes 2, 3, and 5 may indicate the presence of markedly spherocytic red blood cells. This can be differentiated from paroxysmal nocturnal hemoglobinuria because lysis of the spherocytes is unaffected by heating the serum.
5. Inactivating the serum in test tube No. 3 at 56°C destroys the hemolytic system. Therefore, lysis present in this test tube rules out the possibility of a positive test for paroxysmal nocturnal hemoglobinuria.
6. When the patient has received blood transfusions, less lysis occurs because of the presence of normal red blood cells from the transfusion.

SERUM VISCOSITY TEST

Viscosity is the property of a fluid that resists the force causing it to flow. In a protein solution, the viscosity depends on the concentration of the protein. The relative viscosity of serum is determined by comparing it with the viscosity of distilled water and is normally in the range of 1.4 to 1.8. In certain pathologic states associated with qualitative and/or quantitative protein disorders, the serum viscosity is increased. This increase is found most often in Waldenström's macroglobulinemia, less often in multiple myeloma, and rarely in other disorders. The severity of the clinical abnormalities is often better correlated with the viscosity of the serum than with the level of the protein involved. Therefore, therapy may be followed by serum viscosity measurements.

REFERENCE

Fahey, J.L., Barth, W.F., and Solomon, A.: Serum hyperviscosity syndrome, JAMA, *192*, 464, 1965.

REAGENTS AND EQUIPMENT

1. Water bath, 37°C.
2. Vacuum tubing.
3. Aspirator.
4. Laboratory stand with clamp.
5. Sodium chloride, 0.85% (w/v).
6. Distilled water.
7. Ostwald viscometer (Fig. 138).

SPECIMEN

Collect approximately 12 ml of whole blood and allow it to clot. This test requires 5 ml of serum.

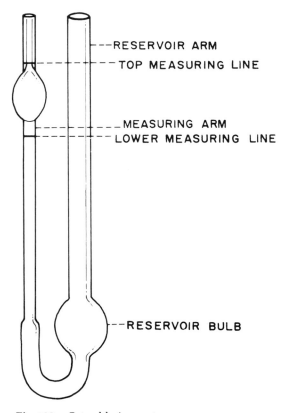

Fig. 138. Ostwald viscometer.

PRINCIPLE

The patient's serum is placed in a viscometer, and the time required for the serum to flow from one mark to a second mark is measured. This time is then compared with the time required for distilled water to flow the same distance in the viscometer.

PROCEDURE

1. Centrifuge the clotted blood at 2,500 RPM for 10 minutes. Remove the serum and centrifuge a second time. Place serum in clean test tube.
2. Rinse the Ostwald viscometer well with 0.85% sodium chloride.
3. Suspend the viscometer in a 37°C water bath by means of a laboratory stand.
4. Pipet 5 ml of patient's serum into the reservoir bulb through the reservoir arm.

5. Allow several minutes for the serum to reach 37°C. At this time, remove any air bubbles in the serum by gently blowing through the aspirator attached to the top of the measuring arm.
6. Using the aspirator, draw the serum up into the measuring arm above the highest line.
7. As soon as the serum is even with the top measuring line, start the stopwatch.
8. Time the passage of serum between the two measuring lines; as soon as the upper border of the serum is even with the lower measuring line, stop the watch. Record the flow time of the serum.
9. Remove the serum and rinse the viscometer with 0.85% sodium chloride.
10. Repeat the preceding procedure, steps 3 through 7, using 5 ml of distilled water in place of the patient's serum.
11. Calculate the results as shown below:

$$\text{Relative serum viscosity} = \frac{\text{Flow time of serum}}{\text{Flow time of distilled water}}$$

DISCUSSION

1. The flow time of distilled water is usually about 59 seconds.
2. The viscometer, when it is not in use, should be sealed with Parafilm.

METHEMOGLOBIN TEST

Methemoglobin is a form of hemoglobin in which the ferrous ion has been oxidized to the ferric state and is, therefore, incapable of combining with or transporting the oxygen molecule. A small amount of methemoglobin is continuously being formed in the red blood cell but, in turn, is reduced by the red blood cell enzyme systems. Methemoglobin is normally present in the blood in a concentration of 1 to 2%. Increased amounts may be found in both hereditary and acquired disorders. The hereditary form of methemoglobinemia is found in disorders in which (1) the red blood cell reducing systems are abnormal and unable to reduce the methemoglobin back to oxyhemoglobin, or (2) in the presence of hemoglobin M, where the structure of the polypeptide chains making up the hemoglobin molecule is abnormal, there is a tendency toward oxidation, and a decreased ability to be reduced back to oxyhemoglobin. The acquired causes of methemoglobinemia are mainly due to certain drugs and chemicals, such as aniline, nitrates, nitrites, and some sulfonamides.

REFERENCE

Dacie, J.V., and Lewis, S.M.: *Practical Hematology,* 5th ed., Churchill Livingstone, New York, 1975.

REAGENTS AND EQUIPMENT

1. Phosphate buffer, pH 6.8.
    Solution 1
Monobasic potassium phosphate (KH₂PO₄)	9.1 g
Distilled water	1,000 ml

    Solution 2
Dibasic sodium phosphate (Na₂HPO₄)	9.5 g
Distilled water	1,000 ml

    For the phosphate buffer, pH 6.8, mix:
Solution 1	50.8 ml
Solution 2	49.2 ml

2. Potassium cyanide solution.
Potassium cyanide	50 g
Distilled water	1,000 ml

3. Potassium ferricyanide solution.
Potassium ferricyanide	50 g
Distilled water	1,000 ml

4. Sterox SE solution.
Sterox SE	10 ml
Distilled water	1,000 ml

5. Test tubes, 13 × 125 mm.

SPECIMEN

Fresh whole blood or anticoagulated whole blood, using EDTA, heparin, or ammonium-potassium oxalate as the anticoagulant.

PRINCIPLE

Whole blood is diluted with a phosphate buffer solution and sterox SE to prevent turbidity. Methemoglobin has a maximum absorbance on the spectrophotometer at a wavelength of 640 nm. The diluted blood is read at this wavelength, and the reading is noted (D_1). Potassium cyanide is added to this solution, converting the methemoglobin to cyanmethemoglobin, and read on the spectrophotometer (D_2). The change in optical density is proportional to the amount of methemoglobin present. Potassium ferricyanide, which converts hemoglobin to methemoglobin, is added to a second dilution of the blood, and its spectrophotometer reading is noted (D_3). Potassium cyanide is added, which converts the methemoglobin to cyanmethemoglobin, and the spectrophotometer reading is noted (D_4). The percentage of methemoglobin present in the blood is then calculated.

PROCEDURE

1. Pipet 4 ml of phosphate buffer solution into a test tube.
2. Add 6 ml of sterox SE solution to the preceding test tube.
3. Pipet 0.2 ml of whole blood into the preceding test tube and mix well. Label test tube No. 1.
4. Place 5.0 ml of the diluted blood solution from test tube No. 1 into a second test tube and label No. 2.
5. Prepare a blank solution by mixing 1 ml of phosphate buffer with 3 ml of sterox SE solution.
6. Read test tube No. 1 in a spectrophotometer at a wavelength of 640 nm, using the blank solution to set optical density at 0. Record the optical density of the solution (D_1).
7. Add one drop of potassium cyanide solution to test tube No. 1, mix, and

read, as in step 6. Record the optical density (D_2).

8. Add one drop of potassium ferricyanide solution to test tube No. 2, mix, and allow to sit for 5 minutes. Read on the spectrophotometer, as in step 6. Record the optical density (D_3).

9. Add one drop of potassium cyanide solution to test tube No. 2, mix, and read, as in step 6. Record the optical density (D_4).

10. Calculation of results:

$$\text{Percent of methemoglobin} = \frac{D_1 - D_2}{D_3 - D_4} \times 100$$

DISCUSSION

Sulfhemoglobin is not measured at any time during this procedure. Therefore, if an appreciable amount of sulfhemoglobin is present, the total hemoglobin reading will be low.

MALARIA SMEARS

Blood smears should be taken from patients suspected of having malaria at 6- to 8-hour intervals. It is not necessary to wait until the patient has fever and chills.

REFERENCE

Miale, J.B.: *Laboratory Medicine: Hematology*, 6th ed., The C.V. Mosby Company, St. Louis, 1982.

REAGENTS AND EQUIPMENT

1. Giemsa staining solution.
   Liquid Giemsa stain   5.0 ml
   Distilled water   95.0 ml
2. Glass slides.
3. Coplin jar.

SPECIMEN

Several thick and thin blood smears.

PROCEDURE

1. Make two or three routine blood smears from fingertip blood or blood anticoagulated with EDTA or ammonium-potassium oxalate. Air-dry the smears.

2. Make two or three thick smears by placing one large drop of blood on a glass slide. Using the corner of a second slide, carefully spread the drop of blood over an area the size of a dime. Allow the smears to air-dry for about 30 minutes.

3. Fix the thin smears with methanol for a few seconds. Do not fix the thick smears.

4. Place the smears in a coplin jar containing Giemsa staining solution for 30 minutes.

5. At the end of 30 minutes, rinse the smears in running tap water and allow to air-dry.

6. Examine the smears microscopically, using the oil immersion objective (100×). The red blood cells on the thick, unfixed smears will be destroyed, making examination easier. It is important to identify correctly the species of malaria *(Plasmodium malariae, vivax, falciparum, or ovale)* when present so that proper medication can be given (Figs. 139, 140, 141, 142).

DISCUSSION

1. *Plasmodium vivax* generally shows all stages of development present in the blood. The ring forms are usually large, and there may be two or more rings present in a red blood cell. The chromatin dot in the early trophozoite may appear singly or, at times, two may be present. The trophozoites are frequently quite ameboid, which is a characteristic of this malaria type. There may be 12 to 24 merozoites present. The infected red blood cells are usually enlarged and may be irregularly shaped. Schüffner's granules may also be found. These granules, which fill the red blood cell, appear as orange- to pink-

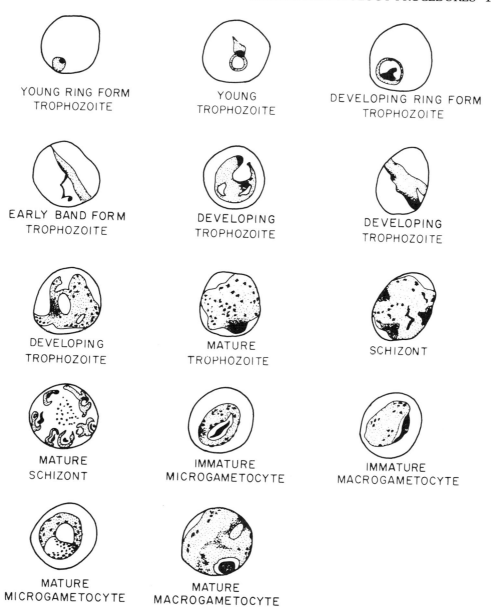

Fig. 139. *Plasmodium malariae.* (Modified from Seiverd, C.E.: *Hematology for Medical Technologists*, Lea & Febiger, Philadelphia, 1972.)

colored stippling. (These granules may not be visible when normal staining times are used. To detect these granules, allow the smears to stain for 3 hours.)

2. In *Plasmodium falciparum* infections, ring forms and gametocytes are generally the only stage(s) seen on the peripheral blood smear. The ring forms present are generally small and delicate and may have one or two chromatin dots. Multiple ring forms in a single red blood cell is a very common finding. The gametocytes in this type of malaria are very characteristic, showing a crescent or sau-

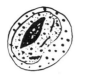

MICROGAMETOCYTE   MACROGAMETOCYTE

Fig. 140. *Plasodium vivax.*

MICROGAMETOCYTE   MACROGAMETOCYTE

Fig. 141. *Plasmodium falciparum.*

MICROGAMETOCYTE   MACROGAMETOCYTE

Fig. 142. *Plasmodium ovale.*

sage shape. The red blood cells may show Maurer's spots, which are irregular, orange- to pink-staining granules that may be present in varying numbers.

3. In *Plasmodium malariae*, all stages of development may be present on the peripheral blood smear. The ring forms generally contain only one chromatin dot, and only one ring form is usually found in the red blood cell. Most often, the schizont will contain 6 to 12 merozoites. Generally, an abundant amount of hematin granules is present, and the red blood cells may contain a fine stippling (Ziemann's dots).

4. *Plasmodium ovale* infection is rarely encountered. All stages of development may be present on the peripheral blood smear. Like *P. malariae*, usually only one ring form per red blood cell is present, and these ring forms contain only one chromatin dot. There are 6 to 12 merozoites present in the schizont. The infected red blood cells may be enlarged, and some may be oval-shaped. Schüffner's dots may also be present.

5

Coagulation

HEMOSTASIS AND COAGULATION

Hemostasis is the process that retains the blood within the vascular system. When a blood vessel is injured, the hemostatic process is designed to repair the break and arrest hemorrhage. The most immediate response to bleeding is vasoconstriction, which decreases the blood flow through the injured blood vessel. Platelets then clump together and adhere to the injured vessel in this area to form a plug and further inhibit bleeding. The coagulation factors present in the blood interact, forming a fibrin meshwork, or clot, to stop the bleeding completely. Slow lysis of this clot begins, and final repair to the injured site takes place.

Hemostasis and coagulation are highly complex mechanisms that, even today, are only partially understood. Only a simplified breakdown of the clotting mechanism is presented here. A basic knowledge of this subject is a necessary tool before carrying out coagulation procedures.

Coagulation

The complexity of the coagulation process has been made more difficult by the large number of different names given to the 12 coagulation factors. To avoid this confusion, an international committee (the International Committee on Nomenclature of Blood Clotting Factors) has established a nomenclature for these clotting factors. Each of the 12 factors has been given a Roman numeral. Listed in Table 10 are the numbers assigned by this committee, along with their most commonly used names. Factor VI, accelerin, is no longer considered one of the coagulation factors.

The interaction of these coagulation factors is shown in Figure 143. The coagulation process is divided into two systems: the *intrinsic system* and the *extrinsic system*. All factors required for the intrinsic system are contained within the blood. The extrinsic system relies on thromboplastin (factor III), which is released from the damaged cells and tissues.

With the exception of calcium and platelet phospholipid, the coagulation factors are proteins. The process of coagulation is a series of biochemical reactions in which an inactive proenzyme is converted to an active enzyme, which, in turn, activates another proenzyme.

STAGE 1—THE GENERATION OF PLASMA THROMBOPLASTIN

In the intrinsic system, the exact stimulus that activates the coagulation mechanism is unknown but is thought to be associated with endothelial injury. Activation of the clotting sequence in vitro is brought about by surface contact with glass, kaolin, Celite, or other negatively charged substances. Initially, a small amount of factor XII is activated. The resulting factor XIIa converts prekallikrein (termed the *Fletcher factor*) to kallikrein

TABLE 10.   COAGULATION FACTORS

FACTOR	NAME
I	Fibrinogen
II	Prothrombin
III	Tissue thromboplastin, thrombokinase
IV	Calcium
V	Proaccelerin, labile factor
VII	Proconvertin, stable factor
VIII	Antihemophilic A factor (AHF), antihemophilic globulin (AHG)
IX	Antihemophilic B factor (AHB), plasma thromboplastin component (PTC), Christmas factor
X	Stuart factor, Stuart-Prower factor
XI	Plasma thromboplastin antecedent (PTA)
XII	Hageman factor, contact factor
XIII	Fibrin stabilizing factor, fibrinase

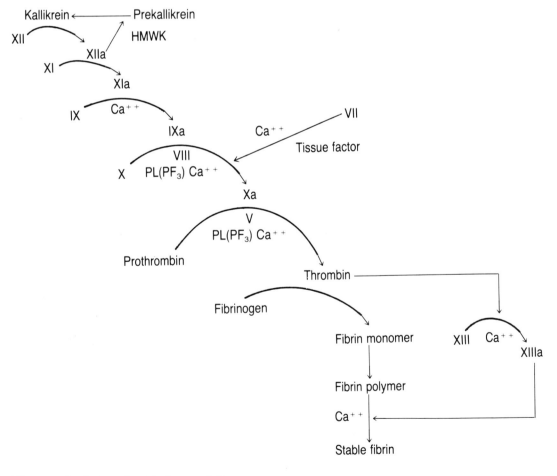

Fig. 143. Intrinsic and extrinsic coagulation process.

in the presence of a high molecular weight kininogen (HMWK) (termed the *Fitzgerald factor*). This formation of kallikrein is thought to be the major pathway for the activation of factor XII. Factor XIIa then converts factor XI to XIa. HMWK is also thought to be required in the activation of factor XI. Factor IX is activated by the enzymatic action of XIa and calcium ions to form IXa. Factor IXa then forms a complex with phospholipid, calcium ions, and factor VIII to convert factor X to Xa. In the extrinsic system, tissue thromboplastin (factor III), calcium ions, and factor VII convert factor X to Xa. (This complex is also capable of activating factor IX.) Activated factor X (Xa) forms a complex with factor V, phospholipid, and calcium ions, which may be termed *plasma thromboplastin*.

STAGE 2—THE FORMATION OF THROMBIN FROM PROTHROMBIN

Plasma thromboplastin converts prothrombin to thrombin. This is accomplished in two steps. In the first step, prethrombin 2 is formed, along with a fragment, termed *fragment 1•2*. In the second step, prethrombin 2 is converted to thrombin. The thrombin that is formed acts on fragment 1•2 to form fragment 1 and fragment 2. Fragment 1 will compete with prothrombin for the tissue thromboplastin complex and, therefore, have a slight inhibitory effect on the prothrombin to thrombin conversion.

STAGE 3—THE FORMATION OF FIBRIN FROM FIBRINOGEN

Fibrin formation occurs by the action of thrombin on fibrinogen. The fibrinogen molecule consists of three polypeptide chains. Thrombin splits off two small peptides on each side of the fibrinogen molecule (Fig. 144). Fibrinopeptide A is released from the alpha chain first by the action of thrombin. Next, fibrinopeptide B is released from the beta chain (by the action of thrombin) to produce the fibrin monomer. These fibrin monomers then polymerize to form a fibrin polymer that is soluble in 5 M urea. (Fibrinopeptides A and B are negatively charged and must be removed from the fibrinogen molecule for polymerization to take place; otherwise, the molecules would repel each other.) Factor XIII, activated by thrombin and calcium, then converts the fibrin polymer to a more stable state by changing the hydrogen bonds to covalent bonds. The resulting fibrin is insoluble in 5 M urea.

It should be noted that the extrinsic and intrinsic systems as described are separated only for the purpose of evaluation. In truth, tissue thromboplastin probably activates both systems, and both the extrinsic and intrinsic mechanisms are involved in activating factor X. In the extrinsic system, only 10 to 20 seconds are required for clotting. A period of 2 to 3 minutes is needed for the formation of thrombin in the intrinsic system.

The Coagulation Factors

The coagulation factors may be divided into four functional groups based on their properties. The *fibrinogen group* consists of factors I, V, VIII, and XIII. They are consumed during the process of coagulation and are, therefore, absent in serum and present in plasma. These factors are not adsorbed out by barium sulfate. Factors V and VIII are susceptible to denaturation and are reduced in quantity in stored

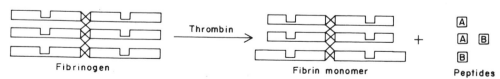

Fig. 144. Action of thrombin on fibrinogen.

plasma. Vitamin K is not necessary for the synthesis of these factors. There is an increased concentration of the factors in this group during an inflammatory response and in pregnancy. The *prothrombin group* includes factors II, VII, IX, and X. Vitamin K is necessary for their synthesis in the liver. Coumarin drugs, which inhibit vitamin K, cause a decrease in these factors. Factors VII, IX, and X are not consumed during the coagulation process and are, therefore, present in serum as well as plasma. All four factors are adsorbed out of plasma by barium sulfate. They are stable and are well preserved in stored plasma. The *contact group* is composed of factors XI and XII. These factors are not consumed during coagulation, do not depend on vitamin K for their synthesis, and are not adsorbed out of the plasma by barium sulfate. These two factors are relatively stable. The *kinin group* includes prekallikrein (Fletcher factor), high molecular weight kininogen (HMWK) (Fitzgerald factor), and kallikrein. These factors are involved in the activation of the coagulation process and also function in the activation of plasminogen (in the fibrinolytic process).

Factor I (fibrinogen) is synthesized in the liver but does not need vitamin K for its production. It is a plasma protein with a molecular weight of 340,000. The normal plasma level is approximately 200 to 400 mg per dl, depending on the procedure used. A minimum of 60 to 100 mg per dl are required for normal coagulation. Fibrinogen has a half-life of 3 to 4 days. It is relatively stable to heat and storage but may be irreversibly precipitated at 56°C. A fraction of fibrinogen, cryofibrinogen, may precipitate at 4°C but goes back into solution upon warming.

Factor II (prothrombin) is synthesized in the liver and needs vitamin K for its maintenance. It is almost entirely consumed in the coagulation process so that little remains in the serum. It is an alpha-2 globulin with a molecular weight of approximately 69,000. Prothrombin is heat-stable and has a half-life of 24 to 48 hours. It readily forms thrombin in the presence of plasma thromboplastin.

Factor III (tissue thromboplastin) is a high molecular weight lipoprotein found in most of the body tissues, with increased concentrations in the lungs and brain. It is not, however, found in platelets. It is probably the phospholipid content of tissue thromboplastin that makes platelets unnecessary in stage I of the coagulation process.

Factor IV (calcium) in the ionized state is necessary for coagulation. The exact mechanism by which calcium acts in the coagulation process is not known. The fact that it is essential for coagulation makes possible the use of anticoagulants, which merely bind up the calcium and, therefore, completely inhibit coagulation. It is unlikely, however, that a bleeding tendency is ever caused by a deficiency of calcium because clinical tetany occurs with higher levels of calcium than are necessary for coagulation.

Factor V (proaccelerin) is synthesized in the liver but does not need vitamin K for its production. It is a globulin with a molecular weight of over 300,000. Factor V is unstable and deteriorates rapidly at room temperature. It is more stable in citrated plasma than in oxalated plasma. Little, if any, factor V is present in serum. It has a half-life in the plasma of approximately 15 hours. Factor V is sensitive to thrombin, and if all of this factor is not used up in the generation of plasma thromboplastin, it is generally destroyed by any thrombin present.

Factor VII (proconvertin) is synthesized in the liver and requires vitamin K for its production. It is a beta globulin with a molecular weight of 60,000. Although it is stable at 4°C for 2 or more weeks, it is slightly heat-labile. It has a half-life of only 5 hours, which means that it disappears rapidly from the blood when production is halted (as in therapy with coumarin drugs). High levels of factor VII are present in both stored plasma and serum, and factor VII activity may actually increase during the coagulation process.

Factor VIII (antihemophilic A factor) does not require vitamin K for its production. The exact site of production is not totally understood but is thought by some to be produced by the reticuloendothelial cells in the liver. Its electrophoretic ability suggests it to be an alpha-2 or beta globulin, and it is thought to have a high molecular weight. Citrated plasma treated with aluminum hydroxide may have an appreciable amount of factor VIII activity removed. It is heat-labile, has a half-life of about 10 hours, and is unstable in citrated plasma. The molecular structure of factor VIII is not completely known. Currently, it may be thought of as a molecule made up of several functional parts: (1) *Factor VIII:C* refers to the coagulant portion of the molecule and represents the ability of the factor VIII molecule to correct coagulation abnormalities associated with hemophilia A. (2) *Factor VIII:Ag* is the factor VIII-related antigen. This is the protein that is detected by various immunoassays. (3) *Factor VIII:R* is that part of the molecule which makes possible platelet aggregation in the presence of ristocetin. (4) *Factor VIII:vW* is the characteristic of the factor VIII molecule that is required for normal platelet adhesion in hemostasis. It is also termed the *von Willebrand factor*.

Factor IX (antihemophilic B factor) is synthesized in the liver and requires vitamin K for its production. It is stable at 4°C for several weeks. Factor IX is a beta globulin. It has a half-life of approximately 25 hours and is present in serum.

Factor X (Stuart factor) is an alpha globulin. It is synthesized in the liver and requires vitamin K for its production. It is relatively heat-stable and is stable for several weeks to 2 months when stored at 4°C. It has a half-life of approximately 40 hours.

Factor XI (plasma thromboplastin antecedent) is a beta-2 globulin with a high molecular weight. The exact site of synthesis is not known. It is relatively stable at room temperature and has a half-life of approximately 45 hours.

Factor XII (Hageman factor) migrates between the beta and gamma globulins on electrophoresis. The actual site of production is not known. It is stable in that it can be stored (in oxalated plasma) at 4°C for almost 3 months. It is relatively heat-stable and remains in serum after 30 minutes at 60°C.

Factor XIII (fibrin-stabilizing factor) is a transglutaminase and has a high molecular weight. Its site of production is not known. Little factor XIII is present in the serum, the major portion being adsorbed to fibrin. It is heat-stable.

Fletcher factor (prekallikrein) is a single chain gamma globulin. It is produced in the liver but is not dependent on vitamin K for its production. It is present in serum and is not adsorbed out of the plasma by barium sulfate.

Fitzgerald factor (high molecular weight kininogen) is a single chain, alpha-globulin that may be acted on by kallikrein to yield kinin. It has a half-life of 6.5 days and is present in serum. It is produced in the liver and is not vitamin K-dependent. It is present in barium sulfate-adsorbed plasma.

Hemostasis

Platelets maintain capillary integrity. In the absence of platelets, red blood cells migrate through the vessel walls in large numbers. In addition, platelets play a major role in the hemostatic process.

Immediately following an injury, the small blood vessels in the area will constrict. There is not much evidence, however, to indicate that this is important in the stoppage of bleeding. In very small wounds or punctures, the site may be closed merely by the elasticity of the skin. The major function of the platelets takes place in the process of hemostasis. Within 1 to 2 seconds after injury to a blood vessel, the hemostatic process begins and proceeds as outlined below. The exact sequence of these events, however, in vivo is somewhat unclear.

1. Platelet adhesion. *Platelet adhesiveness* is defined as the ability of platelets to attach to nonplatelet surfaces. In the first step of hemostasis, the platelets come in contact with the injured tissue. They adhere to the exposed collagen, the basement membrane, and/or to microfibrils. Calcium ions are necessary for platelet adhesion when collagen is not present. It is also thought that certain plasma factors, such as the von Willebrand factor (a subunit of coagulation factor VIII), are also required for platelet adhesion. At this time, the platelet will also change from its disklike shape to a spiny sphere. The volume of the platelet does not change, and the spiny projections are thought to enable the platelet to adhere to other cells and tissue.

2. *Platelet aggregation* is the ability of the platelets to attach to one another. Primary platelet aggregation is reversible and may be caused by adenosine diphosphate (ADP) and other aggregating agents. Secondary platelet aggregation is irreversible and follows primary aggregation. It is caused by agents that are capable of causing the release of platelet ADP and/or the production of prostaglandins and related substances by the platelet.

3. Platelet release reaction. During primary platelet aggregation, the platelet granules cluster in the center of the platelet. The microtubules of the platelet then fuse with the platelet granules (dense bodies and the alpha granules), enabling the contents of the granules to be secreted to the outside *(exocytosis)* through openings in the membrane. Two release reactions have been described for this process.

Release I requires weak stimulation and causes release of the contents of the dense bodies. In *release II*, the contents of the alpha granules and the dense bodies will be released.

4. It is believed that the platelets produce various prostaglandins and thromboxanes that aid in the release reaction and platelet aggregation. Thromboxane A_2 is thought to be a very strong inducer of the platelet release reaction.

5. When platelet factor 3 becomes available from the platelet and with the coagulation factors present in the area, the blood coagulation process begins, and the platelet plug becomes strengthened by the fibrin formation.

6. Clot retraction occurs once the plasma clots in the presence of the platelets. The clot will shrink to about 25% of its original volume. This response depends on the reaction between adenosine triphosphate (ATP) and *thrombosthenin*, a contractile protein from the platelet.

Platelet Factors

The platelet factors have been given Arabic numbers and are designated as platelet factors 1 through 10. They are either derived from the platelet or are associated with platelets. Of these 10 factors, only platelet factors 2, 3, and 4 are unique to the platelet.

Platelet factor 1 refers to plasma coagulation factor V. *Platelet factor 2* is a globulin and is found in the hyalomere portion of the platelet. It inhibits antithrombin III, increases platelet aggregation, and accelerates the action of thrombin or fibrinogen. *Platelet factor 3* is a lipoprotein that is found in the platelet granules and membrane. It is required in two steps of the coagulation process: (1) It interacts with factors VIII and IXa to activate factor X, and (2) it interacts with factor V and prothrombin to form thrombin. *Platelet factor 4* is a glycoprotein, is thought to be stored in the alpha granules, and is extruded during the platelet release reaction. It aids in ADP-induced platelet aggregation and inhibits the anticoagulant effect of heparin. *Platelet factor 5* is platelet fibrinogen. *Platelet factor 6* is a plasmin inhibitor that is associated with platelets. Little information is known about *platelet factor 7* (cothromboplastin), *platelet factor 8* (antithromboplastin factor), and *platelet factor 9* (accelerator globulin stabilizing factor). *Platelet factor 10*, serotonin, is found in the dense body. The platelet factor 10 terminology is rarely used for this substance.

LIMITING MECHANISMS OF HEMOSTASIS AND COAGULATION

Under normal physiologic conditions, coagulation does not occur. When injury does occur, it is imperative that blood coagulation remain localized at the site of injury. The fact that blood is flowing through the circulation has a limiting effect on the development of blood clots. In the area of injury, the flowing blood will move any coagulants present away from the site of injury. These coagulants will be diluted in the blood and can be inactivated by inhibitors present in the plasma or removed from the circulation by the liver. When injury does occur, the platelets localize at the site. The coagulation factors tend to adsorb onto the platelet surface. As fibrin forms, it tends to encapsulate the clot, thus restricting the coagulants to the inside of the clot. In addition, as soon as the coagulation process is begun, fibrinolysis is initiated to ultimately break down the clot that is formed.

Fibrinolysis

Normally, the fibrinolytic system keeps the vascular system free of deposited fibrin or fibrin clots. *Fibrinolysis* occurs when plasminogen is converted into plasma (Fig. 145), which, in turn, dissolves the fibrin (or fibrinogen) into smaller fragments termed *fibrin (fibrino-*

$$\text{Plasminogen} \xrightarrow{\text{Activators}} \text{Plasmin}$$

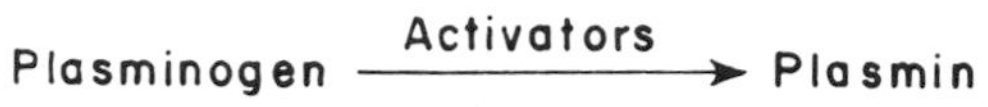

Fig. 145. Formation of plasmin.

gen) degradation products (or *fibrin split products*) (Fig. 146). In addition, inhibitors to the plasminogen activators are present in the blood to help control fibrinolysis.

There are three recognized components in the fibrinolytic system:

1. *Plasminogen* is a beta-globulin found in the plasma in a concentration of approximately 17 to 23 mg per dl. It is most probably produced in the liver. It adheres to and forms complexes with fibrinogen and fibrin, and when a clot forms, large amounts of this substance are adsorbed within the fibrin mass (clot).

2. *Plasminogen activators* are a group of proteolytic enzymes that are specific for the activation of plasminogen. They are found in the lysosomes

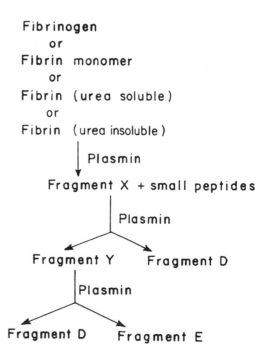

Fig. 146. Degradation of fibrinogen and fibrin by plasmin.

of most cells and in the vascular endothelium, with the highest concentration in the blood vessels of the microcirculation. They are also present in trace amounts in the plasma. The plasminogen activator present in urine is termed *urokinase*. The concentration of these substances are generally increased during anoxia, exercise, and stress.

3. *Plasminogen proactivators* are precursors of plasminogen activators. There may be one or more plasma proteins, which will react with factor XIIa to form plasminogen activators. One such substance, it has been suggested, is the same as prekallikrein.

Inhibitors of fibrinolysis are termed *antiplasmins*. At least five plasma proteins are known that neutralize free plasmin. The two antiplasmins of major importance are thought to be alpha-2-antiplasmin (the most important) and alpha-2-macroglobulin. The antiplasmins are thought to be synthesized in the liver. Generally, there are 10 times the amount of antiplasmin activity than plasmin activity in the plasma.

FIBRINOLYTIC PROCESS

In vivo, the plasminogen activator develops most probably from the interaction of factor XIIa with plasma proactivators. Plasmin is thus formed from the available plasminogen by action of the plasminogen activators. When the fibrin forms, the plasminogen, activated to plasmin, will be found in two forms: (1) free in the plasma (may also be termed the *soluble form*) and (2) adsorbed to fibrin (*gel form*). The plasmin that is free in the plasma is most probably destroyed by the plasma antiplasmins. The adsorbed plasmin is not affected by the plasma antiplasmins (the antiplasmins may be unable to diffuse through the clot) and is, therefore, free to carry out its function (break down the fibrin and any fibrinogen present). (It is in-teresting to note that plasminogen activators in vivo are quickly adsorbed into the clot when they are present during clot formation. Once a clot is formed, however, the plasminogen activators can only enter the thrombi very slowly.) The plasmin, in stepwise fashion, initially breaks down fibrin into one large fragment (fragment X) and several smaller peptides (Fig. 146). Further action by plasmin breaks fragment X into fragment Y and fragment D. Fragment Y is further degraded to fragment E and a second fragment D. Fragments D and E are relatively resistant to further breakdown by plasmin.

Fibrin degradation products are removed from the blood by the liver, kidney, and reticuloendothelial system and have half-lives of about 9 hours. (Fragments X and Y and fibrin monomers form soluble complexes that will form precipitates and gels in vitro in the presence of protamine sulfate and alcohol. This has been termed *paracoagulation* and is the basis for certain coagulation tests.) Most fibrin degradation products, especially fragment Y, are inhibitors of coagulation and are strong antithrombins. Fragments Y and D inhibit fibrin polymerization, whereas fragment E is thought to be an inhibitor of thrombin. Also, the products of fibrin degradation are thought to impair platelet function.

There is much evidence that both the coagulation and fibrinolytic systems are in equilibrium. As a general rule, fibrinolysis increases whenever coagulation increases.

Antithrombins

The *antithrombins* constitute a group of activities or substances that inactivate thrombin. Originally, six antithrombins were described and designated with Roman numerals. Of these, only two are currently considered to have physiologic significance: antithrombins I and III.

Antithrombin I is a term that refers to the ability of fibrin to adsorb thrombin. During the coagulation process, large amounts of thrombin can be adsorbed onto the fibrin that has formed, neutralizing thrombin and making it unavailable for the fibrinogen to fibrin conversion. *Antithrombin II* is considered to be the same as antithrombin III.

Antithrombin III is an alpha-2-glycoprotein that is produced in the liver. When thrombin is present, antithrombin III attaches to the thrombin, forming a complex, and progressively inactivates the thrombin. Heparin, when present, also forms a complex with antithrombin III and increases the inhibitory characteristics of antithrombin III. In this way, the anticoagulant action of heparin in normal blood is brought about by activation of antithrombin III. Heparin serves as the catalyst, increasing the rate of thrombin neutralization by antithrombin III. Decreased amounts of antithrombin III present in the blood will cause a failure to respond to heparin therapy and will also cause hypercoagulation of the blood. Antithrombin III also inactivates factor Xa and, to a lesser degree, factors IXa, XIa, XIIa, kallikrein, and plasmin.

Antithrombins IV and *V* are not well understood and are of questionable significance.

Antithrombin VI represents the anticoagulant actions of fibrinogen degradation products (see the previous section entitled Fibrinolysis).

Other Inhibitors of Coagulation

Alpha-2-macroglobulin is also considered an antithrombin. It is a glycoprotein whose site of production is unknown. It acts progressively to inhibit thrombin and has a slower action than antithrombin III. It is an antiplasmin and also inactivates kallikrein.

Alpha-2-antitrypsin is an alpha globulin. It is a strong inhibitor of factor XIa. It also inactivates plasmin. It acts as a weak, progressive antithrombin, but this characteristic is thought to be of little significance.

C'-1-inactivator is a major plasma inhibitor of factor XIIa and kallikrein and also inhibits factor XIa.

Factor XIa inhibitor, as its name implies, inhibits factor XIa in a time- and temperature-dependent manner.

Alpha-2-antiplasmin forms a complex with plasmin and inactivates plasmin.

Protein C is a newly identified glycoprotein thought to be involved in the coagulation mechanism. It is vitamin K-dependent and is considered to be an anticoagulant. When activated by thrombin, protein C inhibits blood coagulation, most probably inactivating factor V. Normal plasma contains a protein that inhibits activated protein C.

Other coagulation inhibitor substances have been described, but they are less significant than the above inhibitors.

COAGULATION SCREENING PROCEDURES

The activated partial thromboplastin time, prothrombin time, thrombin time (or quantitative fibrinogen), bleeding time, platelet count, and clot retraction constitute a satisfactory *coagulation screen* to perform on the bleeding patient or on one who is suspected of having a bleeding disorder. The best single laboratory test available is the *activated partial thromboplastin time*. This procedure detects deficiencies present in the intrinsic coagulation system, except for platelets and factor XIII. The *prothrombin time* is the method of choice for detecting disorders in the extrinsic system. The *thrombin time* is useful as a test for functional fibrinogen and to test the conversion of fibrinogen to fibrin. It is also sensitive to the presence of thrombin-inhibitors such as heparin. The most widely used screening tests for platelets are the *platelet count*, the *bleeding time*, and the *clot retraction*.

Once it has been established from the results of the coagulation screen that the patient has a coagulation disorder, the exact factor deficiency or abnormality should be identified. The activated partial thromboplastin time with substitutions is an excellent test to proceed with. The results of this test, in conjunction with the results of the prothrombin time, generally identify the factor deficiency if it is present in stage 1 or 2 of the coagulation process. If a factor VII deficiency is suspected, the prothrombin time with substitutions and the Stypven time may be performed. Once the factor(s) deficiency has been identified, a factor assay should be performed. A functional platelet abnormality may be further studied by utilizing the test for platelet factor 3 availability, the prothrombin consumption, the platelet adhesiveness test, or the platelet aggregation procedure. The euglobulin clot lysis time and the test for fibrin split products may be employed to detect the presence of increased fibrinolysis.

In monitoring anticoagulant therapy, the prothrombin time is generally employed when the patient is receiving coumarin drugs. Heparin therapy is usually followed by use of the activated partial thromboplastin time.

REQUIREMENTS FOR ACCURATE COAGULATION TESTS

To obtain the most consistently accurate results in coagulation studies, certain procedures must be adhered to.

Collection of the Specimen

1. The anticoagulant of choice for coagulation studies is 0.109 M sodium citrate. In the past, 0.1 M sodium oxalate was used. Because of the increased lability of factors V and VIII in sodium oxalate, however, it is now used only in rare instances.
2. The ratio of anticoagulant to blood (primarily the plasma portion) is important. Patient blood that has a high hematocrit will contain less plasma. As a result, when the blood has been centrifuged, the plasma fraction will contain an increased concentration of anticoagulant (sodium citrate),

leading to prolonged clotting time results on patients with hematocrits of 50% or higher. (During testing, as calcium is added to the test plasma, it will combine with the excess anticoagulant present instead of being available for the coagulation process.) Therefore, whenever a patient's hematocrit is greater than 50% or less than 20%, the amount of sodium citrate in the collection (Vacutainer) tube should be decreased (or increased) according to the hematocrit reading. The following formula may be followed for determining the proper amount of sodium citrate to use (when the final volume in the tube is 5.0 ml, and 0.5 ml of 0.109 M sodium citrate is normally used).

$$\text{Amount of sodium citrate} = \frac{\text{Patient's plasma volume} \; (100 - \text{hematocrit}) \times 0.5}{\text{Normal plasma volume (60)}}$$

For example, when a patient has a hematocrit of 55%, 0.38 ml of 0.109 M sodium citrate should be placed in the tube and blood added to give a final volume of 5.0 ml.

3. A clean venipuncture is absolutely necessary. If there is any contamination of the blood with tissue thromboplastin, false results will occur. For routine coagulation procedures, the Vacutainer blood collection system is adequate. When obtaining a blood specimen for nonroutine, specialized coagulation procedures, a two-syringe technique should be applied. Using two disposable syringes, withdraw approximately 2 ml of blood into the first syringe. Quickly and carefully disconnect this syringe from the needle (leaving the needle in the patient's vein) and connect the second syringe to the needle. Proceed with the venipuncture, discarding the blood in the first syringe. (Prior to performing

the two-syringe venipuncture, make certain that the first syringe is easily removed from the needle but fits snugly enough so that blood will not leak out at the connection.) When testing for "contact" abnormalities (factors XI and XII and platelet function studies), plastic syringes should be used.

4. Heparinized syringes should never be used for coagulation studies. Heparin has an inhibitory effect on thrombin and, therefore, causes prolonged clotting times.

Preparation of the Plasma Sample

1. Before centrifuging the blood specimen, check each tube with applicator sticks (two) for the presence of clots. Because the tubes should be centrifuged with their tops on, an alternative method is to check the tube for clots after the plasma has been removed.

2. Unless otherwise noted, coagulation testing should be completed within 4 hours of obtaining the specimen from the patient. Once the blood has been centrifuged, however, the red blood cells no longer have a buffering effect on the plasma, and all coagulation testing should be completed within 2 hours. Once the plasma is removed from the cells, it should be placed in a stoppered test tube unless testing is to be performed immediately. Exposure of the plasma to air results in a pH change of the plasma, which may result in invalidly prolonged clotting times.

3. To preserve the labile factors, the blood specimen should be placed on ice immediately after it is withdrawn from the patient. One inexpensive, commercially available ice bath for use in the laboratory is the Kryorack (Streck Laboratories, Inc., Omaha, Nebraska), which contains an aqueous solution within a sealed unit (see Fig. 147) (available in various sizes). This unit, when placed at freezer temperatures ($-18°C$) for 8 hours, maintains a temperature of less than 8°C for 8 hours at room temperature. The tubes do not come in contact with water or ice, affording a more convenient method of refrigerating plasma than the conventional cup or tray of crushed ice.

4. Hemolyzed plasma should not be used for coagulation studies. It tends to give shortened clotting times. Also, lipemic or icteric plasma samples should, in general, not be tested on instruments designed to detect clots by optical density methods.

Performance of Coagulation Tests

1. As a general rule, all coagulation tests should be performed as soon as possible after the patient specimen has been received in the laboratory.

2. Glassware must be scrupulously clean and free of dirt, dust, and scratches. Whenever possible, disposable test tubes should be used. At no time should chromic acid be used to clean the glassware. The acid is thought to change the structure of the glass and tends to prolong the formation of a clot. Detergents containing organic solvents may leave a film on the glassware and prolong clot formation. Mercury contamination also

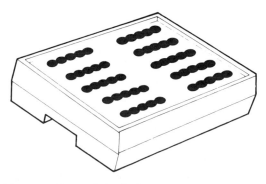

Fig. 147. Kryorack ice bath.

leads to prolonged results. Coagulation glassware should never be used for any other test in the laboratory. When testing for "contact" abnormalities such as platelet studies and factors XI and XII, plastic test tubes must be used.

3. Pipets used for coagulation studies should have a large bore, permitting complete and rapid pipetting. Automatic pipets, of which numerous different types are available, are recommended.

4. Most coagulation studies are carried out at 37°C. It should be noted that specimens incubated in dry heat take slightly longer to reach 37°C than those incubated in a water bath. It is essential, when required, that the specimens and reagents reach the proper temperature of 37°C before proceeding with the test. Overheating or prolonged heating at 37°C, however, may lead to destruction of some of the coagulation factors and, therefore, a prolonged clotting time. The temperature of the incubator should not fluctuate more than ±0.5°C.

5. Timing of the tests is extremely important. Many of the procedures are timed to within one tenth of a second, so that the initial starting and stopping of the stopwatch must be done precisely.

6. The majority of coagulation procedures use a normal control plasma, which is generally purchased in the dried form. When the control plasma is reconstituted with distilled water, it should be allowed to sit for approximately 15 minutes (or according to the manufacturer's directions) and then be gently rotated so that it will be mixed. The control plasma should never be shaken vigorously.

7. Many coagulation procedures employing citrated plasma specimens tend to yield shorter clotting times than the same tests performed on oxalated plasma specimens. For this reason, citrated control plasma specimens should always be used when sodium citrate is employed as the anticoagulant.

8. There are four general techniques in widespread use for reading the end point of most coagulation procedures. The tilt tube method requires gentle tilting of the tube back and forth at the rate of about once per second until a fibrin web is formed. The Nichrome wire loop technique employs the use of a wire loop that is passed through the mixture at the rate of two sweeps per second until a formed clot adheres to the loop. (In these first two techniques, a light source without glare is important. A black background also facilitates the end point readings.) The third and fourth procedures employ the use of automation. In these methods, a clot is detected either by use of a moving probe immersed in the mixture that is triggered by clot formation or by the change in optical density of the mixture when a clot forms.

BLEEDING TIME

The bleeding time is used primarily as a screening test for platelet function. The intrinsic and extrinsic coagulation mechanisms play only a minor role in the bleeding time. The number of platelets present (platelet count) and their ability to form a platelet plug directly affect the bleeding time. Prolonged bleeding times are generally found when the platelet count is below 50,000 per μl, and where there is platelet dysfunction, such as in von Willebrand's disease. Three procedures are currently in use for determining the bleeding time: The Duke method, the Ivy method, and the Mielke method. The Duke method is the easiest to perform but probably yields the least accurate results. The procedure of choice is the Mielke method.

Duke Method

REFERENCE

Duke, W.W.: The pathogenesis of purpura haemorrhagica with especial reference to the part played by the blood platelets, Arch. Intern. Med., *10*, 445, 1912.

REAGENTS AND EQUIPMENT

1. Sterile, disposable lancet.
2. Circular filter paper.
3. Stopwatch.
4. Alcohol sponges.

PRINCIPLE

A standardized puncture of the earlobe is made, and the length of time required for bleeding to cease is recorded.

PROCEDURE

1. Cleanse the earlobe with an alcohol sponge and allow to dry.
2. Make a relatively deep puncture with the sterile blood lancet and start the stopwatch.
3. Using the circular filter paper, blot the blood every 30 seconds. Do not allow the filter paper to touch the wound.
4. When bleeding ceases, stop the watch and record the bleeding time. The normal bleeding time is 1 to 3 minutes and borderline is 3 to 6 minutes.

DISCUSSION

1. If bleeding continues for more than 10 minutes, discontinue the test and apply pressure to the wound. It is advisable to repeat the procedure or to perform another bleeding time according to Ivy's method.
2. An alternative procedure requires the holding of a glass slide behind the earlobe for support. Make a puncture with the sterile blood lancet. Start the stopwatch, discard the glass slide, and proceed with the test as previously described.

Ivy Method

REFERENCE

Ivy, A.C., Nelson, D., and Beecher, G.: The standardization of certain factors in the cutaneous "venostasis" bleeding time technique, J. Lab. Clin. Med., *26*, 1812, 1940.

REAGENTS AND EQUIPMENT

1. Blood pressure cuff.
2. Sterile, disposable blood lancet, capable of making a wound 1 mm wide and 3 mm deep.
3. Stopwatch.
4. Circular filter paper.
5. Alcohol sponges.

PRINCIPLE

Two standardized punctures of the forearm are made, and the length of time required for bleeding to cease is recorded.

PROCEDURE

1. Place a blood pressure cuff on the patient's arm above the elbow. Increase the pressure to 40 mm Hg and hold this exact pressure for the entire procedure.
2. Cleanse an area on the volar surface of the forearm with an alcohol sponge and allow to dry.
3. Choose an area approximately three finger widths below the bend in the elbow. Hold the skin tightly by grasping the underside of the arm firmly. Make two skin punctures, 3 mm deep, avoiding any subcutaneous veins. Start the stopwatch.
4. Blot the blood from each puncture site on a separate piece of circular filter paper every 30 seconds. The filter paper should not touch the wound at any time.
5. When bleeding ceases, stop the watch and release the blood pressure cuff.
6. Record the bleeding times of the two

puncture sites and report the average of the two results. The normal bleeding time is 1 to 7 minutes, with bleeding times of 7 to 11 minutes considered borderline.

DISCUSSION

1. If bleeding continues for more than 15 minutes, the procedure should be discontinued and pressure applied to the wound sites. The bleeding time should be repeated on the other arm. If bleeding has again not ceased within 15 minutes, the results are reported as greater than 15 minutes.
2. The greatest source of variation in this test is largely due to difficulty in performing a standardized puncture. This usually leads to erroneously low results. On the other hand, if a small vein is punctured, the bleeding time will be prolonged. Therefore, if the bleeding time is less than 1 minute or greater than 7 minutes, the procedure should be repeated using the other arm.

Mielke Method

A modification of the Ivy bleeding time has been described by Mielke and associates (Mielke, C.H., Kaneshiro, I.A., Maher, J.M., Weiner, J.M., and Rapaport, S.I.: The standardized normal Ivy bleeding time and its prolongation by aspirin, Blood, 34, 204, 1969). In this procedure, a Bard-Parker or similar disposable blade is employed, along with a rectangular polystyrene or plastic template that contains a standardized slit. The blade is placed in a special handle containing a gauge to standardize the depth of the incision. The slit in the template will standardize the length of the incision. The same procedure that was described for the Ivy bleeding time is employed, utilizing the blood pressure cuff. Two incisions, 9 mm long and 1 mm deep, are made. The average of the two bleeding times is reported. Normal values for this procedure are 2.5 to 10 min-

utes. It should be noted, however, that small scars may be caused by this method.

Simplate Method

The bleeding time, utilizing the Simplate bleeding time device (manufactured by General Diagnostics, Division of Warner-Lambert Company), is a modification of the Ivy procedure and gives results similar to those obtained in the Mielke test. The Simplate contains a spring-loaded blade within a white plastic case. When the tear-away tab (Fig. 148) is removed, the trigger may be depressed, and the edge of the blade (5 mm in length) will spring 1 mm forward out from the housing. The incision made is 5 mm long and 1 mm deep. A Simplate bleeding time device is also available in the form of two blades in one housing (for duplicate testing).

REFERENCE

General Diagnostics: *Simplate Bleeding Time Device,* General Diagnostics, Morris Plains, New Jersey, 1978.

REAGENTS AND EQUIPMENT

1. Blood pressure cuff.
2. Simplate bleeding time device.
3. Stopwatch.
4. Circular filter paper.

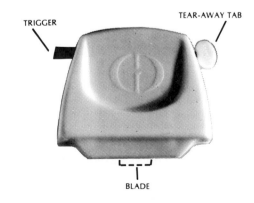

Fig. 148. Simplate bleeding time device.

5. Alcohol sponges.
6. Butterfly bandage.

PRINCIPLE

A uniform incision, 5 mm long and 1 mm deep, is made on the forearm, and the length of time required for bleeding to cease is recorded.

PROCEDURE

1. Place a blood pressure cuff on the patient's arm above the elbow. Increase the pressure to 40 mm Hg and hold this exact pressure for the entire procedure.
2. Cleanse an area on the volar surface of the forearm with an alcohol sponge.
3. Remove the tear-away tab on the Simplate and place it firmly on the forearm, either perpendicular or parallel to the fold of the elbow. (Make certain the area is free of scars, surface veins, and bruises.)
4. Depress the trigger and start the stopwatch. Remove the device approximately 1 second after making the incision. (The incision should be made within 30 to 60 seconds after the blood pressure cuff has been inflated to 40 mm Hg.)
5. Blot the blood from the puncture site on a clean section of the filter paper every 30 seconds. The filter paper should not touch the wound at any time.
6. When bleeding ceases, stop the watch and release the blood pressure cuff. Record the results. The normal range for this procedure is 2.3 to 9.5 minutes.
7. Place a butterfly bandage over the puncture site, and advise the patient to keep the bandage in place for 24 hours.

DISCUSSION

1. Some patients may receive slight scarring at the incision site and should be so informed prior to performing this procedure.

COAGULATION TIME OF WHOLE BLOOD

In the past, the Lee and White clotting time was used as a screening test to measure all stages in the intrinsic coagulation system and to monitor heparin therapy. Today, however, it is a very time-consuming test, has poor reproducibility, is sensitive to only severe factor deficiencies, and is insensitive to high doses of heparin. It is, therefore, of limited use in today's laboratory. In the coagulation of blood in this procedure, most of the time is consumed in the production of the prothrombin activator (plasma thromboplastin). It requires only a matter of seconds to convert prothrombin to thrombin and fibrinogen to fibrin. Therefore, moderate deficiencies in stages 2 and 3 of the coagulation process do not significantly prolong the clotting time. The coagulation time is influenced mainly by defects in stage 1 of the clotting process. Severe hemophilia, afibrinogenemia, and severe fibrinolytic states cause a prolonged clotting time. The presence of an anticoagulant, such as heparin, also causes an abnormally long clotting time.

There are a number of modifications of the in vitro test for the coagulation time of whole blood. They are all based on the same principle and the same basic techniques. The size of the tubes, the amount of blood used, and the temperature at which the determination is performed are the main variables between the different modifications employed. Each of the modified tests, therefore, shows a slight variation in the normal values. Once a technique is chosen, the test must be run under those same conditions each time. The normal values for the test described below are 5 to 15 minutes.

Lee and White Method

REFERENCE

Lee, R.I., and White, P.D.: A clinical study of the coagulation time of whole blood, Am. J. Med. Sci., *145*, 495, 1913.

REAGENTS AND EQUIPMENT

1. Water bath, 37°C.
2. Glass test tubes, 13 × 100 mm.
3. Stopwatch.
4. Syringe (10 ml) and 20-gauge needle.

SPECIMEN

Fresh whole blood, 4 ml.

PRINCIPLE

The coagulation time of whole blood is the length of time required for a measured amount of blood to clot under certain specified conditions.

PROCEDURE

1. Label three 13 × 100-mm test tubes, No. 1, No. 2, and No. 3.
2. Perform a clean, untraumatic venipuncture using a 20-gauge needle and withdraw 4 ml of blood. Start the stopwatch as soon as the blood enters the syringe.
3. After obtaining 4 ml of blood from the patient, remove the needle from the syringe, and carefully place 1 ml of the blood in test tube No. 3, then 1 ml in tube No. 2, and lastly, 1 ml in tube No. 1. The last 1 ml of blood may be discarded.
4. Place the three test tubes in a 37°C water bath.
5. At exactly 5 minutes, tilt test tube No. 1 gently to a 45° angle. Repeat this procedure every 30 seconds, until the test tube can be completely inverted without spilling the contents (that is, until the blood is completely clotted).
6. Record the time it took the blood in test tube No. 1 to clot.

7. Thirty seconds after the blood in test tube No. 1 is clotted, proceed with tube No. 2, and repeat the preceding procedure, tilting the test tube every 30 seconds, until a clot is formed. Record the results. Repeat this procedure for test tube No. 3.
8. Since agitation and handling speed up coagulation, the coagulation time is determined by the clotting time of test tube No. 3.

DISCUSSION

1. It is important to place exactly 1 ml of whole blood in each tube. Amounts greater than 1 ml prolong the clotting time. Less than 1 ml of blood in the test tube yields a shortened clotting time.
2. Poor venipuncture technique, causing hemolysis or tissue thromboplastin to mix with the blood, shortens the clotting time.
3. Incubation at 37°C is important if the normal values for the test have been determined using this technique. Temperatures lower than 37°C retard the clotting time.
4. Bubbles entering the syringe when the blood sample is being obtained increase the rate of coagulation. Unnecessary agitation of the blood shortens the coagulation time.
5. At the completion of the Lee and White clotting time, it is suggested that one test tube remain in the 37°C water bath to be checked after 2 and 4 hours for clot retraction. Also, the tube may be allowed to remain in the water bath overnight and checked the next day for abnormal clot lysis.
6. The Lee and White clotting time may also be performed using siliconized glass test tubes in place of the plain glass test tubes used in the previously described method. Using the same procedure, the normal clotting time (using siliconized tubes and tilting the tubes every 5 minutes) is 20

to 60 minutes. This method is more sensitive to coagulation deficiencies than the unsiliconized test tube procedure. Because of the time involved, however, it is not a practical method for the routine hematology laboratory.

7. The activated clotting time is a modification of the whole blood clotting time and is performed by adding an activator such as Celite or silica to the test tubes. This causes maximum activation of factor XII, a shorter clotting time, and is much more sensitive to factor deficiencies and for monitoring heparin therapy.

CLOT RETRACTION

When blood coagulation is complete, the clot normally undergoes contraction, where serum is expressed from the clot, and the clot becomes denser. Thrombosthenin, released by the platelets, is responsible for clot retraction. In addition, the number of platelets present also affects the clot retraction time. If the platelet count is below 100,000 per μl, poor clot retraction may occur. In rare instances where the platelet count is normal, there may be poor clot retraction due to an abnormality present in the platelets. Normally, clot retraction begins within 30 seconds after the blood has clotted. At the end of 1 hour, there should be appreciable clot retraction and almost complete retraction by the end of 4 hours. Clot retraction should be complete within 24 hours. An abnormal clot retraction time is found in Glanzmann's thrombasthenia.

REFERENCE

Cartwright, G.E.: *Diagnostic Laboratory Hematology*, Grune & Stratton, Inc., New York, 1963.

REAGENTS AND EQUIPMENT

1. Water bath, 37°C.
2. Glass test tubes, 13 × 100 mm.

SPECIMEN

One of the tubes containing 1 ml of whole blood, used in the Lee and White clotting time, or 3 ml of whole fresh blood, placed in a 13 × 100-mm glass test tube.

PRINCIPLE

Whole fresh blood is placed in a 37°C water bath and inspected at 1, 2, 4, and 24 hours for the presence of a retracted clot.

PROCEDURE

1. If a Lee and White clotting time was not performed, obtain 3 ml of blood and dispense carefully into a 13 × 100-mm glass test tube.
2. Place the test tube of blood in the 37°C water bath and allow the blood to clot.
3. As soon as the blood has clotted, inspect the clot at 1, 2, 4, and 24 hours for the formation of a retracted clot. The clot should be firm and retracted from the sides of the tube. It generally occupies a little more than half of the original volume.
4. If a Lee and White clotting time was performed, use one of the three tubes of blood and check for clot retraction at 1, 2, 4, and 24 hours after the blood clotted.
5. Results are reported as the length of time it took for the clotted blood to retract. As an alternative method, the results may be reported as normal, if clot retraction has occurred at 2 to 4 hours; poor, if retraction occurs after 4 hours and within 24 hours; and nil, if no retraction occurs after 24 hours.

DISCUSSION

1. Clot retraction should be almost complete within 4 hours. Normally, the clot will retract from the walls of the test tube until the red blood cell

mass occupies approximately 50% of the total volume of blood in the tube. In abnormal states, there may be variable degrees of retraction or no retraction at all.

2. Shaking or jarring of the test tube of blood should be avoided. This may lead to a shortened clot retraction time.

3. Clot retraction varies inversely with the plasma fibrinogen concentration. That is, if the plasma fibrinogen level is elevated, clot retraction may be poor.

4. Clot retraction may be affected by the red blood cell mass. In blood containing a large mass of red blood cells, the degree of retraction is limited because of the large volume of red blood cells within the clot. In anemic states, the reverse occurs, and the degree of clot retraction is increased.

5. Generally there is a small amount of what is termed *red blood cell fallout* during clot retraction. This is seen as a few red blood cells at the bottom of the tube that have fallen from the clot. The significance of an increased amount of red blood cell fallout is not known. When the fibrinogen level is slightly decreased, however, there will be an increased number of free red blood cells at the bottom of the tube. Whenever red blood cell fallout is increased, a notation on the patient's report should be made.

CLOT LYSIS

The clot used in the clot retraction procedure should be kept at 37°C and examined at the end of 8, 24, 48, and 72 hours for clot lysis. Normally, there is no clot lysis before 72 hours. If the clot that was initially formed becomes fluid in less than 72 hours, abnormal clot lysis is present. The time at which lysis was observed is reported as the clot lysis time. If no lysis occurred, the results are reported as, "no clot lysis after 48 and 72 hours."

PROTHROMBIN TIME

The prothrombin time is a useful screening procedure for deficiencies in factors II, V, VII, and X. Deficiencies in factor I, although rare, may also be detected. This test may be used to follow the course of anticoagulant therapy in patients receiving coumarin drugs. Factors II, VII, IX, and X are inhibited by the coumarin drugs, with factor VII showing decreased activity first. Common causes of a prolonged prothrombin time are vitamin K deficiency, certain liver diseases, specific coagulation deficiencies, and coumarin drug therapy. The normal prothrombin time is generally 11 to 13 seconds. These values, however, differ according to the method and reagents used in the performance of the test. Therefore, each laboratory should determine its own set of normal values.

Quick's One-Stage Prothrombin Time Method

REFERENCE

Quick, A.J.: *Bleeding Problems in Clinical Medicine*, W.B. Saunders Company, Philadelphia, 1970.

REAGENTS AND EQUIPMENT

1. Water bath, 37°C.
2. Thromboplastin-calcium chloride mixture.
3. Normal plasma control.
4. Test tubes, 13 × 100 mm.
5. Stopwatch.

SPECIMEN

Citrated plasma: one part 0.109 M sodium citrate to nine parts whole blood.

PRINCIPLE

The calcium in whole blood is bound by sodium citrate, thus preventing coagulation. Tissue thromboplastin, to which calcium has been added, is mixed with the plasma, and the clotting time is noted.

normal range for the test as performed in your laboratory.

PROCEDURE

1. Centrifuge anticoagulated blood at 2,500 RPM for 10 minutes as soon as possible after blood collection.
2. Remove the plasma from the cells immediately and place on ice.
3. Pipet 0.2 ml of thromboplastin-calcium mixture into the appropriate number of 13 × 100-mm test tubes. Warm the test tubes in the incubator for at least 1 minute, until they have reached 37°C. The incubation period for this mixture is not critical once it reaches 37°C.
4. Incubate the plasma for approximately 2 to 3 minutes, until it reaches 37°C. Plasma should be incubated for no longer than 5 minutes after reaching 37°C.
5. Forcibly blow 0.1 ml of patient's plasma into the test tube containing 0.2 ml of thromboplastin-calcium mixture and simultaneously start the stopwatch.
6. Mix the contents of the tube, and if the tilt method is being used, remove the tube from the water bath and wipe dry. Gently tilt the tube back and forth until a clot forms, at which point the timing is stopped.
7. If the Nichrome wire loop method is preferred, pass the wire loop through the mixture at the rate of two sweeps per second until a formed clot adheres to the loop.
8. Each test and control plasma should be performed in duplicate. The results should agree with each other within ±0.5 seconds when the prothrombin time is below 30 seconds. Duplicate tests on a prothrombin time above 30 seconds will not agree as closely.
9. Average the two results and report the patient's results along with the

DISCUSSION

1. The prothrombin time may also be performed by a semiautomated method using the fibrometer or by a more completely automated method employing optical density readings.
2. A normal plasma control should be run with each group of tests performed. In addition, a normal and an abnormal plasma control should be run each time a new bottle of thromboplastin-calcium mixture is opened. The abnormal control should be in the range of about 25 seconds (20 to 30 seconds) or in the same range as the majority of patients on oral anticoagulant therapy.
3. When reconstituting the thromboplastin-calcium solution, mix well. Excessive shaking does not affect this solution.
4. Generally, the thromboplastin-calcium mixture is a suspension and not a homogeneous solution. It is, therefore, imperative that the suspension be well mixed whenever it is used.
5. Patients receiving coumarin drugs for thromboembolic disorders generally have prothrombin times of 20 to 30 seconds, or 1.5 to 2.5 times their normal prothrombin time.
6. Normal plasma control values must fall within the laboratory's normal range. If the control results fall outside of this range, there is something wrong with the equipment, reagents, or techniques used, and the test must be repeated.
7. If the patient is receiving heparin, the prothrombin must be drawn at least 4 hours after the last injection, or the results obtained for the prothrombin time will be invalidated.

ACTIVATED PARTIAL THROMBOPLASTIN TIME

The *activated partial thromboplastin time (APTT)* is the single most useful procedure available for routine screening of coagulation disorders in the intrinsic system. It measures those coagulation factors present in the intrinsic system except for platelets and factor XIII. (Factor VII is not measured because it is in the extrinsic system.) The APTT is also the method of choice for monitoring heparin therapy. The normal range for the APTT may vary widely from one laboratory to another and is dependent on the reagents used and the clot detection method employed. It is, therefore, very important that each laboratory determine its own normal range for the specific lot number and type of reagents used. Generally speaking, the normal mean value for the APTT will usually fall between 30 and 40 seconds.

REFERENCE

Proctor, R.R., and Rapaport, S.I.: The partial thromboplastin time with kaolin, Am. J. Clin. Path., 36, 212, 1961.

REAGENTS AND EQUIPMENT

1. Water bath, 37°C.
2. Calcium chloride, 0.025 M.
   Anhydrous calcium   1.38 g
      chloride
   Distilled water   500 ml
3. Partial thromboplastin containing an activator (commercially available).
4. Normal control plasma.
5. Test tubes, 13 × 100 mm.
6. Stopwatch.

SPECIMEN

Citrated plasma: one part 0.109 M sodium citrate to nine parts whole blood. Immediately after blood collection, place the tube of blood in a cup of crushed ice and deliver it to the laboratory.

PRINCIPLE

The calcium in whole blood is bound by the anticoagulant to prevent coagulation. The plasma, after centrifugation, contains all intrinsic coagulation factors except calcium and platelets. Calcium, a phospholipid substitute for platelets (partial thromboplastin), and an activator (to ensure maximal activation), are added to the plasma. The time required for the plasma to clot is the activated partial thromboplastin time.

PROCEDURE

1. Centrifuge the anticoagulated blood at 2,500 RPM for 10 minutes as soon as possible after the blood has been collected.
2. Remove the plasma from the cells immediately and place on ice.
3. Incubate a sufficient amount of 0.025 M calcium chloride at 37°C.
4. Pipet 0.2 ml of normal control plasma (or patient's plasma) into a 13 × 100-mm test tube.
5. Pipet 0.2 ml of the partial thromboplastin (containing activator) into the test tube containing the control (or patient's) plasma.
6. Mix the contents of the tube quickly and place in a 37°C water bath for 3 minutes.
7. After exactly 3 minutes, blow in 0.2 ml of the prewarmed calcium chloride and simultaneously start the stopwatch.
8. Mix the test tube once, immediately after adding the calcium chloride. Allow the test tube to remain in the water bath while gently tilting the tube every 5 seconds. At the end of 20 seconds, remove the test tube from the water bath. Quickly wipe off the outside of the test tube with a clean gauze so that the contents of the tube can be clearly seen.
9. Gently tilt the test tube back and forth until a clot forms, at which point the timing is stopped.
10. Control and patient plasma specimens must always be run in duplicate, and the two results averaged to

obtain the final value. The two results should check within ±1.5 seconds of each other. If they do not, another test should be performed. When the clotting time is prolonged, however, duplication of results is more difficult, and the allowable range of variation is wider. In certain abnormal states, clot formation is markedly prolonged. If formation of the clot has not started by the end of 2 minutes, the test may be stopped and the results reported as greater than 2 minutes.

11. Report the patient's results along with the normal range for the test as determined for the laboratory. (Normal control results must always fall within the normal range; otherwise, something is wrong with reagents, equipment, or the technique being used, and the entire test must be repeated.)

DISCUSSION

1. When the APTT is abnormally prolonged, there may be a deficiency in one of the coagulation factors, or there may be an inhibitor(s) present in the patient's plasma. To differentiate between these two abnormal states, perform, in duplicate, as described previously, an APTT, mixing 0.1 ml of normal control plasma with 0.1 ml of patient's plasma (in place of the usual 0.2 ml of patient's plasma). If the results are closer to the value received for the normal plasma control, the problem is probably due to a deficiency of one of the coagulation factors. (The APTT gives normal results when there is a 50% concentration of the coagulation factors present.) If, however, the results received are closer to the original results (using 0.2 ml of the patient's plasma), the defect is thought to be due to an inhibitor(s) present in the patient's plasma.

2. The partial thromboplastin time (without an activator) is performed in exactly the same way as the APTT, using partial thromboplastin without an activator. The normal results for the PTT performed in this way are generally 40 to 100 seconds, with a result of 120 seconds or longer being considered abnormal. The activator in the APTT allows for maximum activation of the contact factors and gives more consistent and reproducible results.

3. The APTT does not test for factor VII or platelets. It detects deficiencies in factors I, II, V, VIII, IX, X, and is also sensitive to circulating anticoagulants or inhibitors. The test is somewhat insensitive to deficiencies in factors XI and XII, the contact factors.

4. The PTT and APTT are much more sensitive to coagulation factor deficiencies than is the whole blood clotting time.

5. If the partial thromboplastin becomes frozen before use (for example, in shipment during the winter), the results of the PTT may be prolonged by as much as 15 or more seconds.

6. If there are sufficient stopwatches available, it is possible to do more than one test at a time by starting each of the 3-minute incubations at 2-minute intervals.

7. The APTT should be performed within 2 hours of blood collection to avoid invalidly prolonged results.

8. An abnormally shortened APTT may be caused by partial clotting of the blood as a result of difficulty in obtaining the blood sample. There may or may not be a clot present in the tube of blood. In circumstances such as this, it is advisable to obtain a new blood sample.

9. A normal plasma control should be run with each group of tests performed. In addition, a normal and an

abnormal plasma control should be run each time a new bottle of reagent is opened. The abnormal control should generally be in a range somewhere between 50 and 70 seconds.

PLASMA RECALCIFICATION TIME
(Plasma Clotting Time)

The plasma recalcification time is a measure of the overall intrinsic coagulation process. In the procedure outlined here, a deficiency in platelets or platelet activity is not detected. The normal plasma recalcification time on platelet-poor plasma is 90 to 250 seconds. A decrease in any of the clotting factors present in the intrinsic system will cause a prolonged clotting time.

REFERENCES

Briggs, R., and MacFarlane, R.G.: *Human Blood Coagulation and Its Disorders*, Blackwell Scientific Publications, Oxford, 1962.

Eli Lilly and Company: ART coagulation test advocated in pre-surgery cases, Clinical Laboratory Forum, 5, 4, 1970.

Miale, J.B.: *Laboratory Medicine: Hematology*, 6th ed., C.V. Mosby Company, St. Louis, 1982.

REAGENTS AND EQUIPMENT

1. Water bath, 37°C.
2. Calcium chloride, 0.025 M.
Anhydrous calcium chloride	1.38 g
Distilled water	500 ml
3. Sodium chloride, 0.85% (w/v).
4. Normal platelet-poor control plasma.
5. Test tubes, 13 × 100 mm.
6. Stopwatch.

SPECIMEN

Citrated plasma: one part 0.109 M sodium citrate to nine parts whole blood; or oxalated plasma: one part 0.1 M sodium oxalate to nine parts whole blood.

PRINCIPLE

Platelet-poor plasma is mixed with sufficient calcium chloride to neutralize the effects of the anticoagulant, and the clotting time is then recorded.

PROCEDURE

1. Immediately after collection, centrifuge blood at 2,500 RPM for at least 20 minutes to obtain a platelet-poor plasma.
2. Incubate, at 37°C for 2 to 3 minutes prior to each test, each of the following in separate test tubes:
   A. Patient's platelet-poor plasma
   B. Normal platelet-poor control plasma
   C. Calcium chloride, 0.025 M
   D. Sodium chloride, 0.85%
3. Into a 13 × 100-mm test tube in the 37°C water bath pipet 0.1 ml of 0.85% sodium chloride and 0.1 ml of patient's plasma. Mix.
4. Blow in 0.1 ml of 0.025 M calcium chloride and simultaneously start a stopwatch.
5. Allow the tube to remain in the 37°C water bath for 90 seconds, tilting the test tube gently every 30 seconds.
6. After 90 seconds, remove the test tube from the water bath and gently tilt. Stop the watch as soon as a clot forms, and record the results.

DISCUSSION

1. The plasma recalcification time varies according to the number of platelets present in the plasma. As the number of platelets increases, the plasma recalcification time shortens. Therefore, it is important to centrifuge the blood in the prescribed manner.
2. The plasma recalcification time may be performed on platelet-rich plasma, in which case the normal range is 90 to 120 seconds. Plasma specimens containing a standard

number of platelets, however, are difficult to obtain.

3. A modification of the plasma clotting time is called the *activated recalcification time* and employs the use of 0.1 ml of platelet-rich plasma, 0.1 ml of 0.03 M calcium chloride, and 0.1 ml of 1% Celite as an activator. The normal clotting time in this procedure is less than 50 seconds.

THROMBIN TIME

The thrombin time tests the third stage of coagulation, the conversion of fibrinogen to fibrin. It measures the availability of functional fibrinogen. The normal thrombin time for this procedure is 15 to 20 seconds. Prolonged times are found when the fibrinogen level is below 100 mg per dl, when the function of fibrinogen is impaired, and in the presence of thrombin-inhibitors such as heparin or fibrin-split products. The thrombin time is a most sensitive test in detecting heparin inhibition. The thrombin time may be normally prolonged in the newborn and in multiple myeloma (the abnormal globulin interferes with the polymerization of fibrin).

REFERENCE

Rapaport, S.I., and Ames, S.B.: Clotting factor assay on plasma from patients receiving intramuscular or subcutaneous heparin, Am. J. Med. Sci., *234*, 678, 1957.

REAGENTS AND EQUIPMENT

1. Stock thrombin (100 units per 1 ml). Reconstitute one vial of Bovine Thrombin, Topical, 5,000 NIH units (Parke, Davis & Company, Detroit, Michigan.) with 5 ml of saline diluent. Add 100 mg of barium sulfate and incubate at 37°C for 20 minutes. Centrifuge at 2,500 RPM for 5 minutes. Carefully remove the supernatant and add it to 20 ml of 0.85% sodium chloride and 25 ml of glycerin. This mixture, stored at 0°C, is stable for several months.

2. Tris buffer, pH 7.35.
   Sigma 121 Primary Standard   6 g
     Biochemical Buffer
   Sodium chloride   6.6 g
   Hydrochloric acid, 0.1 N   440 ml
   Dilute to 1,000 ml with distilled water. Store at 4°C.

3. Normal control plasma.
4. Water bath, 37°C.
5. Nichrome wire loop.
6. Stopwatch.
7. Test tubes, 13 × 100 mm.

SPECIMEN

Plasma obtained from whole blood collected in sodium oxalate, sodium citrate, or EDTA.

PRINCIPLE

A measured amount of thrombin is added to plasma. The length of time for a fibrin clot to form is recorded as the thrombin time.

PROCEDURE

1. Centrifuge blood at 2,500 RPM for 10 minutes to obtain platelet-poor plasma.

2. Immediately before use, prepare working thrombin solution by diluting 0.1 ml of stock thrombin with 0.9 ml of Tris buffer. Incubate at 37°C. (This solution is stable for 20 minutes at 37°C.)

3. Incubate a sufficient amount of Tris buffer at 37°C.

4. Place 0.2 ml of patient's plasma or normal control into a 13 × 100-mm test tube.

5. Add 0.2 ml of Tris buffer to the tube, mix, and allow to incubate for 1 minute.

6. At the end of 1 minute, pipet 0.2 ml of working thrombin solution into the tube, simultaneously starting the stopwatch.

7. With a Nichrome wire loop, sweep

through the mixture, two times per second, until a clot is formed. Stop the watch and record the thrombin time.

8. Run a normal control with each series of thrombin times. Each specimen must be tested in duplicate.

DISCUSSION

1. Duplicate tests performed on the same plasma sample should check within ±1.5 seconds of each other.
2. Whenever thrombin is used, plastic or siliconized pipets should be employed to pipet the thrombin.
3. The concentration of thrombin in the working thrombin solution should be at a concentration that gives a clotting time of 15 to 20 seconds on normal plasma. When the stock thrombin solution is first prepared, it may be necessary to use a 1:12 or greater dilution when preparing the working thrombin mixture. As the stock solution ages, the reverse is true, and a dilution of 1:8 or less with Tris buffer may be required.
4. If the thrombin time is greater than 25 seconds, repeat the procedure, using a 1:1 mixture of the patient's plasma and normal control to test for inhibitors. If inhibitors are present, the thrombin time will not be shortened.

FIBRINOGEN TITER

A deficiency in fibrinogen is a rare occurrence. When it does occur, however, it may produce severe hemorrhage, and little time should be lost in diagnosing the problem. A lack of fibrinogen may be caused by a congenital defect, and it may also be found in certain obstetric and surgical cases. A chronic deficiency of fibrinogen may occur in such cases as liver disease, where production may be defective. Elevated fibrinogen levels are normally found in pregnancy, near term or after delivery. The fibrinogen titer is useful in detecting a deficiency in fibrinogen and in detecting an alteration in the conversion of fibrinogen to fibrin. The normal fibrinogen titer is 1:128 to 1:256. A titer below 1:64 is abnormal.

REFERENCES

Biggs, R., and MacFarlane, R.G.: *Human Blood Coagulation and Its Disorders*, Blackwell Scientific Publications, Oxford, 1962.

Schneider, C.L.: Rapid estimation of plasma fibrinogen concentration and its use as a guide to therapy of intravascular defibrination, Am. J. Obstet. Gynecol., 64, 141, 1962.

Tocantins, L.M., and Kazal, L.A.: *Blood Coagulation, Hemorrhage and Thrombosis*, Grune & Stratton, Inc., New York, 1964.

REAGENTS AND EQUIPMENT

1. Water bath, 37°C.
2. Glass test tubes, 13 × 100 mm.
3. Sodium chloride, 0.85% (w/v).
4. Pipets, 1 ml, plastic.
5. Thrombin (100 units per 1 ml). Reconstitute one vial of Bovine Thrombin, Topical, 5,000 NIH units (Parke, Davis & Company, Detroit, Michigan) with 5 ml of saline diluent. Add 100 mg of barium sulfate and incubate at 37°C for 20 minutes. Centrifuge at 2,500 RPM for 5 minutes. Carefully remove the supernatant and add it to 20 ml of 0.85% sodium chloride and 25 ml of glycerin. This mixture, stored at 0°C, will be stable for several months.
6. Control plasma from a normal individual.

SPECIMEN

Citrated plasma: one part 0.109 M sodium citrate to nine parts whole blood or oxalated plasma: one part 0.1 M sodium oxalate to nine parts whole blood. Citrated blood is recommended because oxalated plasma may yield lower titration results.

PRINCIPLE

Thrombin is added to serial dilutions of the patient's plasma. The fibrinogen titer is the highest plasma dilution in which a visible fibrin clot forms.

PROCEDURE

1. Centrifuge the control and patient's blood at 2,500 RPM for 10 minutes and remove the plasma.
2. Number consecutively two sets of eight, 13 × 100-mm test tubes and place in two rows in a test tube rack. One set of test tubes is for the control plasma and one set for the patient's plasma.
3. Pipet 0.5 ml of 0.85% sodium chloride into each of the 16 test tubes.
4. Pipet 0.5 ml of normal plasma into test tube No. 1 of the control set. Serially dilute the control plasma by mixing test tube No. 1 and transferring 0.5 ml of the diluted plasma to test tube No. 2. Mix test tube No. 2 and pipet 0.5 ml to tube No. 3, and so on. Discard 0.5 ml of the dilution from test tube No. 8.
5. Pipet 0.5 ml of the patient's plasma into test tube No. 1 of the patient's test tubes and serially dilute as described in step 4.
6. Add 0.1 ml of thrombin solution to each of the 16 tubes and mix.
7. Place the test tubes in a 37°C water bath for 15 minutes.
8. At the end of 15 minutes, observe each test tube for the presence of a clot.
9. The highest dilution in which a clot is visible is reported as the fibrinogen titer (Table 11).

DISCUSSION

1. When checking the test tubes for clot formation, tilt the tubes gently.
2. The results of the normal control should fall within the normal range. If not, the thrombin may be unsatis-

TABLE 11. PLASMA DILUTIONS FOR THE FIBRINOGEN TITER

TEST TUBE NUMBER	DILUTION
1	1:2
2	1:4
3	1:8
4	1:16
5	1:32
6	1:64
7	1:128
8	1:256

factory. The test should be repeated with a new mixture of thrombin.
3. Whenever thrombin is used, plastic or siliconized pipets should be employed to pipet the thrombin.
4. It is advisable to keep the test tubes in the 37°C water bath and check for lysis of the clots at 1, 2, and 24 hours after the fibrinogen titer has been read. Lysis of the clots is indicative of increased fibrinolysis.
5. When reading the fibrinogen titer, if the first few test tubes (lower dilutions) contain no clot, but there is clot formation in the last tube(s) (higher dilutions), the presence of a circulating anticoagulant is indicated.

QUANTITATIVE FIBRINOGEN

The following procedure is a method for determining the amount of fibrinogen in a plasma. Although it is a quantitative method, it can be included in the coagulation screen in place of the thrombin time. This procedure is quick and easy to perform.

The normal value for this test is 200 to 400 mg per dl.

REFERENCE

Dade Diagnostics, Inc., American Hospital Supply Corporation: *Data-Fi Fibrinogen Determination Reagents*, Dade Division, American Hospital Supply Corporation, Miami, Florida, 1982.

REAGENTS AND EQUIPMENT

1. Data-Fi Thrombin Reagent, approximately 100 NIH units. Reconstitute with 1.0 ml of distilled water. (This reagent is good for 8 hours after reconstituting when it is stored at room temperature or 4°C.)
2. Data-Fi Fibrinogen Calibration Reference. Reconstitute with 1.0 ml of distilled water. (After reconstitution, this reagent is good for 4 hours when it is stored at 4°C.) Do not shake this reagent.
3. Owren's Veronal Buffer (pH 7.35). This reagent is stable indefinitely at room temperature or at 4°C.
4. Dade Ci-trol Normal (citrated normal plasma) or SNP (standardized normal plasma.). Reconstitute with 1.0 ml of distilled water and mix gently. If citrated plasma is employed, use Ci-trol Normal; with oxalated plasma, use SNP.
   Note: Reagent numbers 1, 2, 3, and 4 are available from Dade Diagnostics, Inc., American Hopsital Supply Corporation, Miami, Florida.
5. Test tubes, 12 × 75 mm.
6. Pipets, 1.0 ml, 2.0 ml, 0.2 ml, and 0.1 ml.
7. Water bath, 37°C.
8. Stopwatch.
9. Wire loop (or fibrometer or Mechrolab Clot-Timer).
10. Double log graph paper.

SPECIMEN

Citrated plasma: one part 0.109 M sodium citrate to nine parts whole blood; or oxalated plasma: one part 0.1 M sodium oxalate to nine parts whole blood.

PRINCIPLE

A measured amount of thrombin is added to plasma, and the clotting time is noted. This result is compared with clotting times of plasma specimens containing known amounts of fibrinogen. From this information, the amount of fibrinogen in mg per dl in the unknown sample can be determined.

PROCEDURE

1. The first time this procedure is set up and each time a new lot number of thrombin is used, a new calibration curve must be set up as outlined below.
   A. Label two 12 × 75-mm test tubes, 1:5.
   Label two 12 × 75-mm test tubes, 1:15.
   Label two 12 × 75-mm test tubes, 1:40.
   B. Place 1.6 ml of Owren's Veronal Buffer in each of the preceding test tubes labeled 1:5; 0.8 ml of Owren's Veronal Buffer into each of the 1:15 labeled test tubes; 2.8 ml of Owren's Veronal Buffer into the two test tubes labeled 1:40.
   C. Add 0.4 ml of the Fibrinogen Calibration Reference to both of the test tubes labeled 1:5. Mix both test tubes. Transfer 0.4 ml from the 1:5 dilution into each of the test tubes labeled 1:15. Mix the 1:15 dilutions. Again, transfer 0.4 ml of the 1:5 dilution into each of the test tubes labeled 1:40. Mix the 1:40 dilutions.
   D. Reconstitute Thrombin Reagent with 1.0 ml of distilled water. Mix well. Keep at room temperature.
   E. Pipet 0.2 ml of the 1:5 diluted Fibrinogen Calibration Reference into each of two 12 × 75-mm test tubes. (One 0.2-ml sample from each of the 1:5 dilutions.)
   F. Incubate the two test tubes at 37°C for at least 2 minutes but no longer than 5 minutes.
   G. Pipet 0.1 ml of Thrombin Reagent into the first test tube and immediately start the stopwatch.
   H. While keeping the test tube in the water bath, immediately begin running the wire loop through the

mixture. At the first sign of fibrin formation, stop the stopwatch and record the result. Repeat steps E through H for the duplicate specimen. Average the two results. If the clotting times are too far apart, however, repeat steps E through H again, or set up two more dilutions and repeat.

I. Repeat steps E through H for the 1:15 and 1:40 dilutions.

J. Using double log graph paper, draw a fibrinogen curve as shown in Figure 149.

K. Use Ci-trol Normal (or SNP) to check the preceding curve. Reconstitute the Ci-trol Normal with 1.0 ml of distilled water. Allow to sit for 10 to 15 minutes. Mix gently. Dilute the Ci-trol Normal 1:10; place 0.9 ml of Owren's Veronal Buffer into a 12 × 75-mm test tube and add 0.1 ml of Ci-trol Normal. Mix well. Determine the clotting time on duplicate samples of the diluted Ci-trol Normal, following steps E through H. Using the previously drawn fi-

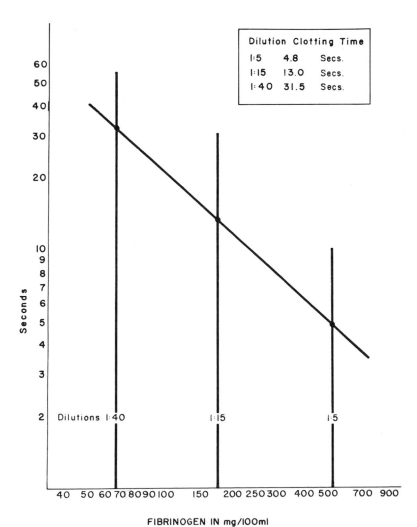

Dilution	Clotting Time	
1:5	4.8	Secs.
1:15	13.0	Secs.
1:40	31.5	Secs.

Fig. 149. Curve for quantitative fibrinogen procedure.

brinogen curve, determine the fibrinogen value in mg per dl for the Ci-trol Normal. This result should fall within the ranges given for that lot number of Ci-trol Normal.

2. Centrifuge the blood at 2,500 RPM for 10 minutes to obtain platelet-poor plasma.

3. Reconstitute Thrombin Reagent with 1.0 ml of distilled water. Mix carefully.

4. Reconstitute Ci-trol Normal (or SNP) with 1.0 ml of distilled water. Allow to sit for 10 to 15 minutes. Mix gently.

5. Make a 1:10 dilution of both the plasma and Ci-trol Normal: place 0.9 ml of Owren's Veronal Buffer into appropriately labeled 12 × 75-mm test tubes (one test tube for the Ci-trol Normal and one test tube for each specimen to be tested). Add 0.1 ml of Ci-trol Normal to the control test tube and 0.1 ml of patient plasma to each of the appropriately labeled patient test tubes. Mix carefully.

6. Pipet 0.2 ml of the diluted Ci-trol Normal into each of two 12 × 75-mm test tubes.

7. Incubate these tubes at 37°C for at least 2 minutes but no longer than 5 minutes.

8. Pipet 0.1 ml of Thrombin Reagent (kept at room temperature) into the first test tube and immediately start the stopwatch.

9. While keeping the test tube in the water bath, immediately begin running the wire loop through the mixture. At the first sign of fibrin formation, stop the stopwatch and record the result.

10. Repeat steps 7 through 9 for the duplicate specimen. Average the two results. Both clotting times should agree with each other within 1.5 seconds. If they do not, repeat steps 7 through 9.

11. Repeat steps 7 through 10 for each patient specimen.

12. Determine the fibrinogen concentration for the Ci-trol Normal and each patient specimen by referring to the previously prepared fibrinogen curve. The Ci-trol Normal result should agree within the ranges given for that lot number of Ci-trol Normal. If it does not, the cause must be found and the entire test repeated on all of the specimens.

DISCUSSION

1. This test should be performed as soon as possible after the blood has been obtained from the patient. The plasma may be stored at 4°C for up to 72 hours, however, with little loss of fibrinogen.

2. When the fibrinogen value is below 50 mg per dl, the plasma should be diluted 1:5 (0.2 ml of plasma added to 0.8 ml of Owren's Veronal Buffer) or 1:2 (0.4 ml of plasma added to 0.4 ml of Owren's Veronal buffer). Perform the fibrinogen in duplicate as outline above, average the results, and determine the fibrinogen value from the curve. Divide these results by two (for the 1:5 dilution) or five (for the 1:2 dilution). If no clot forms with the 1:2 dilution, report a result of less than 15 mg per dl.

3. When the fibrinogen value is above 800 mg per dl, the plasma should be diluted 1:20 (0.1 ml of plasma added to 1.9 ml of Owren's Veronal Buffer). Perform the fibrinogen in duplicate as outlined above, average the results, and determine the fibrinogen value from the curve. Multiply these results by two.

4. In the presence of significant levels of fibrin degradation products (above 100 μg per ml) or heparin (above 0.6 USP units per ml), the test results will be invalidly low.

PROTHROMBIN CONSUMPTION TEST

The prothrombin consumption test is merely a prothrombin time carried out on serum. It tests mainly for the coagulation factors present in stage 1 of the intrinsic system, namely, factors VIII, IX, and platelet factor 3, which are necessary for plasma thromboplastin formation. The normal prothrombin consumption for the procedure outlined below is above 20 seconds but should be determined for each laboratory. Clotting times of 18 to 20 seconds are borderline, and abnormal results show a clotting time of less than 18 seconds. An abnormal prothrombin consumption is found in factors VIII, IX, and platelet factor 3 deficiencies. Deficiencies in factor XI or XII, although of less importance, will be detected because they are also necessary components of stage 1 and needed for plasma thromboplastin generation. If, however, the blood is allowed to clot before proceeding with the test, factor XI and XII deficiencies will not be detected, other than by a prolonged clotting time.

REFERENCE

Lenahan, J.G., and Smith, K.: *Hemostasis*, General Diagnostics, Morris Plains, New Jersey, 1979.

REAGENTS AND EQUIPMENT

1. Water bath, 37°C.
2. Simplastin-A. (This reagent supplies fibrinogen, thromboplastin, calcium, and an optimum amount of factor V. It is available from General Diagnostics, Morris Plains, New Jersey). Reconstitute according to the directions in the package insert.
3. Test tubes, 13 × 100 mm.
4. Stopwatch.

SPECIMEN

Whole blood, 1 to 3 ml, placed in a plain glass test tube (unsiliconized). A normal control blood sample should be obtained at the same time the patient's blood is collected.

PRINCIPLE

When the formation of plasma thromboplastin is normal, all but trace amounts of prothrombin are converted to thrombin. If a prothrombin time is then performed on the serum, with the addition of fibrinogen (and thromboplastin-calcium reagent), the resulting prothrombin time should be prolonged due to decreased amounts of prothrombin. When plasma thromboplastin formation is defective, however, prothrombin conversion to thrombin is decreased, and there is an excess of prothrombin present in the serum. When fibrinogen, thromboplastin, and calcium are added to this serum, therefore, a shortened clotting time results.

PROCEDURE

1. As soon as the patient and control blood specimens are drawn, place them in a 37°C water bath and observe for clotting.
2. Incubate the blood at 37°C for 2 hours after the blood has clotted.
3. Centrifuge the blood at 2,500 RPM for 5 minutes.
4. Remove the serum from the clot. At this point, the serum may be refrigerated for a maximum of 2 hours.
5. Pipet 0.2 ml of Simplastin-A into each of four 13 × 100-mm test tubes and place in the 37°C water bath for 2 minutes.
6. Pipet 0.1 ml of control or patient's serum into one of the preceding test tubes, simultaneously starting the stopwatch.
7. With a Nichrome wire loop, sweep through the mixture at a rate of two sweeps per second. As soon as a fine web or clot forms, stop the watch and record the results.
8. Repeat steps 6 and 7, performing duplicate clotting times on the patient and control serum specimens. Results on the normal control serum must be above 20 seconds for the test to be considered valid.

DISCUSSION

1. In drawing blood, contamination with tissue thromboplastin must be avoided. If this occurs or serum is hemolyzed, the specimen must be redrawn.
2. In place of Simplastin-A, fibrinogen reagent (1.0 ml) may be mixed with thromboplastin-calcium reagent (2.0 ml). The normal results obtained when using these reagents will generally be slightly longer than when the Simplastin-A is used.
3. A severe deficiency in prothrombin yields a normal prothrombin consumption time. Also, a normal result is obtained when there are deficiencies present in more than one factor, such as in Owren's disease (factor V and VIII deficiencies), when one of the decreased factors is present in stage 2 of the coagulation process. Therefore, if the prothrombin time is abnormal, a prothrombin consumption should not be performed.
4. In the presence of thrombocytopenia (decreased platelet count) or abnormally functioning platelets, the prothrombin consumption test need not be performed because platelets are necessary for plasma thromboplastin formation.

FIBRIN STABILIZING FACTOR

Factor XIII, known as the fibrin stabilizing factor, is responsible for converting the fibrin clot to a more stable form. It is thought to exist in the plasma in an inactive form and is activated by thrombin during the fibrinogen-to-fibrin conversion. When factor XIII is present, the fibrin clot formed is insoluble in 5 M urea and should not dissolve in the urea when left standing for 24 hours. A deficiency in this factor is very rare.

REFERENCES

Losowsky, M.S., Hall, R., and Goldie, W.: Congenital deficiency of fibrin-stabilising factor, Lancet, 2, 156, 1965.

Dacie, J.V., and Lewis, S.M.: *Practical Hematology,* 5th ed., Churchill Livingstone, New York, 1975.

REAGENTS AND EQUIPMENT

1. Urea, 5.0 M.

   Urea (desiccator-dried, reagent grade) 300.30 g

   Distilled water 900 ml

   Dissolve urea, and dilute to 1,000 ml with distilled water. Stable at room temperature for several months.
2. Calcium chloride, 0.025 M.

   Anhydrous calcium chloride 1.38 g

   Dilute to 500 ml with distilled water.
3. Normal control plasma.
4. Test tubes, 13 × 100 mm.
5. Water bath, 37°C.

SPECIMEN

Citrated plasma: one part 0.109 M sodium citrate to nine parts whole blood.

PRINCIPLE

The patient's plasma is clotted by the addition of calcium chloride. Urea (5 M) is added to the clot. If factor XIII is not present in the patient's plasma, the clot is dissolved in less than 24 hours by the urea.

PROCEDURE

1. Pipet 0.2 ml of patient's plasma into each of two test tubes. Repeat, pipetting 0.2 ml of normal control plasma into each of two additional test tubes.
2. Add 0.2 ml of 0.025 M calcium chloride to the four test tubes.
3. Incubate the resulting fibrin clots at 37°C for 30 minutes.
4. Loosen the clots from the sides of the test tubes by gently tapping the sides of the tube.
5. Transfer one of the patient's clots and one of the normal control clots to the respective test tubes containing 5 ml

of 5 M urea. Transfer both the remaining patient clot and the normal control clot to a third test tube containing 5 ml of 5 M urea.

6. Allow the mixtures to stand at room temperature.

7. Check the clots at the end of 1, 2, 3, and 24 hours, and note if the clots have dissolved.

8. Report the length of time it took for the patient's clot to dissolve after urea was added. If the clot is still present at the end of 24 hours, report that the clot was insoluble after 24 hours.

DISCUSSION

1. In the absence of factor XIII, the clot usually dissolves within 2 to 3 hours. The test tube containing the normal plasma clot should remain intact for 24 hours, as should the mixed clot of the patient and normal control. If the mixed clot is dissolved, it may be due to some other mechanism, such as fibrinolysis, rather than a deficiency in factor XIII.

2. Monochloroacetic acid (1%, w/v) may be used in place of the 5 M urea for performance of this test.

3. A positive control (a clot that will dissolve in 5 M urea) may also be performed along with the patient test using thrombin and EDTA plasma. Add 10 NIH units of thrombin (0.5 ml of 20 NIH units per ml of thrombin) to 0.5 ml of EDTA plasma. Place the resultant clot in 5.0 ml of 5 M urea. This clot should be dissolved within 24 hours due to the lack of calcium that is necessary for the action of factor XIII.

HICKS-PITNEY TEST

The Hicks-Pitney test is a modification of the thromboplastin generation test. It is a rapid screening test for disorders of thromboplastin generation and detects deficiencies in factors V, VIII, IX, X, XI, and

XII. The test does not, however, distinguish between these defects. If the patient's prothrombin time is normal, a deficiency in factor V or X may be ruled out.

Hicks and Pitney Method

REFERENCE

Hicks N.D., and Pitney, W.R.: A rapid screening test for disorders of thromboplastin generation, Br. J. Haematol., 3, 227, 1957.

REAGENTS AND EQUIPMENT

1. Water bath, 37°C.
2. Calcium chloride, 0.025 M.
   Anhydrous calcium chloride   1.38 g
   Distilled water   500 ml
3. Normal control plasma (plasma substrate).
4. Partial thromboplastin (platelet substitute). (Commercially available.)
5. Sodium chloride, 0.85% (w/v).
6. Test tubes, 13 × 100 mm.
7. Stopwatch.

SPECIMEN

Citrated plasma: one part 0.109 M sodium citrate to nine parts whole blood. Collect one test tube each from the patient and a normal control.

PRINCIPLE

The patient's diluted plasma is mixed with a platelet substitute and calcium chloride. The ability of the patient's plasma to form thromboplastin is measured by adding this generation mixture to normal plasma and determining the clotting time. Normally, sufficient thromboplastin is generated in 3 to 5 minutes to clot a normal plasma in 7 to 12 seconds.

PROCEDURE

1. Centrifuge the patient and control blood specimens at 2,500 RPM for 10 minutes immediately after collection.

2. Remove the plasma and place in respective test tubes in crushed ice.

3. Dilute the control plasma and the patient's plasma 1:10 with 0.85% sodium chloride (0.1 ml of plasma in 0.9 ml of 0.85% sodium chloride). Place both diluted plasma specimens on ice.

4. Add 3 ml of 0.025 M calcium chloride to a 13 × 100-mm test tube and incubate at 37°C.

5. Place five 13 × 100-mm test tubes in the 37°C water bath and pipet exactly 0.1 ml of undiluted normal control plasma (plasma substrate) into each test tube.

6. Prepare the control generation mixture in a 13 × 100-mm test tube in the 37°C water bath by the following procedure:
   A. Pipet 0.5 ml of diluted normal control plasma into the test tube.
   B. Add 0.5 ml of partial thromboplastin.
   C. Incubate for 2 minutes.
   D. Add 0.5 ml of 0.025 M calcium chloride and simultaneously start a stopwatch. If a clot forms in this generation mixture at any time, it should be removed so that it will not interfere with pipetting.

7. When 55 seconds have elapsed on the stopwatch, pipet 0.1 ml of the generation mixture. With the other hand, pipet 0.1 ml of the 0.025 M calcium chloride.

8. When 1 minute has elapsed on the stopwatch, blow the 0.1 ml of generation mixture into one of the test tubes containing 0.1 ml of plasma substrate. Immediately blow the 0.1 ml of calcium chloride into the tube and simultaneously start a second stopwatch.

9. Determine the clotting time of this mixture by the tilt tube method. If clotting has not occurred within 40 to 45 seconds, have a second person continue tilting the tube until clotting occurs. Record the results. If the clotting time is greater than 60 seconds, record as over 60 seconds.

10. Repeat steps 7, 8, and 9 at 1-minute intervals for all five test tubes containing the 0.1 ml of plasma substrate. (Start the second clotting time when 1 minute and 55 seconds have elapsed on the first stopwatch.) Do not stop the first stopwatch at any time during this procedure.

11. If any of the five test tubes has a clotting time of 7 to 12 seconds within the 5-minute incubation of the generation mixture, the test is considered to be normal. If the control test run on the plasma substrate is abnormal, the entire test must be repeated.

12. Place five 13 × 100-mm test tubes in the 37°C water bath. Pipet exactly 0.1 ml of undiluted normal control plasma (plasma substrate) into each tube.

13. Prepare the patient's generation mixture in a 13 × 100-mm test tube in the 37°C water bath by the following procedure:
    A. Pipet 0.5 ml of diluted patient's plasma into the test tube.
    B. Add 0.5 ml of platelet substitute to the tube.
    C. Incubate for 2 minutes.
    D. Add 0.5 ml of 0.025 M calcium chloride and simultaneously start a stopwatch. If a clot forms in this generation mixture at any time, it should be removed so that it will not interfere with pipetting.

14. Repeat steps 7 through 10 as described for the control specimen. Failure of any of the five clotting times to clot in less than 12 seconds using the patient's generation mixture indicates a deficiency in factor VIII, IX, XI, or XII if the prothrombin time is normal. It may also indicate the presence of an anticoagulant.

THROMBOPLASTIN GENERATION TEST

The thromboplastin generation test measures the efficiency with which plasma thromboplastin is formed. It detects factor VIII and factor IX deficiencies and is able to distinguish between the two disorders. Factor XI and XII deficiencies may be detected but cannot be differentiated from each other. If the patient's platelets are used in the test, a platelet abnormality may also be detected.

REFERENCE

Biggs, R., and Douglas, A.S.: The thromboplastin generation test, J. Clin. Path., 6, 23, 1953.

REAGENTS AND EQUIPMENT

1. Barium sulfate, powdered.
2. Water bath, 37°C.
3. Calcium chloride, 0.025 M.
   Anhydrous calcium   1.38 g
      chloride
   Distilled water   500 ml
4. Thromboplastin-calcium chloride mixture.
5. Sodium chloride, 0.85% (w/v).
6. Partial thromboplastin (platelet substitute). (Available commercially.)
7. Ice bath (crushed ice).
8. Test tubes, 13 × 100 mm.
9. Stopwatch.

SPECIMEN

One test tube of clotted blood and one test tube of oxalated blood (one part 0.1 M sodium oxalate to nine parts whole blood) from both a normal patient (to be used as control) and from the patient to be tested.

PRINCIPLE

The patient's diluted serum and adsorbed plasma are mixed with calcium chloride and a substitute platelet factor. This constitutes the patient's thromboplastin generation mixture. The amount of plasma thromboplastin formed by the patient's coagulation factors is measured by the ability of this mixture to clot a normal plasma (which mainly supplies prothrombin and fibrinogen). The patient's generation mixture is incubated for a total of 6 minutes. At 1-minute intervals during this time, samples of the generation mixture are added to a normal plasma, and the clotting time is determined. Normally, there will be enough thromboplastin generated during these 6 minutes to clot normal plasma in 12 seconds or less. When an abnormal result is obtained, normal adsorbed plasma (source of factors I, V, VIII, XI, XII) and normal serum (source of factors VII, IX, X, XI, XII) are substituted, one at a time, to determine which corrects the patient's defect. If the prothrombin time is normal, factors I, II, V, VII, and X are assumed to be normal. Therefore, deficiencies in factors VIII, IX, XI, or XII may be detected.

PROCEDURE

1. Preparation of patient and normal control plasma. (Source of factor VIII.)
   A. Centrifuge the normal control and patient's anticoagulated blood specimens at 2,500 RPM for 10 minutes within 15 minutes of collection.
   B. Remove the plasma and pipet 1.0 ml of each plasma into a separate 13 × 100-mm test tube containing 100 mg of barium sulfate. Place the remaining patient's plasma in the refrigerator in case it is needed for future tests. Refrigerate the remaining control plasma for use as the plasma substrate.
   C. Stir the plasma-barium sulfate mixtures with a glass rod for 10 minutes. Refrigerate for 10 minutes.
   D. Centrifuge the two mixtures at 2,500 RPM for 10 minutes. Remove the adsorbed plasma spec-

imens and place in respective test tubes in crushed ice.

E. Perform a prothrombin time on each of the adsorbed plasma specimens. The prothrombin times should be greater than 3 minutes. If not, readsorb the plasma.

F. Refrigerate the adsorbed plasma specimens.

2. Preparation of the patient and normal control serums. (Source of factor IX.)

A. When the patient and normal control blood specimens have clotted, place the test tubes in a 37°C water bath for 2 hours.

B. At the end of 2 hours, centrifuge the clotted blood specimens at 2,500 RPM for 5 minutes. Remove the serum specimens and place in respective test tubes in crushed ice.

3. Test.

A. Dilute the normal control and patient's adsorbed plasma 1:5 with 0.85% sodium chloride (0.1 ml of adsorbed plasma and 0.4 ml of 0.85% sodium chloride). Place in respective test tubes in crushed ice.

B. Dilute the normal control and patient's serum 1:10 with 0.85% sodium chloride (0.1 ml of serum and 0.9 ml of 0.85% sodium chloride). Place the respective test tubes in crushed ice.

C. Pipet approximately 5 ml of 0.025 M calcium chloride into a 13 × 100-mm test tube and place in the 37°C water bath.

D. Place six 13 × 100-mm test tubes in the 37°C water bath and pipet exactly 0.1 ml of plasma substrate (unadsorbed and undiluted control plasma) into each test tube.

E. Prepare the control generation mixture. Add the following solutions to a 13 × 100-mm test tube in the 37°C water bath:

1) 0.3 ml of diluted adsorbed control plasma.

2) 0.3 ml of partial thromboplastin.

3) 0.3 ml of diluted control serum.

4) 0.3 ml of 0.025 M calcium chloride.

Start a stopwatch at exactly the same time the last reagent (calcium chloride) is added to the mixture. If a clot forms in this generation mixture at any time, it should be removed so that it will not interfere with pipetting.

F. When 55 seconds have elapsed on the stopwatch, pipet 0.1 ml of the generation mixture. With the other hand, pipet 0.1 ml of 0.025 M calcium chloride.

G. When 1 minute has elapsed on the stopwatch, blow the 0.1 ml of generation mixture into one of the test tubes containing 0.1 ml of plasma substrate. Immediately blow the 0.1 ml of calcium chloride into the same test tube and simultaneously start a second stopwatch.

H. Determine the clotting time of this mixture by the tilt tube method. If clotting has not occurred within 40 to 45 seconds, have a second person continue tilting the test tube until clotting occurs. Record the results. If the clotting time is greater than 60 seconds, record as over 60 seconds.

I. Repeat steps F, G, and H at 1-minute intervals for all six test tubes containing the 0.1 ml of plasma substrate. (Start the second clotting time when 1 minute and 55 seconds have elapsed on the first stopwatch.) Do not stop the first stopwatch at any time during this procedure.

J. If any of the six test tubes has a

clotting time of 12 seconds or less within the 6-minute incubation period of the generation mixture, the test is considered to be normal. If the control test performed on the plasma substrate is abnormal, the entire test must be repeated.

K. Place six 13 × 100-mm test tubes in the 37°C water bath and pipet exactly 0.1 ml of plasma substrate (unadsorbed and undiluted control plasma) into each tube.

L. Prepare the patient's generation mixture. Add the following solutions to a 13 × 100-mm test tube in the 37°C water bath:

1) 0.3 ml of diluted adsorbed patient's plasma.
2) 0.3 ml of partial thromboplastin.
3) 0.3 ml of diluted patient's serum.
4) 0.3 ml of 0.025 M calcium chloride.

Start a stopwatch at exactly the same time the last reagent (calcium chloride) is added to the mixture. If a clot forms in this generation mixture at any time, it should be removed so that it will not interfere with pipetting.

M. Repeat steps F through J.

N. If none of the test tubes has clotted in less than 12 seconds using the patient's generation mixture, proceed to step 4, Substitutions. If any of the preceding six test tubes has a clotting time of 12 seconds or less, the results are normal, and step 4 of this procedure may be omitted.

4. Substitutions.

A. Pipet 0.1 ml of plasma substrate into each of six 13 × 100-mm test tubes and place in a 37°C water bath.

B. Prepare a generation mixture. Add the following solutions to a 13 × 100-mm test tube in the 37°C water bath:

1) 0.3 ml of diluted adsorbed control plasma.
2) 0.3 ml of partial thromboplastin.
3) 0.3 ml of diluted patient's serum.
4) 0.3 ml of 0.025 M calcium chloride.

Start a stopwatch at exactly the same time the last reagent (calcium chloride) is added to the mixture. Remove the clot, if formed.

C. Repeat steps F through J, as described previously in step 3, Test.

D. Repeat step A and prepare another generation mixture as follows:

1) 0.3 ml of diluted adsorbed patient's plasma.
2) 0.3 ml of partial thromboplastin.
3) 0.3 ml of diluted control serum.
4) 0.3 ml of 0.025 M calcium chloride.

Start the stopwatch. Remove the clot, if formed.

E. Repeat steps F through J, as described previously in step 3, Test.

5. Interpretation of results. See Table 12.

DISCUSSION

1. Abnormal platelet activity may be detected using the patient's platelets in place of partial thromboplastin in the patient's generation mixture. If this procedure is employed, a prolonged clotting time, using the patient's serum, platelets, and adsorbed plasma, must be followed up by a substitution test, using partial thromboplastin in the patient's generation mixture. Correction of the generation clotting time by partial thromboplastin indicates defective platelet activ-

TABLE 12. INTERPRETATION OF THE THROMBOPLASTIN GENERATION TEST

FACTOR DEFICIENCY	CLOTTING TIME CORRECTED BY ADSORBED PLASMA	NORMAL SERUM	PROTHROMBIN TIME
VIII	yes	no	normal
IX	no	yes	normal
XI or XII	yes	yes	normal
anticoagulant	no	no	may be normal

ity. The patient's platelets for this procedure may be prepared as follows:

A. Centrifuge oxalated blood for 10 minutes at 1,000 RPM immediately after collection.

B. Transfer the platelet-rich plasma to a siliconized or plastic test tube and note the volume of the plasma.

C. Centrifuge the platelet-rich plasma at 3,000 RPM for 15 minutes. A platelet button will be formed.

D. Pour off the supernatant plasma and refrigerate until 20 minutes before use.

E. Resuspend the platelets in 0.85% sodium chloride and centrifuge at 3,000 RPM for 15 minutes.

F. Pour off the supernatant sodium chloride and resuspend the platelets in a volume of 0.85% sodium chloride equal to one third of the original plasma volume.

2. The presence of circulating anticoagulants may give abnormal results in this test.

3. Oxalated plasma must be used if the plasma is to be adsorbed by barium sulfate. If citrated plasma is employed, aluminum hydroxide must be used as the adsorbing agent.

4. The thromboplastin generation test may also be performed on the fibrometer.

PARTIAL THROMBOPLASTIN SUBSTITUTION TEST

The partial thromboplastin substitution test may be performed if the PTT, or activated PTT (APTT), is abnormal to identify factor deficiencies in stage 1 or 2 of the coagulation process.

REFERENCE

Proctor, R.R., and Rapaport, S.I.: The partial thromboplastin time with kaolin, Am. J. Clin. Path., 36, 212, 1961.

REAGENTS AND EQUIPMENT

1. Water bath, 37°C.
2. Calcium chloride, 0.025 M.

Anhydrous calcium chloride	1.38 g
Distilled water	500 ml

3. Partial thromboplastin containing an activator (platelet substitute with an activator). Obtainable commercially.
4. Citrated normal control plasma.
5. Sodium chloride, 0.85% (w/v).
6. Sodium citrate, 0.1 M.

Sodium citrate ($Na_3C_6H_5O_7 \cdot 2H_2O$)	2.94 g
Distilled water	100 ml

7. Test tubes, 13 × 100 mm.
8. Stopwatch.
9. Adsorbed plasma (rich in factors V, VIII, XI, and XII). Prepare as follows:

A. Add 100 mg of barium sulfate to each 1 ml of fresh oxalated normal plasma.

B. Stir this mixture for 10 minutes at room temperature and refrigerate, or place on ice for an additional 10 minutes.

C. Centrifuge at 2,500 RPM for 10 minutes and remove the supernatant plasma.

D. Dilute the adsorbed plasma 1:5 with 0.85% sodium chloride (one part adsorbed plasma to four parts 0.85% sodium chloride).

As an alternative and recommended

procedure, adsorbed plasma reagent may be obtained commercially.

10. Aged serum (rich in factors VII, IX, X, XI, and XII). Prepare as follows:
    A. Incubate a tube of clotted normal blood at 37°C for 3 hours.
    B. Add one part 0.1 M sodium citrate to nine parts whole blood to the preceding test tube.
    C. Allow the test tube to incubate for 2 additional hours at 37°C.
    D. Centrifuge for 10 minutes and remove the serum.
    E. The serum may be used immediately, or stored at −20°C.
    F. Prior to use, dilute the aged serum 1:5 with 0.85% sodium chloride (one part aged serum to four parts 0.85% sodium chloride).

The aged serum reagent may be obtained commercially.

SPECIMEN

Citrated plasma: one part 0.109 M sodium citrate to nine parts whole blood.

PRINCIPLE

An APTT is performed on the patient's plasma diluted 1:1 with:
1. Adsorbed plasma, rich in factors V, VIII, XI, and XII.
2. Aged serum, rich in factors VII, IX, X, XI, and XII.
3. Sodium chloride, 0.85%.
4. Normal control plasma.

The test is also performed on undiluted patient's plasma. A clue as to the specific coagulation defect may be obtained by noting which reagent, adsorbed plasma, or aged serum corrects the APTT. If a prothrombin time, which measures factors I, II, V, VII, and X, is also performed, further information as to the exact factor deficiency may be obtained. The APTT may then be repeated, diluting the patient's plasma 1:1 with plasma specimens deficient in one specific factor. The factor-deficient plasma, unable to correct the APTT,

is a further check as to the exact coagulation deficiency.

PROCEDURE

1. Centrifuge the patient's citrated blood at 2,500 RPM for 10 minutes immediately after the blood has been collected.
2. Remove the plasma from the cells immediately and place on ice.
3. Incubate sufficient 0.025 M calcium chloride at 37°C.
4. Maintain the partial thromboplastin with activator at room temperature.
5. Perform the APTT (as described previously in the Coagulation section, Activated Partial Thromboplastin Time) on the following plasma specimens, using the dilutions indicated and record the results. Each plasma must be tested in duplicate and the two results averaged.
   A. Patient's plasma.
   B. Normal control plasma.
   C. Patient's plasma diluted 1:1 with 0.85% sodium chloride.
   D. Normal control plasma diluted 1:1 with 0.85% sodium chloride.

If any of the preceding patient tests are abnormal (all control values should be normal), proceed with the following dilutions, performing an APTT on:
   E. Patient's plasma diluted 1:1 with the normal plasma control.

If the patient's activated PTT is corrected by the normal control plasma, proceed with the following dilutions, performing an activated PTT on:
   F. Patient's plasma diluted 1:1 with adsorbed plasma.
   G. Normal control plasma diluted 1:1 with adsorbed plasma.
   H. Patient's plasma diluted 1:1 with aged serum.
   I. Normal control plasma diluted 1:1 with aged serum.

6. Record the results on a chart similar to the one on page 216.

	Normal control plasma, 0.1 ml	Patient's plasma, 0.1 ml
Normal control plasma, 0.1 ml		
Patient's plasma, 0.1 ml		
0.85% sodium chloride, 0.1 ml		
Adsorbed plasma, 0.1 ml		
Aged serum, 0.1 ml		

7. Interpretation of results. See Table 13.

DISCUSSION

1. If a factor deficiency is noted, the APTT should be performed, using the specific factor-deficient plasma indicated, in a 1:1 dilution with the patient's plasma. When the deficient factor(s) has been positively identified, appropriate specific factor assays may then be performed.

2. For the patient's APTT to be considered as corrected, the corrected values must fall close to the normal plasma control value, but will not necessarily fall within the normal range because the plasma has been diluted.

PROTHROMBIN TIME WITH SUBSTITUTIONS

The prothrombin time substitution test may be performed along with the APTT when the prothrombin time is prolonged to detect a possible factor VII deficiency.

REFERENCE

Dade Reagents, Inc.: *Coagulation Procedures*, Dade Reagents, Inc., Miami, Florida, 1966.

REAGENTS AND EQUIPMENT

1. Water bath, 37°C.
2. Thromboplastin-calcium chloride mixture.
3. Citrated normal control plasma.
4. Adsorbed plasma. (See the section entitled Partial Thromboplastin Substitution Test [Reagents and Equipment].)
5. Aged serum. (See the section entitled Partial Thromboplastin Substitution Test [Reagents and Equipment].)
6. Sodium chloride, 0.85% (w/v).
7. Test tubes, 13 × 100 mm.
8. Stopwatch.

SPECIMEN

Citrated plasma: one part 0.109 M sodium citrate to nine parts whole blood.

PRINCIPLE

A prothrombin time is performed on the patient's plasma diluted 1:1 with aged serum and 1:1 with adsorbed plasma. Together with the results obtained from the APTT, it is possible to detect a factor VII deficiency.

PROCEDURE

1. Centrifuge the patient's citrated blood at 2,500 RPM for 10 minutes immediately after collection.

TABLE 13. PROBABLE COAGULATION DEFICIENCIES BASED ON PROTHROMBIN TIME AND APTT TEST RESULTS

APTT	PT	ADSORBED PLASMA APTT	AGED SERUM APTT	PROBABLE DEFICIENCY
N	N	N	N	No deficiency found
A	N	C	C	XI or XII
A	N	NC	C	IX
A	A	NC	C	X
A	A	C	NC	V
A	N	C	NC	VIII
A	A	NC	NC	II

APTT = Activated partial thromboplastin time. PT = Prothrombin time. N = Normal result. A = Abnormal (prolonged) result. C = Corrected. NC = Not corrected.

2. Remove the plasma from the cells immediately and place on ice.

3. Pipet 0.2 ml of thromboplastin-calcium mixture into the appropriate number of 13 × 100-mm test tubes. Warm the test tubes in the 37°C water bath.

4. Perform the prothrombin time on the following plasma specimens using the dilutions indicated, and record the results. Each plasma must be tested in duplicate and the two results averaged.

   A. Patient's plasma.

   B. Normal control plasma.

   If the prothrombin time on the patient's plasma is abnormal, perform a prothrombin time on the following dilutions:

   C. Patient's plasma diluted 1:1 with 0.85% sodium chloride.

   D. Normal control plasma diluted 1:1 with 0.85% sodium chloride.

   E. Patient's plasma diluted 1:1 with normal control plasma.

   F. Patient's plasma diluted 1:1 with adsorbed plasma.

   G. Normal control plasma diluted 1:1 with adsorbed plasma.

   H. Patient's plasma diluted 1:1 with aged serum.

   I. Normal control plasma diluted 1:1 with aged serum.

5. For simplicity, record the results on a chart similar to the one that follows:

	Normal control plasma (1 part)	Patient's plasma (1 part)
Normal control plasma (1 part)		
Patient's plasma (1 part)		
0.85% sodium chloride (1 part)		
Adsorbed plasma (1 part)		
Aged serum (1 part)		

6. For an interpretation of results, refer to Table 14.

DISCUSSION

1. For the patient's prothrombin time to be considered as corrected, the corrected result should fall within a lower range, close to the results received for the normal plasma control, but it will not necessarily fall within the normal range because the plasma has been diluted.

ASSAY FOR FACTOR VIII (VIII:C)

Test results for the assay for factor VIII are expressed as percentages, in relation to the amount of activity of the factor present in a normal plasma pool or in a plasma containing known concentrations of the factor. The normal range is 50 to 200%. A factor VIII deficiency is found in classic hemophilia and von Willebrand's disease.

REFERENCES

Hardisty, R.M., and MacPherson, J.C.: A one-stage factor VIII assay and its use on venous and capillary plasma, Thromb. Diath. Haemorrh., 7, 215, 1962.

Lenahan, J.G., and Smith, K.: *Hemostasis*, General Diagnostics, Morris Plains, New Jersey, 1979.

REAGENTS AND EQUIPMENT

1. Partial thromboplastin containing an activator (platelet substitute with an activator). Obtainable commercially.

2. Water bath, 37°C.

3. Calcium chloride, 0.025 M.

   Anhydrous calcium chloride   1.38 g

   Dilute to 500 ml with distilled water.

4. Factor VIII-deficient substrate. Obtainable commercially.

5. Reference plasma with known factor VIII assay. Obtainable commercially.

6. Imidazole-buffered saline, pH 7.2 to 7.4.

   Imidazole (obtainable from Eastman Co., Rochester, NY)   3.4 g

   Sodium chloride   5.85 g

   Hydrochloric acid, 0.1 N   186 ml

TABLE 14. PROBABLE COAGULATION DEFICIENCIES BASED ON PROTHROMBIN TIME SUBSTITUTION TEST AND APTT SUBSTITUTION TEST RESULTS

| | | PROTHROMBIN TIME | | APTT | | |
| | | ADSORBED PLASMA | AGED SERUM | ADSORBED PLASMA | AGED SERUM | |
APTT	PT					PROBABLE DEFICIENCY
N	N	—	—	—	—	No deficiency found
A	N	—	—	C	NC	VIII
A	N	—	—	C	C	XI or XII
A	N	—	—	NC	C	IX
N	A	NC	C	—	—	VII
A	A	C	NC	C	NC	V
A	A	NC	C	NC	C	X
A	A	NC	NC	NC	NC	II

APTT = Activated partial thromboplastin time. PT = Prothrombin time. N = Normal result. A = Abnormal (prolonged) result. C = Corrected. NC = Not corrected.

Dilute to 1 liter with distilled water.

7. Ice bath.
8. Stopwatch.
9. Test tubes, 13 × 100 mm.
10. 2-cycle semilog graph paper.

SPECIMEN

Citrated plasma: one part 0.109 M sodium citrate to nine parts whole blood. Place the test tube of blood in a cup of ice immediately after collection.

PRINCIPLE

An APTT is performed on factor VIII-deficient substrates containing varying dilutions of the patient's plasma (Table 15). The patient's plasma is used to correct the APTT. The amount of correction by the patient's plasma is then compared with results of the APTT, using a known normal, or reference, plasma in place of the patient's plasma. The factor VIII content of the patient's plasma is expressed as the percentage of normal.

TABLE 15. DILUTIONS FOR FACTOR VIII AND IX ASSAY

DILUTING FLUID (ml)	PLASMA (ml)	DILUTION	PLASMA CONCENTRATION
0.4	0.1	1:5	20 %
0.9	0.1	1:10	10 %
1.9	0.1	1:20	5 %
3.9	0.1	1:40	2.5%

PROCEDURE

1. Centrifuge the patient's blood at 2,500 RPM for 20 minutes immediately after collection. Remove the plasma and place on ice. Proceed with the test immediately.
2. Maintain the partial thromboplastin (with activator) at room temperature.
3. Reconstitute the factor VIII-deficient substrate as directed and place on ice.
4. Incubate sufficient 0.025 M calcium chloride at 37°C.
5. Add imidazole-buffered saline to four 13 × 100-mm test tubes, in the amounts listed in Table 15. Do not add the patient's plasma (or normal reference plasma) until immediately before each test is performed. (The patient's plasma is tested first, and the reference plasma is prepared immediately before use.)
6. Place eight 13 × 100-mm test tubes in the 37°C water bath. (All plasma samples are to be run in duplicate.)
7. Prepare the 1:5 dilution of the patient's plasma.
8. To one of the 13 × 100-mm test tubes in the water bath add:
   A. 0.1 ml of partial thromboplastin.
   B. 0.1 ml of factor VIII-deficient substrate.
   C. 0.1 ml of diluted patient's plasma (1:5 dilution).
9. Quickly mix the contents of the test

tube and set clock No. 1 for 3 minutes.

10. When 1 minute has elapsed on clock No. 1, repeat step 8 for the duplicate plasma specimen.
11. Mix the contents of the test tube and set clock No. 2 for 3 minutes.
12. When 3 minutes have elapsed on clock No. 1, quickly pipet 0.1 ml of 0.025 M calcium chloride into the first test tube, simultaneously starting a stopwatch. Leave the test tube in the 37°C water bath for 30 seconds.
13. After 30 seconds have elapsed on the stopwatch, remove the test tube from the water bath and gently tilt the tube at a rate no faster than once per second.
14. When clotting occurs, stop the watch. This is the end point.
15. When 3 minutes have elapsed on clock No. 2, quickly pipet 0.1 ml of 0.025 M calcium chloride into the second test tube, simultaneously starting a stopwatch. Leave the test tube in the incubator for 30 seconds.
16. After 30 seconds have elapsed on the stopwatch, remove the test tube from the water bath and gently tilt the tube at a rate no faster than once per second.
17. When clotting occurs, stop the watch.
18. Average the preceding two results and record the clotting time for that dilution.
19. Prepare the 1:10, 1:20, and 1:40 dilutions of the patient's plasma immediately before use and repeat steps 8 through 18 for each of the dilutions.
20. Using the reference plasma in place of the patient's plasma, repeat steps 8 through 18 for each plasma dilution, as listed in Table 15.
21. Calculation of results (Fig. 150).
    A. Using two-cycle semilog graph paper, plot each average clotting time in seconds against the plasma concentration in percent-

ages. Use the logarithmic scale for the plasma concentration, plotting 1 to 10% on the first cycle and 20 to 100% on the second cycle. There will be eight points plotted.
    B. Draw a straight line that best connects the four points of the reference plasma. This represents the normal activity curve.
    C. By interpolation, determine from the graph the concentrations of reference plasma that give the same clotting times as the different dilutions of the patient's plasma. Multiply the resulting reference plasma dilutions by the patient plasma dilution factors. See Figure 150 for an example.
    D. Average the four values received for the percent activity of the patient's plasma. This result represents the percent of normal activity of factor VIII (or factor IX) present in the patient's plasma.

DISCUSSION

1. In hemophilia A, it is generally accepted that a factor VIII level of 30 to 35% of normal activity is satisfactory for normal hemostasis.
2. Pooled normal plasma may be used in place of reference plasma. The advantage of reference plasma is that it has previously been assayed and, therefore, contains a known percentage of factor VIII (IX).
3. Factor VIII-deficient substrate may be replaced by plasma known to be deficient in factor VIII. This plasma may be stored at 0°C and thawed immediately before use. A plasma to be used as factor VIII-deficient, however, must have a concentration of 0 to 1% of normal activity of the factor before it is acceptable. Also, even though the plasma is stored at 0°C, it may gradually become deficient in

Concen. of plasma	Ref. plasma (sec.)	Pt's plasma (sec)	Concen. of ref plasma (%)	Dilution factor	% activity of pt's plasma
20%	58	67	10	5	50%
10%	67	76	5.2	10	52%
5%	77	85	2.7	20	54%
2.5%	86	91	1.4	40	56%
					53% activity

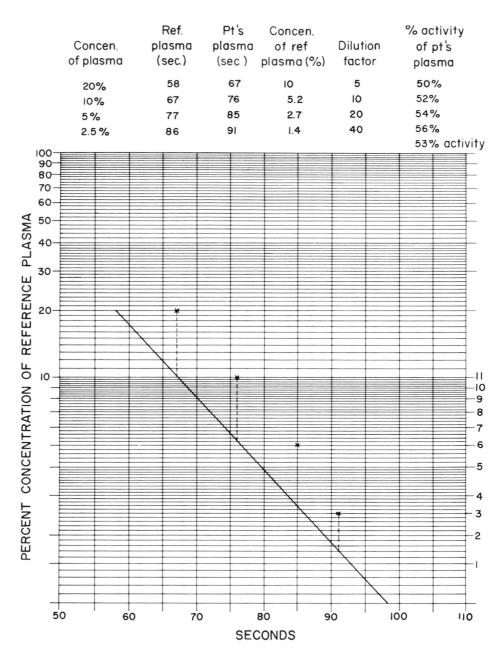

Fig. 150. Calculation of results for factor VIII and IX assay.

additional clotting factors, particularly factor V.

ASSAY FOR FACTOR IX

The assay for factor IX is carried out using a procedure identical to the one described for the factor VIII assay. The only

exceptions that should be noted are: (1) use factor IX-deficient substrate in place of factor VIII deficient substrate. (2) To prepare the percent activity curve, use a reference plasma with a known factor IX assay in place of the factor VIII-assayed reference plasma. The normal range for factor IX is 50 to 200%. Decreased amounts of factor IX are present in Christmas disease (also known as hemophilia B), liver disease, vitamin K deficiency, and in newborns.

ASSAY FOR FACTOR XI

The assay for factor XI is carried out using a procedure identical to the one described for the factor VIII assay. The only exceptions that should be noted are: (1) Use factor XI-deficient substrate in place of factor VIII-deficient substrate. (2) To prepare the percent activity curve, use a reference plasma with a known factor XI assay in place of the factor VIII-assayed reference plasma. The normal range for factor XI is 50 to 150%.

ASSAY FOR FACTOR XII

The assay for factor XII is carried out using a procedure identical to the one described for the factor VIII assay. The only exceptions that should be noted are: (1) Use factor XII-deficient substrate. (2) To prepare the percent activity curve, use a reference plasma with a known factor XII assay in place of the factor VIII-assayed reference plasma. The normal range for factor XII is 50 to 150%.

ASSAY FOR FACTOR V

The test results for factor V assay are expressed in percentages, in relation to the activity of factor V present in a normal plasma or in a plasma containing a known concentration of the factor. The normal range for factor V is 50 to 200%.

REFERENCES

Biggs, R., and MacFarlane, R.G.: *Human Blood Coagulation and Its Disorders*, Blackwell Scientific Publications, Oxford, 1962.

Hardisty, R.M., and Ingram, C.I.C.: *Bleeding Disorders, Investigation and Management*, Blackwell Scientific Publications, Oxford, 1965.

Lenahan, J.G., and Smith, K.: *Hemostasis*, General Diagnostics, Morris Plains, New Jersey, 1979.

REAGENTS AND EQUIPMENT

1. Water bath, 37°C.
2. Thromboplastin-calcium chloride mixture.
3. Imidazole-buffered saline, pH 7.2 to 7.4.
   Imidazole (obtainable from Eastman Co., Rochester, NY) 3.4 g
   Sodium chloride 5.85 g
   Hydrochloric acid, 0.1 N 186 ml
   Dilute to 1 liter with distilled water.
4. Factor V-deficient substrate. (Commercially available.)
5. Reference plasma with known factor V assay. (Commercially available.)
6. Ice bath.
7. Test tubes, 13 × 100 mm.
8. Stopwatch.
9. Two-cycle semilog graph paper.

SPECIMEN

Citrated plasma: one part 0.109 M sodium citrate to nine parts whole blood. Place the tube of blood in a cup of ice immediately after collection.

PRINCIPLE

A prothrombin time is performed on factor V-deficient substrates containing varying dilutions of the patient's plasma. The patient's plasma is used to correct the prothrombin time. The amount of correction by the patient's plasma is compared with the results of the prothrombin time performed on a known reference plasma in place of the patient's plasma. The factor V content of the patient's plasma is expressed as the percentage of normal.

PROCEDURE

1. Centrifuge the patient's blood at 2,500 RPM for 20 minutes immediately after collection. Remove the plasma and place in a cup containing crushed ice.

2. Warm the thromboplastin-calcium mixture to 37°C.

3. Reconstitute the factor V-deficient substrate as directed and place on ice.

4. Add imidazole-buffered saline to four 13 × 100-mm test tubes, in the amounts listed in Table 16. Do not add the patient's plasma (or normal reference plasma) until immediately before each test is performed. (The patient's plasma is tested first, and the reference plasma is prepared immediately before use.)

5. Place eight 13 × 100-mm test tubes in the 37°C water bath. (All plasma samples are to be run in duplicate.)

6. Prepare the 1:5 dilution of the patient's plasma.

7. To one of the 13 × 100-mm test tubes in the water bath, add:
   A. 0.1 ml of factor V-deficient substrate.
   B. 0.1 ml of diluted patient's plasma (1:5 dilution).

8. Add 0.2 ml of the thromboplastin-calcium mixture to the test tube and simultaneously start a stopwatch.

9. Mix the contents of the test tube and stop the watch at the first indication of clot formation. Perform duplicate prothrombin times on each plasma dilution, average the results, and record.

10. Repeat steps 4 through 9, substituting the reference plasma for the patient's plasma.

11. Calculation of results:
    A. Using two-cycle semilog graph paper, plot each average clotting time in seconds against the plasma concentration in percent. Use the logarithmic scale for the plasma concentration. Plot 1 to 10% on the first cycle and 20 to 100% on the second cycle. There will be 10 points plotted.
    B. Draw the straight line that best connects the five points of the reference plasma. This represents the normal activity curve.
    C. By interpolation, determine from the graph the concentrations of reference plasma that give the same clotting times as the different dilutions of patient's plasma. Multiply the resulting reference plasma dilutions by the patient plasma dilution factors. (The calculations are similar to those for the factor VIII assay. See Figure 150 for an example.)
    D. Average the five values received for the percent activity of patient's plasma. This result represents the precentage of normal activity of factor V present in the patient's plasma.

DISCUSSION

1. Pooled normal plasma may be used in place of the reference plasma.

2. Factor V-deficient plasma may be used in place of the factor V-deficient substrate. If this is employed, a prothrombin time greater than 60 seconds should be obtained on the factor V-deficient plasma before it is used. (Factor V-deficient plasma may be prepared by incubating normal plasma at 37°C for 24 hours or by re-

TABLE 16. DILUTIONS FOR FACTOR V ASSAY

TUBE	BUFFERED SALINE (ml)	PLASMA (ml)	DILUTION	PLASMA CONCENTRATION %
1	0.4	0.1	1:5	20
2	0.9	0.1	1:10	10
3	1.9	0.1	1:20	5
4	3.9	0.1	1:40	2.5

frigerating the normal plasma at 4 to 10°C for 2 weeks.)

ASSAY FOR FACTOR II

The assay for factor II may be carried out using a procedure identical to the one described for the factor V assay. The only exceptions to be noted are that a factor II-deficient substrate must be used in place of the factor V-deficient substrate, and a reference plasma with a known factor II assay must be used in place of the factor V-assayed reference plasma. The normal range for factor II is 50 to 150%.

ASSAY FOR FACTOR VII

The assay for factor VII is carried out using a procedure identical to the one described for the factor V assay. The only exceptions to be noted are that a factor VII-deficient substrate must be used in place of the factor V-deficient substrate, and a reference plasma with a known factor VII assay must be used in place of the factor V-assayed reference plasma. The normal range for factor VII is 50 to 150%.

ASSAY FOR FACTOR X

The assay for factor X may be carried out using a procedure identical to the one described for the factor V assay. The only exceptions to be noted are that a factor X-deficient substrate must be used in place of the factor V-deficient substrate, and a reference plasma with a known factor X assay must be used in place of the factor V-assayed reference plasma. Normal values for factor X are 50 to 150%.

STYPVEN TIME

The Stypven time is capable of detecting deficiencies in prothrombin and factors V and X. It, therefore, differs from the prothrombin time in that deficiencies in factor VII are not detected. The normal Stypven time is 20 to 25 seconds.

REFERENCE

Miale, J.B.: *Laboratory Medicine: Hematology,* 6th ed., C.V. Mosby Company, St. Louis, 1982.

REAGENTS AND EQUIPMENT

1. Water bath, 37°C.
2. Stypven brand Russell's viper venom. (Obtainable from Burroughs Wellcome Company, Research Triangle Park, North Carolina.) Prepare according to directions on the package.
3. Calcium chloride, 0.025 M.
   Anhydrous calcium chloride — 1.38 g
   Distilled water — 500 ml
4. Normal plasma control.
5. Test tubes, 13 × 100 mm.
6. Stopwatch.

SPECIMEN

Citrated plasma: one part 0.109 M sodium citrate to nine parts whole blood.

PRINCIPLE

Russell's viper venom (Stypven) is a thromboplastic substance that contains a factor VII-like substance. A prothrombin time using Stypven as a source of tissue thromboplastin and factor VII is performed. Deficiencies in factors V, X, and prothrombin may be detected.

PROCEDURE

1. Centrifuge the patient's blood at 2,500 RPM for 10 minutes as soon as possible after the blood has been collected.
2. Remove the plasma from the cells immediately and place on ice.
3. Incubate each of the following in separate test tubes at 37°C for 3 minutes:
   A. Patient's plasma.
   B. Normal control plasma.
   C. Calcium chloride, 0.025 M.
   D. Russell's viper venom (Stypven).
4. Into a 13 × 100-mm test tube in the 37°C water bath pipet 0.1 ml of

Stypven and 0.1 ml of 0.025 M calcium chloride. Mix.

5. Add 0.1 ml of patient or control plasma and simultaneously start the stopwatch.
6. Record the clotting time, as is done in the one-stage prothrombin time.
7. Each patient and control plasma should be performed in duplicate.

DISCUSSION

1. If the one-stage prothrombin time is normal, the Stypven time need not be performed.
2. In a factor VII deficiency, the prothrombin time would be prolonged and the Stypven time normal.
3. To make the test more specific for factor X and also for factor V, the Stypven time may be performed by the addition of 0.1 ml of bovine charcoal-filtered plasma as a source of factor V. This bovine plasma is obtainable from Colorado Serum Company, Denver, Colorado.

FLETCHER FACTOR

A deficiency of the Fletcher factor may be determined by use of a modification of the activated partial thromboplastin time (APTT).

REFERENCE

Hattersley, P.G., and Hayse, D.: The effect of increased contact activation time on the activated partial thromboplastin time, Am. J. Clin. Path., 66, 479, 1976.

REAGENTS AND EQUIPMENT

1. Water bath, 37°C.
2. Calcium chloride, 0.025 M.
3. Partial thromboplastin (containing a kaolin, silica, or Celite activator). Elagic acid should not be used as an activator in this specific test because it will not correct the APTT in a Fletcher factor deficiency.
4. Normal control plasma.
5. Test tubes, 12 × 75 mm.
6. Stopwatch.

SPECIMEN

Citrated plasma: one part 0.109 M sodium citrate to nine parts whole blood. Immediately after blood collection, place the tube of blood in a cup of crushed ice and deliver it to the laboratory.

PRINCIPLE

Patients with a Fletcher factor deficiency will have a prolonged APTT. If the plasma-partial thromboplastin mixture is incubated for 10 minutes (instead of the routine 3 or 5 minutes) the prolonged APTT will be shortened if the deficiency is due to the Fletcher factor.

PROCEDURE

1. Centrifuge the patient's blood at 2,500 RPM for 10 minutes. Remove the plasma from the cells immediately and place on ice.
2. Perform an APTT on the patient and normal control plasma specimens as outlined previously in the section entitled Activated Partial Thromboplastin procedure. If the patient results are normal, a Fletcher factor deficiency is not considered to be present. If the patient results are prolonged, proceed as follows.
3. Perform an APTT on the patient and normal control plasma specimens as previously outlined, except the plasma-partial thromboplastin mixture should be incubated for 10 minutes before adding calcium chloride and determining the clotting time.
4. Interpretation of results. The APTT performed in step 3 (with the 10-minute incubation) should correct to a normal or almost normal clotting time in the presence of a Fletcher factor deficiency. If the APTT is not corrected by the increased incubation time, a problem other than a Fletcher factor deficiency is assumed to be

present. The normal plasma control should remain within or near the normal range with the 10-minute incubation period.

PROTAMINE TITRATION

When patients undergo open-heart surgery, heparin is used to prevent activation of the coagulation process. At the completion of surgery, protamine is administered to neutralize the effects of the heparin. Protamine in excess, however, is capable of interfering with factor IX activity and with thromboplastin generation. The protamine titration, therefore, is used to estimate the minimum required dose of protamine. All preparations for the protamine titration must be made prior to receiving the patient's blood.

REFERENCE

Perkins, H.A., Osborn, J.J., Hurt, R., and Gerbode, F.: Neutralization of heparin invivo with protamine. A simple method of estimating the required dose, J. Lab. Clin. Med., 48, 223, 1956.

REAGENTS AND EQUIPMENT

1. Sodium chloride, 0.85% (w/v).
2. Protamine sulfate, 1%. Obtain from the hospital pharmacy. (This is the same protamine that is used by the patient.) Store at 4°C.
3. Test tubes, 12 × 75 mm.

SPECIMEN

One 20-ml syringe filled with 15 ml of whole blood.

PRINCIPLE

A specific amount of whole blood is added to varying dilutions of protamine sulfate. At the end of 15 minutes, the test tubes are tilted to determine the lowest concentration of protamine sulfate that causes the blood to clot.

PROCEDURE

1. Prepare a stock protamine solution (1,000 µg per ml): 1 ml of 1% prota-mine sulfate in 9 ml of 0.85% sodium chloride.
2. Prepare the following dilutions in 12 × 75-mm test tubes, according to Table 17.
3. Label eleven 12 × 75-mm test tubes, according to the final concentration of protamine, which will be 100, 50, 45, 40, 35, 30, 25, 20, 15, 10, and 5 µg per ml when the blood is added (Table 18).
4. Transfer 0.1 ml of the protamine sulfate dilution into the preceding set of test tubes.
5. As soon as the blood is collected from the patient, add 1.0 ml of whole blood to each of the test tubes containing 0.1 ml of diluted protamine sulfate. Dispense the blood directly from the syringe into the test tube.
6. Invert each test tube once, to mix, and set a clock for 15 minutes.
7. At the end of 15 minutes, tilt each test tube to determine the smallest amount of protamine sulfate that causes the blood to clot. This may be interpreted as the amount of protamine sufficient to neutralize the heparin in 1 ml of whole blood. Therefore, this amount of protamine sulfate times the patient's total blood volume gives the proper dosage of protamine to be given to the patient to overcome the effects of the heparin.

DISCUSSION

This test may be performed at room temperature or in a 37°C water bath. The same end point will be reached at both temperatures.

TOURNIQUET TEST (CAPILLARY FRAGILITY TEST)

The tourniquet test is a crude measure of capillary fragility. Because platelets function to maintain capillary integrity, the degree of thrombocytopenia will correlate with the tourniquet test, as will the

TABLE 17. CONCENTRATION OF PROTAMINE SULFATE FOR THE PROTAMINE TITRATION PROCEDURE

TEST TUBE NO.	ml of STOCK PROTAMINE SULFATE	ml of 0.85% SODIUM CHLORIDE	CONCENTRATION OF PROTAMINE SULFATE IN μg/ml
1	1.00	0.00	1000
2	0.50	0.50	500
3	0.45	0.55	450
4	0.40	0.60	400
5	0.35	0.65	350
6	0.30	0.70	300
7	0.25	0.75	250
8	0.20	0.80	200
9	0.15	0.85	150
10	0.10	0.90	100
11	0.05	0.95	50

TABLE 18. FINAL CONCENTRATION OF PROTAMINE SULFATE FOR THE PROTAMINE TITRATION PROCEDURE

0.1 ml of PROTAMINE SULFATE FROM TEST TUBE NO.	FINAL CONCENTRATION OF PROTAMINE SULFATE AFTER BLOOD HAS BEEN ADDED (μg/ml)
1	100
2	50
3	45
4	40
5	35
6	30
7	25
8	20
9	15
10	10
11	5

bleeding time. In normal patients, none to very few petechiae are formed during this test. (Petechiae are minute hemorrhages under the skin and appear as small bruises.) A positive tourniquet test (presence of numerous petechiae) will be found in thrombocytopenia purpura, and von Willebrand's disease.

REFERENCE

Cartwright, G.E.: *Diagnostic Laboratory Hematology*, Grune & Stratton, Inc., New York, 1963.

REAGENTS AND EQUIPMENT

1. Stethoscope.
2. Blood pressure cuff.

PRINCIPLE

An inflated blood pressure cuff on the upper arm is used to apply pressure to the capillaries. At the end of 5 minutes, the arm is examined for petechiae. If a patient has thrombocytopenia, there will not be enough platelets present to maintain capillary integrity, and small bruises will form on the arm.

PROCEDURE

1. Apply a blood pressure cuff on the upper arm above the elbow, and take a blood pressure reading.
2. Inflate the blood pressure cuff to a point halfway between the systolic and diastolic pressures. (However, never exceed a pressure of 100 mm Hg.) Maintain this pressure for 5 minutes.
3. Remove the blood pressure cuff.
4. Examine the forearm, hands, and fingers for petechiae. Disregard any petechiae within one-half inch of the blood pressure cuff because this may be due to pinching of the skin by the cuff.
5. The test results are graded roughly as follows:

   1+ = A few petechiae on the anterior part of the forearm.

   2+ = Many petechiae on the anterior part of the forearm.

   3+ = Multiple petechiae over the whole arm and back of the hand.

   4+ = Confluent petechiae on the arm and back of the hand.

DISCUSSION

1. An alternative procedure uses the inflated blood pressure cuff at a pressure of 80 mm Hg, regardless of the patient's blood pressure.
2. The test should not be repeated on the same arm within 7 days.
3. At times, the petechiae may not appear until several minutes after the blood pressure cuff has been removed. If this occurs, these petechiae should be included in the grading of the test results.

TEST FOR PLATELET FACTOR-3 AVAILABILITY

Platelets activated during the coagulation process liberate platelet factor-3, a phospholipid, which is essential for normal blood coagulation. Normal values for this method are determined by the correlation of patient and control results. The patient's platelet-rich plasma should give a clotting time similar in length to that of the normal platelet-rich control plasma. Increased clotting times occur in thrombocytopenia and in defects in platelet factor-3 availability, as found in thrombasthenia and some uremic patients.

REFERENCE

Hardisty, R.M., and Ingram, C.I.C.: *Bleeding Disorders, Investigations and Management*, Blackwell Scientific Publications, Oxford, 1965.

REAGENTS AND EQUIPMENT

1. All glassware in this test must be siliconized or plastic because platelets adhere to glass.
2. Water bath, 37°C.
3. Calcium chloride, 0.025 M.
Anhydrous calcium chloride	1.38 g
Distilled water	500 ml
4. Light kaolin suspension.
Kaolin	0.50 g
Tris buffer, pH 7.35	100 ml

   (For preparation of the Tris buffer, refer to the section entitled Thrombin Time [Reagents and Equipment].)
   Store at 4°C.
   (Celite 505, a 1% suspension in sodium chloride, 0.85%, w/v, may be used in place of the kaolin. This is obtainable from Johns-Manville Products Corporation, New York, New York.)
5. Normal platelet-poor control plasma.
6. Normal platelet-rich control plasma.
7. Reagents and equipment as used for the platelet count.
8. Test tubes, 13 × 100 mm.
9. Stopwatch.

SPECIMEN

Platelet-rich and platelet-poor patient plasma specimens and normal control plasma specimens. Collect blood using a plastic syringe. Mix one part 0.109 M sodium citrate with nine parts whole blood and place in a plastic test tube. Collect two test tubes of blood from both the patient and the normal control.

PRINCIPLE

Equal parts of patient's platelet-rich plasma (PRP) are mixed with normal control platelet-poor plasma (PPP). A second mixture of equal parts of patient's platelet-poor plasma and normal control platelet-rich plasma is made. Kaolin is added to activate the platelets. Calcium chloride is added, and the clotting time of the mixtures is recorded. Platelet counts are performed on the platelet-rich plasma specimens of both the patient and normal control.

PROCEDURE

1. For platelet-rich plasma, centrifuge one test tube each of the patient's and normal control blood at 1,000 RPM for 10 minutes. Remove the plasma from the cells using a plastic transfer pipet. For platelet-poor plasma, centrifuge both the patient's and normal

control blood at 2,500 RPM for at least 20 minutes. Remove the plasma from the cells.

2. Label eight 13 × 100-mm test tubes as shown in Table 19 and pipet the indicated plasma specimens into each test tube.

3. Place test tube No. 1 in the water bath. Add 0.2 ml of the well-mixed kaolin suspension.

4. Set a clock for 27 minutes. (This mixture is to be incubated for 20 minutes.)

5. At 1-minute intervals, repeat step 3 starting with test tube No. 2, then test tube No. 3, and so forth until the kaolin suspension has been added to all eight test tubes in the water bath.

6. When the clock has 7 minutes remaining (20 minutes after kaolin was added to test tube No. 1), add 0.2 ml of 0.025 M calcium chloride to test tube No. 1 and simultaneously start a stopwatch.

7. Using the tilt-tube method, determine the clotting time. It should be approximately 30 seconds.

8. Continue to add 0.2 ml of 0.025 M calcium chloride to each succeeding tube at 1-minute intervals. That is, when the clock has 6 minutes remaining, add calcium chloride to test tube No. 2 and so forth, so that calcium chloride is added to each test tube exactly 20 minutes after the kaolin was added.

9. Average the duplicate results and record.

10. Perform a platelet count on the patient's platelet-rich plasma and the normal platelet-rich control plasma.

TABLE 19. MIXTURES FOR PLATELET FACTOR-3 AVAILABILITY TEST

TEST TUBE NO.	PLATELET-RICH PLASMA	PLATELET-POOR PLASMA
1, 8	0.1 ml control	0.1 ml control
2, 7	0.1 ml control	0.1 ml patient
3, 6	0.1 ml patient	0.1 ml control
4, 5	0.1 ml patient	0.1 ml patient

11. Interpretation of results: the plasma mixtures in test tubes No. 2 and No. 7 and in No. 3 and No. 6 differ only in their source of platelets. If the average clotting times of these two groups agree within 2 to 3 seconds of each other and the platelet counts on the patient's and normal control platelet-rich plasma specimens are within 100,000 to 300,000 per μl, the patient has no significant defect in platelet factor-3 availability. If, however, the clotting times in test tubes No. 3 and No. 6 are more prolonged and differ more widely from test tubes No. 2 and No. 7, this may be due to decreased platelets (thrombocytopenia) in the patient or to defective platelet factor-3 availability. If the platelet count performed on the patient's platelet-rich plasma is within the range of 100,000 to 300,000 per μl, the prolonged clotting time is probably due to defective platelet factor-3 availability. A patient with abnormal platelet function generally has a clotting time about 15 seconds longer than the control.

PLATELET ADHESIVENESS TEST

One of the functions of platelets is their participation in hemostasis, where they adhere to each other and to the walls of damaged blood vessels to form a hemostatic plug. The adhesiveness of blood platelets is measured in vitro by their ability to adhere to glass surfaces. The normal values for this test are 26 to 60% platelet adhesiveness. Decreased values, using the procedure to be described, are found in thrombasthenia, where there is a qualitative disorder in platelets, von Willebrand's disease, and in some cases of myeloid metaplasia and thrombocythemia. Increased platelet adhesiveness has been reported in venous thrombosis, pulmonary embolism, coronary disease, following splenectomy, and in diabetes mellitus.

Salzman Method

REFERENCES

Lenahan, J.G., and Smith, K.: *Hemostasis,* General Diagnostics, Morris Plains, New Jersey, 1979.

Salzman, E.W.: Measurement of platelet adhesiveness, a simple in vitro technique demonstrating an abnormality in von Willebrand's disease, J. Lab. Clin. Med., *62,* 724, 1963.

REAGENTS AND EQUIPMENT

1. A double-ended, 20-gauge, Vacutainer needle.
2. Hypodermic needle, 20 gauge.
3. Vacutainer holder.
4. Vacutainer tubes (two) containing EDTA anticoagulant.
5. Siliconized ML-ML adapter, obtainable from Becton-Dickinson Company, Rutherford, New Jersey.
6. Siliconized 3200 A adapter, obtainable from Becton-Dickinson Company, Rutherford, New Jersey.
7. Polyvinyl tubing (inner diameter of 0.113 inch). (Obtainable from Insultab, Inc., 252 Mishawuum Rd., Woburn, Massachusetts, 01802.)
8. Grease-free, soda-lime-silica glass beads, with an average diameter of 0.0185 inch. (Obtainable from Minnesota Mining Company as "Superbrite," type 070.)
9. Siliconized nylon mesh, with openings of 0.002 inch.
10. Duco cement.
11. Materials necessary for two platelet counts.
12. Glass bead filter.
    A. Cut two pieces of siliconized nylon mesh to fit exactly over the ends of the two siliconized adapters.
    B. Using Duco cement, glue a piece of the nylon mesh to one end of each of the adapters.
    C. Attach one end of the polyvinyl tubing to that end of the adapter to which the nylon mesh is glued (Fig. 151).
    D. Fill the polyvinyl tubing with 1.3 g of glass beads.
    E. After packing the glass beads into the tube, cut the tubing. Allow a little extra unfilled tubing to remain to fit over that end of the second adapter that contains the nylon mesh. (The degree of packing of the glass beads and, therefore, the length of the polyvinyl tubing should be such that it takes 40 to 50 seconds for the blood to be collected through this system.)

SPECIMEN

One tube of whole blood collected according to routine procedure, using the Vacutainer assembly with a 20-gauge needle and drawing the blood directly into an EDTA vacuum tube. A second speci-

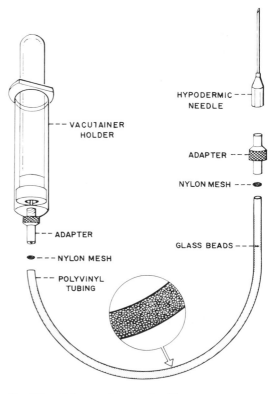

Fig. 151. Salzman glass bead collecting system.

men of blood is collected through the glass bead collecting system directly into an EDTA vacuum tube.

PRINCIPLE

A platelet count is performed on both specimens of blood. The number of platelets in the blood, collected through the glass bead collecting system, will be lower than the number obtained by routine venipuncture. This is due to the adhesiveness of the platelets, which have adhered to the glass beads in the filter system. The results of this procedure are expressed as the percentage of platelets retained in the filter.

PROCEDURE

1. Perform two clean venipunctures at separate sites, with and without the use of the glass bead collecting system. (The blood collection rate through the glass bead collecting system should be 6 to 10 ml per minute.)
2. Perform a platelet count on both blood samples.
3. Calculate the percent of platelet adhesiveness as shown below.

$$\text{Percent of platelet adhesiveness} = \frac{\text{Platelet count without glass beads} - \text{Platelet count with glass beads}}{\text{Platelet count without glass beads}} \times 100$$

DISCUSSION

1. If the glass beads are siliconized, there will be no platelet adhesion.
2. There is no correlation between the patient's platelet count and platelet adhesion.
3. Heparin therapy does not interfere with platelet adhesiveness.
4. It is recommended that each laboratory determine its own set of normal values. Slight differences in technique and the length of the polyvinyl tubes are important factors.
5. E.W. Salzman feels that calcium ions are necessary for platelet adhesion under the conditions of this test. For

this reason, the blood passes through the filter system prior to being anticoagulated.

6. Modifications of this procedure may be utilized to produce more standardized and reproducible results. Becton, Dickinson and Company (Rutherford, New Jersey) market the B-D Platelet Retention Column (similar to the previously described glass bead column but more standardized). Also, use of a constant-flow syringe pump provides a constant rate of blood flow through the column. Whole blood is collected and anticoagulated with heparin. Part of this whole blood is then drawn through the glass bead column at a constant, preset rate by means of an infusion pump and is collected in a tube containing EDTA. Platelet counts are then determined on the whole blood sample drawn through the glass bead column and on the blood sample not drawn through the column. The percent of platelet adhesiveness is then calculated as previously outlined. (The infusion pump, Model #901, is obtainable from Harvard Apparatus Company, Inc., Millis, Massachusetts.)

PLATELET AGGREGATION TEST

There is evidence that adenosine diphosphate (ADP) in the red blood cells or platelets is responsible for the clumping of platelets during the coagulation process and for the formation of a platelet plug in injured blood vessels. Normally, platelets undergo rapid aggregation (clumping) when ADP is added to platelet-rich plasma. In thrombasthenia, the platelets fail to aggregate, and this test may be used to diagnose this disorder. Decreased platelet aggregation may also be found in uremia and macroglobulinemia.

REFERENCE

Dacie, J.V., and Lewis, S.M.: *Practical Hematology*, 5th ed., Churchill Livingstone, New York, 1975.

REAGENTS AND EQUIPMENT

1. Barbitone buffer, pH 7.35 to 7.4.

Sodium diethyl barbiturate, 0.1 M	570 ml
Hydrochloric acid, 0.1 N	430 ml
Sodium chloride	5.67 g

   Dilute with an equal volume of 0.9% sodium chloride before use.
2. Adenosine diphosphate.

Adenosine diphosphate	10 µg
Barbitone buffer	1 ml

   This solution must be made up fresh each day the test is performed.
3. Test tubes, 12 × 75 mm.
4. Water bath, 37°C.
5. Stopwatch.

SPECIMEN

Citrated platelet-rich plasma: one part of 0.109 M sodium citrate to nine parts whole blood. Collect a specimen of blood from a normal control at the same time the patient's blood is obtained.

PRINCIPLE

Adenosine diphosphate is added to platelet-rich plasma, and the specimen is observed for platelet aggregation.

PROCEDURE

1. Centrifuge the patient and control blood specimens at 1,000 RPM for 10 minutes immediately after collection.
2. Pipet 0.2 ml of normal control platelet-rich plasma into a 12 × 75-mm test tube in the 37°C water bath.
3. Incubate for 30 seconds.
4. Pipet 0.1 ml of ADP solution into the test tube and simultaneously start a stopwatch.
5. Agitate the mixture vigorously while keeping it in the 37°C water bath. Examine the mixture every 5 to 10 seconds for macroscopic agglutination. Normal clumping should occur within 30 seconds after the addition of ADP. Record the degree of platelet aggregation (1+, 2+, 3+, 4+) and the time, after the addition of ADP, before clumping occurred.
6. Repeat steps 2 through 5, using the patient's platelet-rich plasma. If no aggregation with the patient's platelets has occurred after 2 minutes, place a small drop of the mixture on a slide. Examine the plasma mixture under the microscope for small clumps of platelets. (This may also serve as a check to determine if there are sufficient platelets in the plasma to give valid results.)

DISCUSSION

1. Failure of the normal control plasma to show normal platelet aggregation may be due to improperly prepared platelet-rich plasma. Therefore, check the plasma microscopically for platelets. If the platelet-rich plasma shows a decrease in platelets, both control and patient blood specimens must be redrawn and the procedure repeated.
2. A more complete procedure for platelet aggregation is outlined in Chapter 7 (the section entitled Bio/Data Platelet Aggregation Profiler).

TESTS FOR INHIBITORS (ANTICOAGULANTS)

Some coagulation abnormalities are caused by inhibitors of specific factors rather than by a deficiency in a specific factor. These inhibitors may be fast-acting or may progressively destroy the factor. The presence of inhibitors is rare but must be properly diagnosed when present. Inhibitors have been observed in certain chronic illnesses such as lupus erythematosus and chronic nephritis, in patients with hemophilia and Christmas disease, in patients with congenital deficiencies of other coagulation factors, and in some women soon after childbirth.

REFERENCES

Hardisty, R.M., and Ingram, C.I.C.: *Bleeding Disorders, Investigation and Management,* Blackwell Scientific Publications, Oxford, 1965.

Lenahan, J.G., and Smith, K.: *Hemostasis,* General Diagnostics, Morris Plains, New Jersey, 1979.

REAGENTS AND EQUIPMENT

1. Water bath, 37°C.
2. Calcium chloride, 0.025 M.

   | Anhydrous calcium chloride | 1.38 g |
   | Distilled water | 500 ml |

3. Partial thromboplastin (platelet substitute).
4. Normal control plasma.
5. Test tubes, 13 × 100 mm.
6. Stopwatch.

SPECIMEN

Citrated plasma: one part 0.109 M sodium citrate to nine parts whole blood.

PRINCIPLE

Inhibitors (sometimes termed *circulating anticoagulants*) may be detected by performing an APTT on the patient's plasma, a normal control plasma, and various dilutions of the patient and normal control plasma at specifically timed intervals. The results are compared with each other. In the presence of an inhibitor, there will be little to no correction in the clotting time when the patient's plasma is mixed with normal plasma. If a factor deficiency exists, the clotting time of the patient's plasma will show significant correction when mixed with normal plasma.

PROCEDURE

1. Place the test tube of blood in a cup containing crushed ice immediately after the blood is drawn.
2. Centrifuge the blood at 2,500 RPM for 10 minutes. Immediately remove the plasma and place the test tube in a cup containing crushed ice.
3. Perform an APTT on each of the following:
   A. Patient plasma.
   B. Normal control plasma.
   C. 1:1 mixture of the patient's plasma and normal control plasma (0.5 ml of patient plasma plus 0.5 ml of normal control plasma).
   D. 9:1 mixture of the patient's plasma and normal control plasma (0.9 ml of patient plasma plus 0.1 ml of normal control plasma).
   E. 1:9 mixture of the patient's plasma and normal control plasma (0.1 ml of patient plasma plus 0.9 ml of normal control plasma).
4. Record the results on a time chart (see below).
5. Incubate the patient and control plasma specimens and mixtures at 37°C.
6. Perform an APTT, in duplicate, on each plasma, control, and plasma-control mixture after 10, 30, and 60

Time (minutes)	Patient's plasma (seconds)	Normal control plasma (seconds)	1:1 Patient plasma and normal control (seconds)	9:1 Patient plasma and normal control (seconds)	1:9 Patient plasma and normal control (seconds)
0					
10					
30					
60					

minutes of incubation at 37°C. Record the results on the time chart (see below).

7. To interpret the results of this procedure, compare the clotting times at the different time intervals. It must be kept in mind, however, that as the plasmas incubate, there is normally a slight increase in the clotting times because of some loss of labile components in the plasma. For this reason, attention must be paid to the clotting times of the normal control plasma. Before the clotting times of the patient's plasma and the patient-control mixture are considered prolonged, the degree of prolongation from the previously run test must be greater than that shown by the normal control plasma. If an inhibitor is present, the clotting times of the patient's plasma will not be corrected (shortened) appreciably by the addition of normal plasma. Generally, in the presence of an inhibitor, the 9:1 mixture of the patient's plasma and normal control shows no significant correction of the clotting time; the 1:1 mixture may show very slight correction; and the 1:9 mixture slightly more correction. It must be kept in mind, however, that some inhibitors act progressively, and it may be a while before the clotting time of the patient plasma-normal control mixtures show the effects of the inhibitor (a prolonged clotting time). It is, therefore, very important to incubate the plasma samples for 60 minutes and note these results. In the presence of a factor deficiency, the clotting time of the patient plasma samples should be corrected by the addition of normal control plasma.

DISCUSSION

1. The prothrombin time may be used in place of the APTT for this procedure in those instances where the original APTT performed on the patient was normal and the original prothrombin time was abnormal.

EUGLOBULIN CLOT LYSIS TIME

The euglobulin clot lysis time is a screening procedure for the measurement of fibrinolytic activity and is more sensitive than the clot lysis time. The euglobulin fraction of plasma contains plasminogen, fibrinogen, and activators capable of transforming plasminogen to its active state, plasmin. Normally occurring inhibitors of this reaction (plasminogen to plasmin) are not present in this fraction of the plasma. Once a clot is formed, clot lysis occurs more quickly in this fraction of the plasma than in whole blood. Increased fibrinolytic activity has been associated with circulatory collapse, adrenalin injections, sudden death, pulmonary surgery, pyrogen reactions, and obstetric complications. Normally, clot lysis does not occur in less than 2 hours but is usually complete within 4 hours. Clot lysis in less than 2 hours is indicative of abnormal fibrinolytic activity.

REFERENCE

Bucknell, M.: The effect of citrate on euglobulin methods of estimating fibrinolytic activity, J. Clin. Path., 11, 403, 1958.

REAGENTS AND EQUIPMENT

1. Calcium chloride, 0.025 M.
   Anhydrous calcium chloride   1.38 g
   Distilled water   500 ml
2. Acetic acid, 1% (v/v).
3. Borate solution, pH 9.0.
   Sodium chloride   9.0 g
   Sodium borate   1.0 g
   Dilute to 100 ml with distilled water.
4. Water bath, 37°C.
5. Test tube, 15 × 125 mm.

SPECIMEN

Oxalated plasma: one part 0.1 M sodium oxalate to nine parts whole blood. Citrated plasma should not be used because the presence of citrate tends to increase fibrinolytic activity.

PRINCIPLE

The plasma euglobulins are precipitated with 1% acetic acid and resuspended in a borate solution. The euglobulins are then clotted by the addition of calcium chloride. The clot is incubated, and the time of lysis is reported.

PROCEDURE

1. Collect blood with a plastic or siliconized syringe. Mix the specimen with the appropriate anticoagulant and immediately place on ice.
2. Centrifuge the blood specimen at 2,500 RPM for 10 minutes and immediately proceed with the test. The procedure must be carried out within 20 minutes of blood collection.
3. Into a 15 × 125-mm test tube, pipet 9.0 ml of distilled water, 0.5 ml of the patient's plasma, and 0.1 ml of 1% acetic acid.
4. Refrigerate the preceding mixture for 30 minutes at 4°C to allow euglobulin precipitation.
5. Centrifuge at 2,500 RPM for 5 minutes.
6. Pour off the supernatant and invert the tube on filter paper to drain.
7. Add 0.5 ml of the borate solution and place in a 37°C water bath.
8. Stir the mixture gently with a glass rod.
9. Add 0.5 ml of 0.025 M calcium chloride to the mixture.
10. Record the time of clot formation.
11. Incubate the test tube in the 37°C water bath and periodically check for clot lysis. When clot lysis begins, check the tube every 5 minutes until the lysis is complete.
12. Report the results as the length of time from clot formation to complete clot lysis.

PROTAMINE SULFATE

The protamine sulfate procedure tests primarily for the presence of fibrin monomers. During stage 3 of the coagulation process, when thrombin acts on fibrinogen, fibrin monomers are formed that then polymerize to form a fibrin clot. Also detected in this procedure are early fibrin- (fibrinogen) split products (fragments X and Y). During the process of fibrinolysis, plasmin breaks down fibrin and fibrinogen to fragments X, Y, D, and E. Under certain pathologic conditions, intravascular coagulation may be stimulated. In these instances, there is widespread appearance of fibrin clots in the blood vessels of the microcirculation. Fibrin monomers are, therefore, present in the plasma. Because of the presence of coagulation, there is stimulation of the fibrinolytic system and the formation of fibrin- (fibrinogen) split products. Rapid detection of the presence of fibrin monomers is an important aid in the diagnosis of disseminated intravascular coagulation. Normally, there should be no fibrin monomers present in the plasma.

REFERENCE

Seaman, A.J.: The recognition of intravascular clotting, Arch. Intern. Med., *125*, 1016, 1970.

REAGENTS AND EQUIPMENT

1. Protamine sulfate, 1%, w/v.
2. Test tubes, 13 × 100 mm.
3. Pipets, 1.0 ml and 0.1 ml.
4. Water bath, 37°C.

SPECIMEN

Citrated plasma: one part 3.1% sodium citrate to nine parts whole blood.

PRINCIPLE

Fibrin monomers and early fibrinogen degradation products present in the plasma precipitate in the presence of a weak solution of protamine sulfate.

PROCEDURE

1. Centrifuge the patient's blood immediately after collection at 2,500 RPM for 10 minutes.
2. Label a 13 × 100-mm test tube with the patient's name.
3. Pipet 1.0 ml of patient's plasma into the above mentioned test tube. Incubate at 37°C for 5 minutes.
4. Add 0.1 ml of 1% protamine sulfate solution to the prewarmed patient plasma. Mix the test tube by tilting. Return to the 37°C water bath and allow to incubate undisturbed for 15 minutes.
5. At the end of the incubation period, remove the test tube from the water bath and carefully examine it for white fibrin threads. During this process, very gently tilt the test tube. Unnecessary mixing of the plasma solution will break up any fibrin threads present, giving a false-negative result. The presence of fibrin threads in the plasma constitutes a positive test for fibrinogen degradation products. An opalescent appearance of the plasma is interpreted as a negative result.

DISCUSSION

1. This test procedure must be performed at 37°C. Lower temperatures cause the plasma to take on an opalescent appearance.

ETHANOL GELATION TEST

The ethanol gelation test is designed to detect the presence of fibrin monomers in the plasma. It is a screening procedure to be utilized as an aid in the diagnosis of disseminated intravascular coagulation and in distinguishing this condition from primary fibrinolysis.

Breen and Tullis Method
(Modified by H. Glueck)

REFERENCES

Breen F.A., Jr., and Tullis, J.L.: Ethanol gelation: A rapid screening test for intra-vascular coagulation, Ann. Intern. Med., 69, 1197, 1968.

Breen, F.A., Jr., and Tullis, J.L.: Ethanol gelation test improved, Ann. Intern. Med., 71, 433, 1969.

REAGENTS AND EQUIPMENT

1. Sodium hydroxide, 0.1 N.
2. Ethyl alcohol, 50% (v/v).
3. Buffered citrated anticoagulant.
   Sodium citrate, 0.109 M   3 parts
   Citric acid, 0.1 M   2 parts
4. Test tubes, 12 × 75 mm.

SPECIMEN

Collect blood using a plastic syringe, and mix nine parts whole blood to one part buffered citrate anticoagulant. Collect normal control blood at the same time the patient's blood is obtained.

PRINCIPLE

During the process of disseminated intravascular coagulation, the level of fibrin monomer (intermediate product of fibrinogen breakdown to fibrin) in the blood increases. The fibrin monomer is precipitated from the plasma by ethyl alcohol and forms a gel or precipitate.

PROCEDURE

1. Centrifuge the buffered citrated blood at 2,500 RPM for 20 minutes to obtain platelet-poor plasma.
2. Into two appropriately labeled 12 × 75-mm test tubes, place nine drops of patient's plasma and control plasma.
3. Add one drop of 0.1 N sodium hydroxide to each test tube.
4. Mix well.
5. Carefully layer 0.15 ml of 50% ethyl alcohol over the mixture in each test tube.
6. Allow the test tubes to sit undisturbed for 1 minute.
7. Inspect the interface (line between the plasma and ethyl alcohol) for a line of precipitation.

8. Precipitation or gel formation constitutes a positive test.

9. If the test is negative after 1 minute, allow the test tubes to sit for 9 additional minutes. At the end of this time, if a precipitate or gel forms, add one more drop of 0.1 N sodium hydroxide and gently shake the test tube. If the precipitate formed is nonspecific, it will disappear. Persistence of the precipitate constitutes a positive test.

DISCUSSION

1. An increased pH above 7.7 causes a delay in precipitate formation. It is, therefore, important to use buffered sodium citrate as the anticoagulant. Sodium oxalate produces too alkaline a pH.

2. The presence of heparin or contamination with a few red blood cells does not alter the results of this test.

FIBRINOGEN DEGRADATION PRODUCTS

Fibrinogen degradation products may be demonstrated in the blood of patients with primary fibrinolysis and during the process of disseminated intravascular coagulation with secondary fibrinolysis.

The Thrombo-Wellcotest procedure described here is a rapid, sensitive test for fibrinogen degradation products present in the blood. The normal level of serum fibrinogen degradation products in the adult is less than 8 μg/ml.

Thrombo-Wellcotest Procedure

REFERENCE

Wellcome Reagents Limited: *Thrombo-Wellcotest. Rapid Latex Test for Detection of Fibrinogen Degradation Products*, Wellcome Research Laboratories, Beckenham, Kent, England, 1981.

REAGENTS AND EQUIPMENT

1. Sample collection tubes (contain thrombin to cause rapid and complete clotting and soya bean enzyme inhibitors to prevent the breakdown of fibrin).

2. Glycine saline buffer.

3. Latex suspension. (The latex particles have been sensitized with an anti-fibrinogen degradation product globulin.)

4. Positive control serum.

5. Negative control serum.

6. Glass test slide.

7. Disposable pipet droppers.

8. Disposable mixing rods.
(Note: All preceding reagents are available from Wellcome Reagents Division, Burroughs Wellcome Company, Research Triangle Park, North Carolina, 27709.)

9. Test tubes, 10 × 75 mm.

SPECIMEN

Using a clean, dry syringe, obtain 2.0 ml of blood from the patient and transfer immediately to the sample collection tube. These tubes may also be used with a Vacutainer system and will draw 2 ml of blood. As soon as the blood is in the tube, mix well by inverting several times.

PRINCIPLE

Whole blood is added to thrombin (to ensure complete clotting) and soya bean enzyme inhibitors (to prevent any breakdown of fibrin). After incubation (to ensure complete clotting), the patient's serum is diluted and mixed with latex particles coated with anti-fibrinogen. If fibrinogen degradation products are present, agglutination of the latex particles will occur.

PROCEDURE

1. As soon as the blood sample arrives in the laboratory, place it in the 37°C incubator for 20 minutes.

2. At the end of the incubation period, ring the clot with an applicator stick and centrifuge for 5 minutes at 2,000 RPM. (Make certain the blood is com-

pletely clotted. If it is not, inquire if the patient is receiving heparin.)

3. Carefully remove the serum and place in a 10 × 75-mm test tube. No red blood cells should be present.

4. Label two 10 × 75-mm test tubes 1:5 and 1:10. Using the graduated dropper from the test kit, place 0.75 ml of the glycine buffer into the test tube labeled 1:5. Using a disposable dropper from the test kit, add five drops of the patient's serum to this test tube. Mix. Using a disposable dropper from the test kit, place four drops of the glycine buffer into the test tube labeled 1:10. Transfer four drops of diluted serum from the test tube labeled 1:5 to the test tube labeled 1:10.

5. Label rings on the glass slide: positive, negative, 1:5, and 1:10.

6. Place one drop of each control serum in the appropriate ring. Transfer one drop of the 1:5 dilution and one drop of the 1:10 dilution to the appropriate ring on the glass slide. (Allow all drops to fall freely from the pipet. Do not touch the pipet to the glass slide during this process.)

7. Mix the latex suspension of the anti-fibrinogen degradation products globulin vigorously. Immediately add one drop to each of the serum dilutions and control specimens.

8. Using a separate applicator stick for each sample, quickly stir each mixture, spreading over the entire area of the ring. Immediately set a clock for 2 minutes.

9. Rotate the slide for exactly 2 minutes, using a backward and forward motion. Examine each mixture for macroscopic agglutination. Determine the presence or absence of agglutination immediately after the 2-minute mixing period. False-positive results may occur after the 2-minute period because of drying effects. The appearance of graininess must not be interpreted as macroscopic agglutination.

10. Interpretation of results (see Table 20). The negative and positive control specimens must show no agglutination and agglutination, respectively.

11. If the 1:10 dilution of the patient's plasma showed agglutination, further dilutions of the patient plasma should be made as described below. If qualitative results only are desired, the result may be reported as >20 μg per ml.

12. Label four 10 × 75-mm test tubes 1:20, 1:40, 1:80, and 1:160. Using the disposable pipet, place four drops of glycine buffer into each of the test tubes. Transfer four drops of the patient's 1:10 dilution into the test tube labeled 1:20. Mix and transfer four drops of the 1:20 dilution to the test tube labeled 1:40. Mix and transfer four drops of the 1:40 mixture to the test tube labeled 1:80. Mix and transfer four drops of the 1:80 dilution to the test tube labeled 1:160.

13. Label the rings on the glass slide for each of the above dilutions and for the negative and positive control specimens.

14. Place one drop of each control serum and one drop from each patient dilution onto the appropriate ring on the glass slide. Repeat steps 7, 8, and 9 above and interpret the results as shown in Table 20.

DISCUSSION

1. If the patient to be tested is receiving heparin, Reptilase-R should be added to the patient's blood in the sample collection tube for clotting to occur. (Add 1.0 ml of distilled water to the Reptilase-R. Pipet 0.2 ml of the reconstituted Reptilase-R to 2 ml of the patient's whole blood. Mix.)

2. This procedure may also be performed using a urine sample. For the

TABLE 20. FIBRINOGEN-DEGRADATION PRODUCTS
(Interpretation of Results)

PLASMA DILUTION	PATIENT RESULTS (− equals no agglutination, + equals agglutination)						
1:5	−	+	+	+	+	+	+
1:10	−	−	+	+	+	+	+
1:20			−	+	+	+	+
1:40				−	+	+	+
1:80					−	+	+
1:160						−	+
Results µg/ml	10	10− 20	20− 40	40− 80	80− 160	160− 320	>320

exact procedure, the reader is referred to the Thrombo-Wellcotest instruction booklet.

3. The sample test tubes may be kept at room temperature.
4. The centrifuged serum sample may be refrigerated for up to 1 week or stored at −20°C for longer before performing the test.
5. False-positive results may occur in patients with rheumatoid arthritis (patients positive for the rheumatoid factor).
6. It is suggested that a positive and negative control be run on each slide. When reading the slide, compare the patient results with the positive and negative controls to interpret the presence of agglutination.

ANTITHROMBIN III

Antithrombin III progressively destroys thrombin. It is thought of as a heparin co-factor in that heparin forms a complex with antithrombin III. The anticoagulant effect of heparin is catalytic, increasing the inhibitory effects of antithrombin III. It will be decreased in thrombotic disease, disseminated intravascular coagulation, and in women taking oral contraceptives. Antithrombin III may be measured by electroimmunoassay, radial immunodiffusion, or by the neutralization of thrombin (described below).

REFERENCES

Lenahan, J.G., and Smith, K.: Hemostasis, General Diagnostics, Morris Plains, New Jersey, 1979.

Zuck, T.F., Bergin, J.J., Raymond, J.M., and Dwyre, W.R.: Implications of depressed antithrombin-III activity associated with oral contraceptives, Surg. Gynecol. Obstet., 133, 609, 1971.

REAGENTS AND EQUIPMENT

1. Barbital acetate buffer, pH 7.32 to 7.52.
   Solution A
   Sodium acetate   9.714 g
   Sodium barbital   14.714 g
   Dilute to 500 ml with distilled water.
   Solution B
   Hydrochloric acid, 0.1 N 5.0 ml
   Sodium chloride,   2.0 ml
     0.85%, w/v
   Distilled water   15.0 ml
   Solution A   5.0 ml
   Working solution
   Solution B   1 part
   Sodium chloride,   4 parts
     0.85%, w/v
2. Stock thrombin (200 units per ml). Reconstitute one vial of Bovine Thrombin, Topical, 1,000 NIH units (Parke, Davis and Co.) with 5.0 ml of 50% glycerol (v/v).
3. Working thrombin reagent (100 units per ml). Mix equal parts of the stock thrombin and the barbital acetate buffer.
4. Fibrinogen (General Diagnostics, Morris Plains, New Jersey). Reconstitute with 1.0 ml of distilled water. (A more concentrated solution of fibrinogen is desired.)

5. Glass test tubes, 12 × 75 mm.
6. Water bath, 37°C.
7. Pipets, 1.0, 0.1, and 0.2 ml.
8. Stopwatch.

SPECIMEN

Whole blood, 5 ml, placed in a plain test tube, 13 × 100 mm in size. A normal control blood from a male donor should be obtained at the same time the patient's blood is collected.

PRINCIPLE

Whole blood is allowed to clot and then incubated at room temperature for 2 hours. During this time, 20 to 30% of the antithrombin III present in the blood will be consumed. The serum is then incubated with a specific amount of thrombin for 6 minutes. During this time, the antithrombin III present will neutralize this thrombin. Fibrinogen is then added to the serum-thrombin mixture, and the clotting time is noted. The lower the concentration of antithrombin III originally present in the patient's plasma, the less thrombin will be neutralized and the shorter will be the clotting time when fibrinogen is added.

PROCEDURE

1. Allow the patient and control blood specimens to clot. Incubate at room temperature for 2 hours.
2. Centrifuge the blood specimens at 2,500 RPM for 10 minutes. Remove the serum and place in appropriately labeled test tubes.
3. Label three 12 × 75-mm test tubes: patient, normal control, and abnormal control.
4. Place 0.6 ml of the normal control and patient sera into the appropriately labeled test tubes. Place 0.6 ml of 0.85% sodium chloride into the abnormal control test tube.
5. Incubate the patient serum test tube at 37°C for 1 minute.
6. Add 0.15 ml of the working thrombin

reagent to the patient serum test tube. Mix. Start the stopwatch.
7. When 5 minutes have elapsed on the stopwatch, place 0.1 ml of the fibrinogen solution in a 12 × 75-mm test tube and place in 37°C water bath.
8. When exactly 6 minutes have elapsed on the stopwatch, add 0.2 ml of the patient's serum-thrombin mixture to the 0.1 ml of fibrinogen. Start the stopwatch. Gently tilt the test tube backward and forward until a clot forms, at which point the timing is stopped. Record the results.
9. Repeat steps 6 through 9 for the normal and abnormal control specimens.
10. Interpretation of results. The abnormal control should yield a clotting time between 4 and 8 seconds. (This control measures the activity of the thrombin solution.) The normal control should give a result greater than 30 seconds, but this result will depend on the normal range for the test as determined for your particular laboratory. Patient results of less than 30 seconds generally indicate a decreased concentration of antithrombin III.

DISCUSSION

1. If hemolysis is present in the patient or normal control serum, the specimen should be recollected. Hemolysis or the presence of red blood cells will cause an increased consumption of prothrombin, causing lower antithrombin III activity in the serum.
2. Following the 2-hour incubation period, the serum may be frozen for up to 24 hours with little loss in antithrombin III activity.
3. The 2-hour incubation period is somewhat critical to more closely standardize the loss of antithrombin III activity.
4. The 6-minute incubation period for

the serum-thrombin mixture is critical. Excessive incubation will inactivate the added thrombin.

COAGULATION TESTING—THE FUTURE

One current trend in coagulation testing appears to be toward more sophisticated methods assaying for actual amounts of the substance present. Many of the components in the coagulation and fibrinolytic systems gain proteolytic activity when they are activated. In this way, they become serine proteases, which may be then assayed by using specific synthetic chromogenic and fluorogenic peptide substrates, thus employing the principles of enzymology.

At present, there are specific chromogenic and fluorogenic substrates available to test for various coagulation factors (factors XIIa, IXa, Xa, and VIIa), kallikrein, thrombin, plasmin, antithrombin III, urokinase, and some platelet factors.

6

Diseases

ANEMIA

Anemia signifies a decreased amount of hemoglobin in the blood and, therefore, a decreased amount of oxygen reaching the tissues and organs of the body. This is responsible for many of the symptoms in an anemic person. Anemia has many different causes, and before effective treatment can be initiated, the exact cause must be found. Numerous tests have been devised and are used in conjunction with the clinical findings to differentiate the various types of anemias.

To detect anemia in the laboratory, the two most important tests are the hemoglobin and hematocrit. An accurate red blood cell count is also most helpful in calculating the red blood cell indices. The anemia may then be classified as normocytic, microcytic, or macrocytic, depending on the values obtained for the mean corpuscular volume (MCV). The presence or absence of hypochromia, as shown by the mean corpuscular hemoglobin concentration (MCHC), is also valuable in diagnosis. Most anemias are normocytic-normochromic, macrocytic-normochromic, or microcytic-hypochromic, depending on the cause.

Examination of the red blood cell morphology on a stained blood smear is a basic tool in evaluating anemia, and it is an opportunity to double-check the results obtained for the red blood cell indices. Further examination of the red blood cell may be made: The shape of the red blood cell may be determined and the presence or absence of sickle cells, spherocytes, target cells, and inclusion bodies noted. In addition, white blood cell and platelet numbers and morphology should be examined. In certain cases, a clue to the cause of the anemia may rest with these cells, for example, in cases of leukemia. Also, in some anemias, there are specific abnormalities present in the white blood cells or platelets in addition to those found in the red blood cells.

The reticulocyte count, or, rather, the recticulocyte production index, is a test performed routinely for anemia diagnosis. It is a relatively accurate reflection of the amount of effective red blood cell production taking place in the bone marrow. In cases where the reticulocyte count is decreased, this may point to defective hemoglobin synthesis, replacement of the normal marrow by tumor cells, or failure of the bone marrow to produce the normal number of cells. On the other hand, increased reticulocyte counts in the presence of anemia may indicate such conditions as increased red blood cell destruction or blood loss. It must be remembered, however, that if effective erythropoiesis is taking place, the reticulocyte count is slightly elevated in proportion to the degree of anemia present.

Examination of bone marrow smears may prove helpful in estimating the relative number of red blood cells and their precursors being produced by the marrow. Normally, 20 to 35% of the nucleated cells present in the marrow are erythroid cells. This figure may be written as the myeloid:erythroid ratio (M/E), which normally is 3:1, or as the erythroid:granulocyte ratio (E/G), which is, therefore, 1:3 in a normal marrow. This figure may then be studied in conjunction with the reticulocyte count. For example, if the relative number of erythroid cells in the marrow is increased, but the reticulocyte count is normal or decreased, there may be a defect in the maturation of the erythroid cells (since the red blood cells are obviously not reaching the peripheral blood). Ineffective erythropoiesis may be said to be occurring. It is also important to note the morphology of the erythroid cells (as well as other cellular elements) and the presence of any tumor cells.

When a bone marrow biopsy is performed in cases of anemia, an iron stain (counterstained with nuclear fast red) should be done on a marrow concentrate smear to determine the percentage of sideroblasts. The presence or absence of ringed sideroblasts should also be noted. An estimation of the marrow iron stores may be determined from a marrow particle smear stained with the Prussian-blue iron stain.

The serum iron and iron-binding capacity (tests usually performed by the chemistry department) are helpful aids in differentiating anemias. The high incidence of iron-deficiency anemia increases the usefulness of this procedure.

A test for the determination of fecal urobilinogen (usually performed by the urinalysis department) measures the total excretion of the breakdown products of heme. Increased amounts of urobilinogen are generally found in hemolytic anemias and in those anemias in which ineffective red blood cell production is present.

The serum bilirubin (performed in the chemistry department) indicates in-creased destruction of red blood cells, as is found in hemolytic anemias.

In addition to the aforementioned laboratory procedures, three other tests concerned with red blood cell production, although not employed routinely, deserve mention here: (1) The plasma iron turnover is a procedure employing the use of radioactive iron (^{59}Fe). A known amount of this isotope is injected into the patient intravenously. Its rate of disappearance from the blood is measured by taking blood samples at regular intervals for 1 to 2 hours and determining the amount of radioactivity remaining. In anemias in which the total red blood cell production is decreased, the ^{59}Fe remains in the blood longer. (2) The red blood cell utilization of iron is a measure of effective erythropoiesis. After injection of the ^{59}Fe, blood samples are collected for a period of 2 to 3 weeks. The radioactivity in the samples is measured, and the amount of ^{59}Fe present in the red blood cells is then calculated. Normally, the ^{59}Fe reappears in the red blood cell as hemoglobin iron within 10 to 14 days after injection. (3) The life span of the red blood cell may also be determined by the use of various radioisotopes. The patient's red blood cells may be tagged with radioactive chromium (^{51}Cr). Blood samples are then measured for radioactivity over a period of 25 to 35 days, and a red blood cell survival curve is plotted on graph paper.

In summary, total erythropoiesis refers to the total production of red blood cells and is measured by the erythroid : granulocytic ratio, the fecal urobilinogen, and the plasma iron turnover. Effective erythropoiesis is the production of red blood cells that reach the circulation or peripheral blood and is measured by the red blood cell utilization of iron, the reticulocyte production index, and the red blood cell life span. In addition, more specific tests have been devised for diagnosing anemias. Many of these procedures have been outlined in Chapter 4, Special Hematology Procedures, and include, among others, hemoglobin electrophoresis, osmotic fragility, autohemolysis, acid-serum test, and Heinz body preparation.

Anemia basically results from one of two causes: (1) decreased red blood cell production or (2) increased red blood cell destruction. In addition, in circumstances where there is an increased plasma volume, laboratory test results (hemoglobin, hematocrit, and red blood cell count) may also show a state of anemia even though the red blood cell mass is normal. Several classifications of anemia have been devised. None of these is completely satisfactory but will be of some help in learning the basics of anemia. A brief outline of the anemias classified according to morphology and cause are given in the following section. These are not complete lists and contain only the more common causes.

Morphologic Classification of Anemias

1. Macrocytic, normochromic red blood cells.
    A. Vitamin B_{12} deficiency, folic acid deficiency.
        1) Pernicious anemia
        2) Sprue
        3) Following gastrectomy
    B. Disease of the liver.
2. Normocytic, normochromic red blood cells.
    A. Defective formation of the blood cells or the presence of tumor cells in the bone marrow.
        1) Aplastic anemia
        2) Leukemia
        3) Hodgkin's disease
        4) Multiple myeloma
        5) Leukoerythroblastosis
        6) Metastatic cancer
        7) Anemia associated with renal disease
        8) Anemia associated with inflammatory disease
    B. Abnormal hemoglobin, increased destruction of red blood cells.

1) Certain acquired hemolytic anemias
2) 11.6 Paroxysmal nocturnal hemoglobinuria
3) Sickle cell anemia
4) Hemolytic disease of the newborn
3. Microcytic, hypochromic red blood cells.
    A. Iron-deficiency anemia.
    B. Thalassemia.
    C. Sideroblastic anemias.

Classification of Anemias According to Cause

1. Decreased production of red blood cells.
    A. Bone marrow damage, infiltration, atrophy.
        1) Leukemias
        2) Leukoerythroblastosis
        3) Aplastic anemia
        4) Lymphoma
        5) Multiple myeloma
        6) Myelofibrosis
    B. Decreased erythropoietin.
        1) Inflammatory process
        2) Renal disease
        3) Hypothyroidism
    C. Deficiency of substances.
        1) Iron deficiency
        2) Vitamin B_{12} deficiency, folic acid deficiency
        3) Vitamin C deficiency
    D. Defect in globin synthesis.
        1) Thalassemia
    E. Defect in heme synthesis.
        1) Sideroblastic anemias
    F. Cirrhosis of the liver
2. Increased red blood cell destruction or loss.
    A. Acute blood loss.
    B. Due to intrinsic defects within the red blood cell.
        1) Hereditary
            a. Spherocytosis, ovalocytosis
            b. Hemoglobinopathies such

as sickle cell disease, hemoglobin C disease.
  c. Enzyme defects such as G-6-PD deficiency, pyruvate kinase deficiency
 2) Acquired
   a. Paroxysmal nocturnal hemoglobinuria
 C. Due to extracorpuscular causes.
  1) Drugs or chemicals
  2) Physical trauma to the red blood cells such as thermal injury
  3) Infection (malaria)
  4) Antibodies
3. Increased plasma volume.
 A. Last trimester of pregnancy.
 B. Hyperproteinemia.

MEGALOBLASTIC ANEMIAS

There are a variety of megaloblastic anemias due to deficiencies of vitamin B_{12} and folic acid. Pernicious anemia is a classic example of this form of anemia.

Pernicious Anemia

Pernicious anemia is most often found in people above 60 years of age and rarely in patients below 40 years of age. This disease is caused by a deficiency in vitamin B_{12}, caused by an inability of the gastric mucosa to secrete the intrinsic factor that is necessary for the absorption of vitamin B_{12}. There is strong evidence at present that this disorder may be an inherited autoimmune disease. Antibodies to intrinsic factor have been found in over half of the cases of pernicious anemia, and antibodies to the parietal cells of the stomach have been found to be present in over 85% of the patients having pernicious anemia. The clinical symptoms evolve slowly over a period of several months. Generally, the person shows weakness and shortness of breath, and the skin takes on a lemon-yellow pallor. Characteristically, the tongue may be raw and red or, more commonly, may be sore, pale and smooth. Gastrointestinal symptoms are usually present in the form of abdominal pain, diarrhea, nausea, and vomiting. There are central nervous system disorders in the degeneration of the white matter in parts of the spinal cord. This is the cause of several neurologic symptoms such as numbness and tingling of the extremities, loss of position sense, muscle weakness, and decreased tendon reflexes. In more advanced cases, the brain may be affected, and the patient may become emotionally unstable or show personality changes.

The peripheral blood smear shows characteristic changes. Pancytopenia is the usual finding. The majority of red blood cells are macrocytic-normochromic, with some oval macrocytes present. There may be a few microcytes and teardrop-shaped red blood cells, and moderate to marked anisocytosis and poikilocytosis is commonly found. Basophilic stippling, Howell-Jolly bodies, and nucleated red blood cells exhibiting karyorrhexis are usually seen. Neutrophils showing hypersegmentation are commonly encountered. These cells may be larger in size than the normal neutrophil. The nuclear chromatin pattern of the granulocytic cells often gives a much looser or more open appearance than normal. The bone marrow contains an increased number of erythroid cells that are characteristically megaloblastic, and the developing granulocytic cells are often larger in size than normal. One of the more consistent findings in pernicious anemia is the lack of free hydrochloric acid in the gastric secretions. The Schilling test (usually performed by the radiology department) is positive in pernicious anemia, and the serum vitamin B_{12} level is decreased. The serum iron level may be normal to elevated, and the serum bilirubin level may show a slight increase.

Other Conditions Caused by Vitamin B_{12} Deficiency

A megaloblastic anemia will result following a total gastrectomy because all of the intrinsic factor-secreting cells have been removed. Vitamin therapy is used to treat this condition. A partial gastrectomy or surgery for a gastric ulcer may or may not leave the patient with a megaloblastic anemia, which, again, is treatable with vitamin therapy.

A dietary deficiency of vitamin B_{12} is rare but may be found in vegetarians who also avoid consuming milk and egg products.

One case of megaloblastic anemia has been reported in a patient who was found to have an abnormal intrinsic factor.

Various diseases of the small intestine may cause a megaloblastic anemia. Normally, vitamin B_{12} is absorbed in the lower ileum, which contains little or no bacteria. When bacteria are present, they compete for the vitamin B_{12}, thus making it unavailable for absorption.

Reversible malabsorption of vitamin B_{12} has occurred in patients taking para-aminosalicylic acid (PAS), colchicine, neomycin, and a few other drugs.

Imerslund's syndrome is inherited as an autosomal recessive trait and manifests itself during the first 2 years of life. These patients are not able to absorb vitamin B_{12}, regardless of whether it is bound to intrinsic factor. They also have persistent proteinuria. The megaloblastic anemia is treated with vitamin B_{12}.

In Zollinger-Ellison syndrome, there is impaired vitamin B_{12} absorption but no megaloblastic anemia.

Patients on hemodialysis will have decreased vitamin B_{12} concentrations that are treatable with the administration of vitamin B_{12}.

Vitamin B_{12} deficiency will also be found in carriers of the fish tapeworm, *Diphyllobothrium latum*, because the organism lodges in the ileum and takes up the host's vitamin B_{12}. Treatment consists of expulsion of the organism and vitamin B_{12} therapy.

Folate Deficiency

Folic acid deficiency manifests itself in a manner similar to vitamin B_{12} deficiency, except that neurologic symptoms are absent.

Dietary deficiencies of folic acid are relatively rare in this country and are found primarily in chronic alcoholics and people with peculiar dietary habits, where relatively few fresh green vegetables or little animal protein is consumed.

The most common cause of folate deficiency occurs during pregnancy. The laboratory findings are generally less abnormal than those found in pernicious anemia, and this condition is treated with folic acid.

Megaloblastic anemia may be found during infancy, occurring most often between 6 and 12 months of age, and is caused by a folic acid deficiency that may be accompanied by a vitamin C deficiency. Laboratory test results show macrocytosis, anisocytosis, and poikilocytosis but in a less severe state than is found in pernicious anemia. The bone marrow shows mild to severe megaloblastic changes and includes the granulocytic alterations. Treatment consists of administration of vitamin C and folic acid.

Megaloblastic anemia is also found in patients with alcoholic cirrhosis of the liver and is almost always due to folic acid deficiency. This is due in part to lack of dietary folic acid and also to abnormal folate metabolism.

Some contraceptive drugs and anticonvulsants such as phenobarbital, diphenylhydantoin (Dilantin), and primidone (Mysoline) will cause a folate deficiency and mild hematologic changes.

Disorders Affecting DNA Synthesis

A number of disorders affect DNA synthesis and produce a megaloblastic anemia. Transcobalamin II deficiency, Form-amino-transferase deficiency, N-methyl tetrahydrafolate transferase deficiency, and dihydrofolate reductase deficiency are all inherited disorders, in addition to orotic aciduria (disorder of pyrimidine metabolism) and Lesch-Nyhan syndrome (disorder of purine metabolism). There are also acquired drug-induced disorders caused by a variety of drugs, including those used in chemotherapy.

Steatorrheas

Three malabsorption disorders have been classified as steatorrheas: *tropical sprue, nontropical sprue (idiopathic steatorrhea),* and *celiac disease.* The last two disorders are now called *gluten-sensitive enteropathies* because they are caused by an abnormal reaction to gluten.

The exact cause of tropical sprue is unknown. At the onset of the disease, there is diarrhea, anorexia, and marked weakness. After several weeks to months, there is a depletion of nutrients, and malabsorption takes place. Following this phase a macrocytic anemia develops, most likely caused by a lack of absorption of folic acid in the beginning and an ensuing lack of vitamin B_{12} as the disease becomes more chronic. Administration of folic acid is used for treatment of the anemia and also appears to improve the intestinal problems.

The gluten-sensitive enteropathies may be inherited and represent an abnormal reaction to gluten, a component of wheat and other grains. These patients show chronic diarrhea and weight loss, with possible hypocalcemia, demineralization of bones, and possible deficiency of vitamin K-dependent coagulation factors. Children with celiac disease generally show an iron deficiency anemia, with about 30% having a folic acid deficiency. Adults usually have a folic acid deficiency. About 40% of adults will also show malabsorption of vitamin B_{12}. Iron absorption is decreased, and iron stores may be low. Treatment includes folate and/or vitamin B_{12}, in addition to iron therapy and a gluten-free diet.

IRON-DEFICIENCY ANEMIA

Iron-deficiency anemia results when the iron stores of the body have been de-pleted, and there is no longer sufficient iron available for normal hemoglobin production. The iron stores become depleted over a long period of time when the iron loss exceeds iron intake.

The normal adult body contains approximately 4,000 mg of iron. About 60% of this total iron is present in the circulating blood, where 1 ml of red blood cells contains approximately 1 mg of iron. The remaining body iron is present as stored iron, mainly in the liver and reticuloendothelial cells of the bone marrow. Each day, 20 to 25 ml of red blood cells are broken down as a result of normal red blood cell aging. During this process, approximately 1 mg of iron is lost (each day) and excreted through the urine, bile, and other secretions. The remaining 19 to 24 mg of iron are reutilized for production of more hemoglobin in the formation of new red blood cells. It can, therefore, be seen that unless there is an increased need for iron, as in childhood, pregnancy, or excessive blood loss, iron-deficiency anemia will not occur. When iron is being utilized by the red blood cells at a faster rate (as during infancy or bleeding) and the dietary intake of iron is not sufficient to keep up with the increased use, the iron stores will then be utilized for hemoglobin iron. When the iron stores become exhausted, iron-deficiency anemia results. The normal adult only absorbs 5 to 10% of the iron in his diet each day.

An increased amount of dietary iron is needed during infancy, childhood, pregnancy, and in women during the childbearing years. The adult male has no increased demands for iron and could live without dietary iron for approximately 6 years before iron-deficiency anemia developed. Therefore, when this anemia is found in men, it is almost always due to chronic blood loss.

Iron-deficiency anemia is characterized by microcytosis, hypochromia, and poikilocytosis of the red blood cells, as seen on the stained blood smear. The reticulocyte count is within the normal range, except following hemorrhage or iron therapy, when it is increased. The platelet count is normal. Frequently, the platelets may appear smaller in size than usual. When the iron stain is employed on bone marrow concentrate smears, the number of sideroblasts is decreased and storage iron is absent. The serum iron is decreased, whereas the total iron-binding capacity is increased.

ANEMIA OF CHRONIC DISORDERS

Anemia of chronic disorders is present in chronic infections. inflammatory diseases, and neoplastic diseases. It is a frequently found anemia, probably second in incidence to iron-deficiency anemia.

Anemia of chronic disorders is generally a mild to moderate anemia that develops during the first or second month of illness. The hematocrit rarely falls below 30%. In severe illness, however, the hematocrit level may decrease further. This usually begins as a normocytic-normochromic anemia. Slight hypochromia may develop, and, more rarely, microcytosis may be found, but not to the degree seen in iron-deficiency anemia. Also, microcytosis occurs after hypochromia is present. In iron-deficiency anemia, microcytosis develops before hypochromia. There may be slight anisocytosis and poikilocytosis. The reticulocyte count is generally normal to decreased. The white blood cell and platelet counts are unaffected by the anemia. The serum iron level is decreased, and the total iron-binding capacity is normal to decreased. The percent saturation is usually decreased. The life span of the red blood cells in this anemia is reduced, whereas the production of red blood cells is normal to only slightly increased. It is suggested, therefore, that the anemia develops because the bone marrow cannot increase red blood cell production enough to compensate for the decreased red blood cell life span. There is also a decrease in the transfer of iron from the reticuloendothelial storage sites to the bone marrow. The anemia of chronic disorders shows no improvement with iron therapy and only improves with correction of the primary disorders.

SIDEROBLASTIC ANEMIA

There are several sideroblastic anemias that may be classified according to whether they are inherited or acquired.

Hereditary sideroblastic anemia is most commonly inherited as a sex-linked recessive trait that occurs in males. The anemia usually manifests itself in adolescence, although it may be present at birth or during infancy. The anemia is generally severe, with hematocrit levels of approximately 20%. The red blood cells are hypochromic and microcytic, with moderate anisocytosis and poikilocytosis. Also, target cells and basophilic stippling are usually present. The white blood cell and platelet counts are generally normal. There is a marked increase of storage iron in the bone marrow, and the serum iron and the percent saturation are increased. The bone marrow generally shows erythroid hyperplasia, and there are many ringed sideroblasts present. This is defective heme synthesis. Patients with this disorder may be treated with pyridoxine. Some patients respond well to this treatment, some respond partially, and a few do not respond at all.

Acquired refractory sideroblastic anemia is more common than the inherited sideroblastic anemia and is a disease found in adults above 50 years of age. There is moderate anemia, with hematocrit levels of approximately 25 to 30%. The red blood cells are generally normocytic to slightly macrocytic. There are usually two red blood cell populations present: a large number of normochromic red blood cells and a smaller group of hypochromic red blood cells. There may be occasional hypochromic red blood cells containing heavy basophilic stippling. The white blood cell and platelet counts are normal, and bone marrow generally shows erythroid hyperplasia along with the presence of ringed sideroblasts. No treatment is generally used for patients showing only moderate anemia. When treatment is required, transfusions, pyridoxine, or androgens are utilized.

A sideroblastic anemia may also develop secondary to such other diseases as leukemia, hemolytic anemia, neoplastic and inflammatory diseases, and uremia. In these circumstances, there are anemia, some hypochromic red blood cells in the peripheral blood, and a few ringed sideroblasts in the bone marrow.

Sideroblastic anemia may also be caused by certain agents or drugs that interfere with heme synthesis. This anemia may be found in alcoholism, lead poisoning, tuberculosis therapy (antituberculosis drugs), and as a result of receiving large doses of chloramphenicol. Drug-induced sideroblastic anemia is reversible, in that when the patient is removed from the causative agent or drug, the sideroblastic anemia disappears.

HEMOCHROMATOSIS

Excessive amounts of iron that accumulate in the blood and tissues is classified as *hemosiderosis* if the iron accumulation in the macrophages causes little parenchymal cell injury. In *hemochromatosis*, however, the iron accumulates in the parenchymal cells and injures the tissues.

Hereditary hemochromatosis is a rare disease and is inherited as an autosomal recessive trait. It is found primarily in middle-aged men. It is caused by a disorder in the absorption of iron. The iron contained in food is absorbed into the system irrespective of the body's requirement for iron. This excess iron is stored in the tissues, to their detriment.

These patients generally show hepatomegaly (enlarged liver) and a bronze-colored skin pigmentation. In about 50% of the cases, there will be splenomegaly, rheumatoid arthritis-type symptoms, and diabetes mellitus (frequently insulin-resistant). Weakness and weight loss are commonly found as a result of the diabetes. Cardiac abnormalities and loss of hair may also result.

Laboratory tests show an increased serum iron level, slightly decreased transferrin, and an increased saturation of transferrin. The patient's hemoglobin, hematocrit, and blood smear are generally normal, as is the test for rheumatoid arthritis. The macrophages in the bone marrow generally show many small, stainable particles of iron. A liver biopsy will generally show the parenchymal cells to be overloaded with iron.

Hemochromatosis is generally treated by the use of phlebotomy procedures, removing 1 pint of blood at regular intervals until the accumulated iron is removed.

Hemochromatosis may also be caused: (1) By increased numbers of blood transfusions, where the iron is usually stored in the macrophages and not in the parenchymal cells of the liver. (2) In association with chronic anemias (termed *erythropoietic hemochromatosis*), such as thalassemia major and intermedia, and sideroblastic anemias, where the clinical symptoms are similar to hereditary hemochromatosis. (3) By an increased dietary intake of iron (exceeding 100 mg per day). (4) By contributory factors such as alcohol abuse and liver disease.

CONGENITAL DYSERYTHROPOIETIC ANEMIAS

The *congenital dyserythropoietic anemias* are so named because the nucleated red blood cells show multinuclearity, karyorrhexis, and bizarre malformations. They are divided into three groups: Type I, Type II (also termed HEMPAS), and Type III.

Type I is rare and thought to be inherited as an autosomal recessive trait. It is a mildly macrocytic anemia and shows marked anisocytosis and poikilocytosis.

Cabot rings and basophilic stippling are often present in the red blood cells of the peripheral blood. The bone marrow shows megaloblastic characteristics of the developing red blood cells, along with binucleated and incompletely separated or multilobed cells. Splenomegaly is often present.

Type II is also termed HEMPAS (hereditary erythroblast multinuclearity with positive acidified serum test) and is the most common form of this anemia. It is inherited as an autosomal recessive trait. Hepatosplenomegaly is generally present, and jaundice may or may not occur. There is usually a normocytic anemia, along with anisocytosis, poikilocytosis, and basophilic stippling. The bone marrow shows multinuclearity of the nucleated red blood cells but shows no megaloblastic changes. The red blood cells show hemolysis in the acid-serum test but do not hemolyze in the sugar-water test. The red blood cells in this disorder contain an antigen on them, termed the HEMPAS antigen. This disorder generally runs a benign course. A splenectomy is only rarely performed.

Type III is rare and is thought to be inherited as an autosomal dominant trait. It is a normocytic to slightly macrocytic anemia and shows as many as 30% multinucleated red blood cells.

ANEMIA OF BLOOD LOSS

The clinical symptoms associated with anemia due to blood loss depend on the severity of the bleeding. The patient's cardiovascular status, his age, and his emotional and physical health also play a part in his response to bleeding.

In acute blood loss, when there is a sudden loss of 25 to 30% of the total blood volume (1,000 to 1,500 ml), most healthy patients show light-headedness and hypotension when they are in an upright position. With a sudden loss of 40 to 50% of the total blood volume, the patient goes into a severe state of shock, with the pos-

sibility of death. Between 30 to 40% blood loss leads to shortness of breath, sweating, loss of consciousness, and decreased blood pressure. The pulse becomes rapid and weak, and urine volume is reduced. Within an hour of acute blood loss, the platelet count increases, and there is a shortened whole-blood coagulation time. After several hours, the white blood cell count becomes elevated, and there is a shift to the left. Within 1 to 2 days following hemorrhage, the reticulocyte count becomes elevated. Immediately after acute blood loss, the hemoglobin, hematocrit, and red blood cell count are generally elevated due to vasoconstriction and change in blood distribution. Dilution of the blood by tissue fluids then takes place as a defense mechanism to compensate for the lost blood. When this occurs, the hemoglobin, hematocrit, and red blood cell count begin to drop. A normocytic-normochromic anemia develops, with slight anisocytosis and poikilocytosis. Following severe bleeding, large polychromatophilic red blood cells and nucleated red blood cells are present in the peripheral blood. The red blood cell count returns to normal within about 6 weeks after hemorrhage.

In chronic blood loss, when bleeding occurs in small quantities over a period of time, iron-deficiency anemia may develop as a result of the depletion of the iron stores. The white blood cell count is generally low, as is the reticulocyte count, and polychromatophilia is present.

LEUKOERYTHROBLASTOSIS

Leukoerythroblastosis has several synonyms: leukoerythroblastic anemia, myelophthisic anemia, and myelopathic anemia, to name a few. It is a condition of anemia caused by space-occupying disorders of the bone marrow.

The most common cause of leukoerythroblastosis is metastatic carcinoma of the breast, prostate gland, lungs, adrenal gland, or thyroid, due to the tendency of the cancer to spread by vascular channels to bone. It is also found secondary to such diseases as Niemann-Pick disease, Gaucher's disease, Schüller-Christian disease, leukemias, and in some cases of Hodgkin's disease and multiple myeloma.

A normochromic-normocytic anemia of varying degrees is present. One distinguishing characteristic of this condition is the increased presence of nucleated red blood cells in the peripheral blood, quite out of proportion to the degree of anemia. Polychromatophilia, basophilic stippling, and reticulocytosis are usually present. The white blood cell count is generally normal to decreased, with a normal distribution of white blood cells. Frequently, however, a few immature granulocytes may be present. The platelet count is normal to moderately decreased with occasional bizarre forms of the platelet present. Examination of the bone marrow usually shows the cause of leukoerythroblastosis.

ANEMIA OF CHRONIC RENAL INSUFFICIENCY

Patients with chronic renal insufficiency generally show anemia due to failure of the kidneys to produce erythropoietin. Many times, there is a direct relationship between the blood urea nitrogen levels and the severity of the anemia. The higher the blood urea nitrogen, the more severe the anemia. If the kidney disorder is due to infection, however, an anemia of chronic disorders is generally present.

In anemia of chronic renal insufficiency, the red blood cells are normocytic-normochromic, and the hematocrit level is generally 15 to 30%. In addition to decreased red blood cell production, hemolysis may also be present due to a plasma factor that has an adverse effect on red blood cell metabolism, causing the formation of burr cells and irregularly contracted and fragmented red blood cells. The reticulocyte count is generally normal but may sometimes be increased. Some macrocytosis may be present in patients in a dialysis program due to loss of folic acid during dialysis. The white blood cell count is usually normal, with slight neutrophilia. The platelet count is normal to slightly increased. In many cases, however, platelet function is impaired, resulting in bleeding from the genitourinary or gastrointestinal tracts. When this occurs, iron-deficiency anemia may develop. The bone marrow generally shows erythroid hyperplasia. When the renal failure becomes acute, however, the bone marrow may show erythroid hypoplasia.

ANEMIA OF ENDOCRINE DISEASES

Anemia is generally present in disorders that affect the thyroid gland, pituitary gland, adrenal gland, and the gonads.

In hypothyroidism, there is generally a mild to moderate normochromic-normocytic anemia. The reticulocyte count is normal, as is the red blood cell survival time. This anemia is usually a result of decreased bone marrow production caused by decreased oxygen requirements. Hypothyroidism, however, may be complicated by an iron-deficiency anemia or a folic acid or vitamin B_{12} deficiency, in which case the red blood cells will be microcytic-hypochromic or macrocytic, respectively. The response of the anemia to therapy is generally slow, and it may take 6 months to 1 year for the hemoglobin to become normal. Anemia is uncommon and does not generally occur in hyperthyroidism.

In Addison's disease, a mild normocytic-normochromic anemia may be present. This may not be readily apparent in the presence of dehydration.

In hypopituitarism, there is generally a moderate normocytic-normochromic anemia present caused by deficiencies of certain glands controlled by the pituitary gland. A loss in other factors of the pituitary gland, such as growth hormone, may also be a cause of the anemia.

A decrease in testosterone secretion in

males will result in decreased red blood cell production, causing a drop in hemoglobin of 1 to 2 g per dl. This is probably because androgens are capable of increasing erythropoietin synthesis.

Anemia is rarely found in *hyperparathyroidism*.

ANEMIA OF LIVER DISEASES

Anemia is a common finding in the presence of cirrhosis of the liver and other liver diseases. There is generally a normocytic to slightly macrocytic anemia present. The MCV is rarely greater than 115 fl. This anemia may be caused by a decreased red blood cell survival, an inability of the bone marrow to respond to the anemia, or an increase in the total blood volume that exaggerates the anemia. In some cases, iron deficiency anemia may result from blood loss. A sideroblastic anemia may develop in cases of chronic alcoholism. The anemia, however, is rarely severe. The bone marrow will show normal cellularity or an increased cellularity with erythroid hyperplasia. The reticulocyte count is often increased but can be decreased as a result of alcohol ingestion. The platelet count may be normal or slightly decreased, as found in cirrhosis of the liver. In hepatitis, obstructive jaundice, and cirrhosis of the liver, there may be changes in the red blood cell membrane lipids. An increase in cholesterol and lecithin levels leads to an increased red blood cell membrane surface, which gives rise to "thin" macrocytes or target cells. In some instances, there will be an increase in the red blood cell membrane cholesterol level, but not the lecithin level. In this circumstance, "spur" cells are formed, which are thorny projections on the red blood cell that are similar to acanthocytes.

APLASTIC ANEMIA

The basic defect in *aplastic anemia* is a failure in the production of the red blood cells, white blood cells, and platelets. Another term used to describe this condition is *pancytopenia*, which is a reduction in all of the formed elements of the blood. Aplastic anemia may occur as a congenital defect *(Fanconi's anemia)*, or it may be acquired as a result of exposure to chemical or physical agents, in association with other diseases, or as a result of an unknown cause *(idiopathic aplastic anemia)*.

Acquired aplastic anemia may occur as the result of exposure to such physical and chemical agents as ionizing radiation, benzene and its derivatives, sulfur or nitrogen mustard compounds, certain antibiotics, antimitotic agents, and antimetabolites. Agents that may occasionally produce a pancytopenia are antimicrobial agents, anticonvulsants, sedatives and tranquilizers, and other drugs to which certain individuals may be sensitive. The clinical course of the disease may show a very rapid onset and a rapid progression to death, or it may have a slow onset and a chronic course. Laboratory tests generally show pancytopenia with low white blood cell, red blood cell, and platelet counts. The red blood cells are usually normocytic and normochromic. In rare cases, the red blood cells may be macrocytic. Varying degrees of anisocytosis and poikilocytosis may be present. Basophilic stippling, polychromatophilia, and nucleated red blood cells are absent from the peripheral blood. Reticulocytes are decreased to absent. There is generally a neutropenia along with a relative lymphocytosis. The bone marrow is hypocellular, with an increase in fat. Relative lymphocytosis may also be present in the bone marrow. Occasionally, biopsies show a normal marrow. This is misleading because there may be small areas in the marrow in which there is residual blood-cell producing activity. A repeat marrow biopsy at another location gives the typical hypocellular picture. The bleeding time and clot retraction are usually abnormal because of the absence of platelets. The serum iron level is increased, and the iron-binding protein is saturated. Erythropoietin levels are greatly increased. Treatment of aplastic anemia involves (1) removal of the causative agent, if known, (2) red blood cell transfusions to maintain a minimum hemoglobin level, (3) platelet transfusions if necessary, (4) prevention of infection, (5) bone marrow transplantation for severe forms of the disease, and (6) corticosteroids, androgens, and splenectomy for those patients with less severe forms of the illness or those who cannot undergo bone marrow transplantation.

Aplastic anemia may also develop several months following the onset of viral hepatitis. The prognosis in these cases is not good and may result in death. Aplastic anemia has also been found as a complication of some mycobacterial infections and following other disorders.

Idiopathic aplastic anemia is an acquired condition whose cause is unknown. The symptoms and laboratory tests are similar to those of acquired aplastic anemia.

Fanconi's anemia, or *familial aplastic anemia*, is a congenital defect, the onset of which occurs between 5 and 10 years of age. Some chromosomal defects have been described, and developmental abnormalities are present. Deposits of melanin are common, which show up as patchy brown pigmentation of the skin. There is generally a normocytic to slightly macrocytic anemia. Target cells may be present, along with nucleated red blood cells and immature white blood cells. The bone marrow may be normocellular to hypercellular in the beginning but will become hypocellular as the disease progresses. Hemoglobin F is generally increased. This disorder is usually treated with androgens and corticosteroids and has about the same prognosis as the acquired form of the disease.

PURE RED BLOOD CELL APLASIA

Pure red blood cell aplasia is a term given to a category of diseases in which red blood cell production is suppressed, with little or no abnormalities found in the white blood cells or platelets.

Congenital erythroid hypoplasia of Diamond-Blackfan is a rare disorder that is characterized by a moderate to severe anemia. It generally manifests itself during the first 2 to 3 months of life. Infants with this disorder generally show pallor and may or may not have splenomegaly and/or hepatomegaly. At diagnosis, the hemoglobin is quite low, 2 to 10 g per dl, and the anemia is normochromic and may be slightly macrocytic. Reticulocytes in the peripheral blood are decreased to absent. The bone marrow is generally normal except for a marked decrease in erythroid cells. Corticosteroid therapy is used in the treatment of this disorder. When patients do not respond to this treatment, blood transfusions are used. This can cause serious complications, however, because of hemochromatosis, where the liver may become severely damaged.

Acute acquired pure red blood cell aplasia (acute acquired erythropoietic hypoplasia) may suddenly occur for a short period during the course of a hemolytic anemia, certain infections, malnutrition, or with various kinds of drug therapy. The erythroblasts in the bone marrow will suddenly disappear, and an anemia soon develops if this condition persists for any length of time. When this condition occurs during drug therapy, removal of the drug is generally followed by a return to normal erythropoiesis.

Chronic acquired pure red blood cell aplasia (chronic acquired erythrocytic hypoplasia) occurs in adults. About one half of the cases of this disorder have been found in patients with a thymoma (thymic tumor). Removal of the tumor, when present, is followed by an improvement in erythropoiesis more than 50% of the time. The anemia of this disorder is generally severe and is normocytic to slightly macrocytic. The white blood cells and platelets are usually normal. Reticulocytes are decreased to absent. The bone marrow shows normal white blood cell and platelet development and a marked decrease in maturing red blood cells. The serum iron level is usually increased, and the iron-binding capacity is saturated. This disorder has been treated with androgens, adrenal steroids, and immunosuppressive drugs.

HEMOLYTIC ANEMIAS

The hemolytic anemias are a group of anemias that are characterized by an increased destruction of red blood cells. In this condition, the bone marrow is able to respond to the red blood cell destruction. These anemias may be divided into those that are inherited and those that are acquired. Generally speaking, the red blood cells in hemolytic anemias that are inherited have intrinsic defects within the red blood cell itself. The acquired hemolytic anemias usually have normal red blood cells that are destroyed by extrinsic factors or agents outside of the red blood cell. Intravascular hemolysis and extravascular hemolysis refer to the site of red blood cell breakdown: within the bloodstream or outside the blood.

Hereditary Spherocytosis

Hereditary spherocytosis, also known as *congenital hemolytic anemia* and *congenital hemolytic jaundice*, is inherited as a non-sex-linked dominant trait. The symptoms of this condition are variable, depending on the severity of the disease. As a general rule, those cases recognized early in the life of the patient are likely to be more severe than those cases where the symptoms appear later in life. Most often, hereditary spherocytosis is diagnosed in childhood, adolescence, or early adult life. The disorder is caused by a defect in the red blood cell membrane. The exact defect present, however, is not known. The red blood cells are hyperpermeable to sodium, and show an increased rate of destruction, and, as the name of the disease implies,

are spherocytic. The most consistent physical finding is splenomegaly. Jaundice is commonly present and increases during hemolytic episodes. The liver is usually enlarged, and the patient may also exhibit pallor, depending on the degree of anemia present.

This disease is usually accompanied by a moderate anemia. The most constant finding in the peripheral blood is spherocytes. These cells have a decreased diameter and an increased concentration of hemoglobin. The number of spherocytes varies from a few to many. Polychromatophilia is present, and the reticulocyte count may be increased to 20% or higher. There are usually a few nucleated red blood cells present in the peripheral blood. This number increases, however, during hemolytic episodes. The white blood cell and platelet counts are usually normal, except during periods of hemolysis, when there is slight leukocytosis and thrombocytosis. The osmotic fragility test is increased, and the autohemolysis test usually shows greater than 20% hemolysis after 48-hour incubation. The serum bilirubin level is elevated, and the urine and stool may contain increased amounts of urobilinogen. Plasma haptoglobin is generally reduced and may be undetectable. The direct Coombs' test is negative. The bone marrow is hypercellular, with an absolute increase in the erythroid cells. These cells usually constitute 25 to 60% of all the marrow cells.

The treatment for this condition is splenectomy. Spherocytosis continues, but the red blood cell survival time is no longer decreased, because the spleen was the agent responsible for the destruction of the red blood cells. The red blood cell count (also hemoglobin and hematocrit) increases, and the bilirubin level returns to normal. The reticulocyte count decreases, and increased red blood cell production is no longer present. The osmotic fragility and autohemolysis tests continue to be increased.

Hereditary Elliptocytosis

Hereditary elliptocytosis is transmitted as an autosomal dominant gene. This condition is characterized by the presence of variable numbers of elliptical, or oval-shaped, mature red blood cells. The nucleated red blood cells and reticulocytes are normal in shape, however.

Approximately 90% of the individuals showing elliptocytosis have no clinical symptoms other than the presence of elliptical red blood cells. The remaining patients with this condition, however, display a hemolytic anemia similar to hereditary spherocytosis. In this case, the osmotic fragility and autohemolysis of the red blood cells are increased. A splenectomy alleviates the hemolytic condition.

Abetalipoproteinemia

Abetalipoproteinemia is characterized by the absence of beta-lipoprotein in the blood. It manifests itself during the first few months of life with growth failure, abdominal distention, and steatorrhea. This disorder also shows acanthocytosis of the red blood cells, retinitis pigmentosa, and neurologic damage. Laboratory tests show a decreased cholesterol level (usually less than 50 mg per dl) and the absence of beta-lipoprotein in the plasma. The blood smear shows large numbers of acanthocytes. The reticulocyte count is normal to increased, and if anemia is present, it is mild. The red blood cell life span may or may not be shortened. There is no definite treatment for this disorder.

Stomatocytosis

Several causes of *stomatocytosis* have been described: (1) red blood cells containing increased amounts of sodium and a decreased amount of potassium, (2) red blood cells lacking the Rh blood group antigens (Rh_{NULL} phenotype), and (3) red blood cells having neither of the above characteristics. Stomatocytes may also be found in acute alcoholism, liver disorders, cardiovascular disease, and in a small percentage of normal individuals.

Stomatocytosis caused by increased sodium and decreased potassium is inherited as an autosomal dominant trait. The anemia is generally mild. The reticulocyte count may be normal to moderately elevated and is usually 10 to 20%. Approximately 10 to 50% of the red blood cells will appear as stomatocytes. The serum bilirubin level will be increased and the haptoglobin decreased, depending on the amount of hemolysis present. The osmotic fragility may be decreased, normal, or increased. Autohemolysis is increased and not completely corrected with glucose and ATP. Red blood cell survival is generally slightly shortened. Splenectomy may or may not aid in the treatment of this disorder.

Rh_{NULL} Disease

Rh_{NULL} disease is inherited and represents an absence of all Rh-Hr antigens on the red blood cell. It is characterized by a mild normocytic-normochromic anemia. The blood smear shows both stomatocytes and spherocytes. The reticulocyte count is generally slightly elevated. The autohemolysis and osmotic fragility are both increased.

High Phosphatidylcholine Hemolytic Anemia

High phosphatidylcholine hemolytic anemia is inherited and represents an imbalance in the membrane phospholipid content of the red blood cell. It usually causes a mild anemia with morphologically normal red blood cells. The anemia may increase in the presence of infection or under conditions of stress.

Glucose-6-Phosphate Dehydrogenase Deficiency

Glucose-6-phosphate dehydrogenase (G-6-PD) deficiency is inherited. It is sex-linked, being carried on the X chromosome. The disease becomes fully expressed in the hemizygous male and the homozygous female.

Glucose-6-phosphate dehydrogenase is an enzyme present in the red blood cell. It plays a major role in the hexose-mono-phosphate shunt. It is concerned with the regeneration of TPNH, necessary for the reduction of oxidized glutathione—a mechanism by which hemoglobin is protected from oxidation. The absence of this enzyme is usually harmless unless the red blood cell is exposed to redox compounds (antimalarial drugs, sulfonamides, nitro-furans, sulfones, analgesics, and antipy-retics). When there is a deficiency of G-6-PD, the red blood cell is unable to generate reduced nicotinamide-adenine dinucleo-tide phosphate (NADP) rapidly enough to combat the effects of oxidizing drugs. The oxidation of hemoglobin to methemoglo-bin is then followed by Heinz body for-mation. There are both quantitatively and qualitatively abnormal forms of the en-zyme, which may be due to a decrease in the enzyme activity or to a qualitative ab-normality of the enzyme.

Upon continual ingestion of a redox compound by a patient deficient in G-6-PD, a hemolytic episode will occur. This condition may be divided into three phases: (1) During the acute hemolytic phase, there is destruction of 30 to 50% of the red blood cells. There is Heinz body formation, and basophilic stippling and polychromatophilia are present on the pe-ripheral blood smear. The serum bilirubin is elevated, as is the reticulocyte count. (2) During the recovery phase (tenth to for-tieth day), the reticulocyte count reaches a peak of 8 to 12%. Macrocytes are present on the peripheral blood smear, and the hemoglobin and hematocrit levels begin to increase to normal. Haptoglobin is absent in the blood, and methemalbumin is pres-ent. Plasma hemoglobin is increased dur-ing the first two stages. (3) The resistant phase begins when the anemia disappears and continues as long as the same dose of the drug is administered. If the drug dos-age is increased, another hemolytic epi-sode will occur.

A few patients continually show chronic anemia, but the majority are not anemic except during a hemolytic episode after exposure to certain drugs. The au-tohemolysis test shows increased he-molysis of red blood cells after 48-hour incubation in patients with glucose-6-phosphate dehydrogenase deficiency. The autohemolysis, however, is partially cor-rected by the addition of glucose or ATP. This deficiency has, therefore, been de-scribed as having type I autohemolysis. The ascorbate-cyanide test is positive for patients with this deficiency.

Pyruvate Kinase Deficiency

Pyruvate kinase is an enzyme in the Embden-Meyerhof pathway and may be the most common cause of hereditary non-spherocytic hemolytic anemia.

Pyruvate kinase deficiency is inherited as an autosomal recessive trait, with mem-bers of both sexes being equally affected. Heterozygous individuals manifest no symptoms, whereas homozygous individ-uals have the clinical disease. The disease may be present at birth. The newborn is jaundiced and may require transfusions or exchange transfusions. In most instances of pyruvate kinase deficiency, however, the disease is first found in infancy or childhood, with some cases not appearing until adulthood. Characteristics of this disorder are jaundice, splenomegaly, ane-mia of varying severity, and occasional dark urine.

The laboratory findings in this disorder show mild to severe anemia with hema-tocrit levels of approximately 18 to 36%. The red blood cells are normochromic and may be slightly macrocytic. The reticulo-cyte count is moderately to markedly in-creased, and the peripheral blood smear shows polychromatophilia and the pres-ence of nucleated red blood cells. There may be slight anisocytosis, and there are generally irregularly contracted red blood cells present. The white blood cell and platelet counts are usually normal. In the autohemolysis test, the type II pattern is found. Mildly affected patients, however, may show a normal autohemolysis test. The bone marrow shows erythroid hyperplasia. The serum bilirubin and fecal urobilinogen levels are increased. The serum haptoglobin is decreased to absent. The red blood cell pyruvate kinase activity is in the range of 5 to 25% of normal.

There is no exact treatment for pyruvate kinase deficiency. Limited use of blood transfusions and splenectomy have been utilized.

Other Red Blood Cell Enzyme Deficiencies

Other red blood cell enzyme deficiencies, not as common as G-6-PD and pyruvate kinase deficiencies, can also cause a hemolytic anemia.

Pyrimidine 5-nucleotidase deficiency causes an abnormality in nucleotide metabolism. Laboratory tests show basophilic stippling, and red blood cell autohemolysis is increased and only poorly corrected with glucose.

Glucosephosphate isomerase deficiency causes an abnormality in anaerobic glycolysis and is the third most common red blood cell enzyme deficiency. It causes a moderately severe anemia. The stained blood smear shows anisocytosis, poikilocytosis, and marked polychromatophilia, and nucleated red blood cells may also be present. The reticulocyte count may be significantly increased, and the autohemolysis test is increased with only partial correction by glucose and ATP. *Triosephosphate isomerase, hexokinase,* and *diphosphoglycerate mutase* are other enzyme deficiencies that have been found to occur and are involved in anaerobic glycolysis.

Several deficiencies in addition to G-6-PD have been found in enzymes required in the hexose monophosphate shunt. These deficiencies are rare but do cause a hemolytic anemia. These deficiencies include *glutathione synthetase, glutathione peroxidase,* and *glutathione reductase.*

Unstable Hemoglobin Disease

Unstable hemoglobin disease is rare and may be caused by any one of a large number of hemoglobin variants, all of which are less stable than normal hemoglobin. They are inherited as autosomal dominant traits and all of the known cases are heterozygous. The severity of the disease varies according to the hemoglobin variant, and there may be no clinical symptoms or the disease may produce a mild, moderate, or severe hemolytic anemia.

The degree of anemia and reticulocytosis present will depend on the severity of the disease. Heinz bodies are characteristically present in the red blood cells because of the instability of the hemoglobin. These may cause a lower than normal MCHC because the hemoglobin present in Heinz bodies is not measured. The stained blood smear generally shows anisocytosis, poikilocytosis, basophilic stippling, polychromatophilia, and sometimes hypochromia. If the anemia is severe, spherocytes and schistocytes may also be present. If the spleen is enlarged, there may be a thrombocytopenia caused by sequestering of the platelets in the spleen. The reticulocyte count will generally be increased. Much care must be taken when performing the reticulocyte count to distinguish the Heinz bodies from true reticulocytes. The heat denaturation test and the isopropanol precipitation test are both positive. Therapy is generally not necessary in cases of mild anemia. When the anemia is more severe, a splenectomy is generally performed.

Normal Hemoglobins and Hemoglobinopathies

The hemoglobin molecule is composed of four heme groups, each attached to a separate polypeptide chain. This polypeptide chain is composed of amino acids attached to each other in a definite characteristic sequence to form a long chain. Each chain is then bent and coiled as a result of further bonding between the amino acids.

Different types of normal hemoglobins have been described and given specific names based on the number and sequence of amino acids composing each polypeptide chain. On the following pages, the normal and more common abnormal hemoglobin forms are discussed briefly.

NORMAL HEMOGLOBINS

The major portion of normal hemoglobin in adult blood is termed *hemoglobin A*. The globin portion of each hemoglobin A molecule is composed of two alpha chains, containing 141 amino acids, and two beta chains, made up of 146 amino acids. The formula for hemolgobin A is: $\alpha_2^A \beta_2^A$, indicating that the molecule is made up of two normal hemoglobin A, alpha chains, and two normal hemoglobin A, beta chains. The concentration of hemoglobin A normally comprises 95% or more of the total adult hemoglobin.

A second type of hemoglobin, *hemoglobin A_2*, is normally found in the adult in a concentration of 1.5 to 3% of the total hemoglobin. Hemoglobin A_2 consists of two alpha^A chains, and two other chains that differ from the beta^A chains by the substitution of 10 amino acids. These two chains, since they differ so greatly from beta^A chains, are termed delta, thus giving hemoglobin A_2 the formula: $\alpha_2^A \delta_2^{A_2}$.

Fetal hemoglobin, *hemoglobin F*, is normally present in high concentrations during fetal life. At birth, at least half of the hemoglobin present in the newborn is hemoglobin F. The concentration of hemoglobin F then falls rapidly and assumes the normal adult level of 2% or less by 1 or 2 years of age. Hemoglobin F is comprised of two alpha chains and two other chains that differ from the beta^A chains and are termed gamma. The formula for hemoglobin F is, therefore: $\alpha_2^A \gamma_2^F$.

In early fetal life, a primitive or embryonal hemoglobin is found, namely, *hemoglobin Gower 1* and *hemoglobin Gower 2*. These two hemoglobins persist for only a short time in the embryo. Hemoglobin Gower 1 is designated $\epsilon_4^{Gower\ 1}$, and hemoglobin Gower 2 is written as $\alpha_2^A \epsilon_2^{Gower\ 2}$.

ABNORMAL HEMOGLOBINS

The structure of abnormal hemoglobins is based on at least four kinds of polypeptide chains, alpha, beta, delta, and gamma, and possibly a fifth chain, epsilon. The synthesis of any given type of chain is under genetic control. The structurally abnormal hemoglobins usually consist of polypeptide chains with a normal number of amino acids but with a single amino acid substitution. For example, if a normal pair of chains has glutamic acid at the sixth position, the abnormal form may have a valine molecule in place of the glutamic acid. Alterations in the amino acid composition of the polypeptide chain usually cause a change in the net charge of the molecule. This property is then employed to detect the presence of different hemoglobins. Using the techniques of electrophoresis, blood is placed on a medium in an electric field. The difference in the net charge of the hemoglobin molecule determines its mobility and the speed with which it migrates. Most of the abnormal hemoglobins that have been discovered are now detected by this method.

Hemoglobin S is an abnormal hemoglobin that causes sickling of the red blood cells under conditions of reduced oxygen concentration. It shows an amino acid substitution in the beta chains and is written as $\alpha_2^A \beta_2^{6\ val}$, indicating a substitution of valine at the sixth position in the normal beta chain. Hemoglobin S is confined to blacks and, in the homozygous state, causes sickle cell anemia. An individual heterozygous for hemoglobin S shows the sickle cell trait.

Hemoglobin C ($\alpha_2^A \beta_2^{6\ lys}$) is found primarily in blacks and only rarely in whites. It is, many times, inherited in combination with hemoglobin S and may also be found in the homozygous or heterozygous state. When hemoglobin C is present, the red blood cells appear as target cells, or, less often, hemoglobin crystals may be demonstrated within the red blood cell.

Hemoglobin D shows several varieties of abnormal hemoglobin that are indistinguishable from each other by electrophoretic methods. Both alpha and beta chain abnormalities have been reported. The electrophoretic mobility of hemoglobin D is the same as hemoglobin S, although red blood cells containing hemoglobin D show no sickling at a reduced oxygen concentration.

Hemoglobin E ($\alpha_2^A \beta_2^{26 \text{ lys}}$) shows the same electrophoretic mobility as hemoglobin A_2 and is sometimes associated with thalassemia. In the homozygous state, many target cells are present.

Hemoglobins have also been found that contain no alpha chains. For example: *hemoglobin H* consists of four beta chains: β_4^A; and *hemoglobin Bart's* is comprised of four gamma chains: γ_4^F.

Hemoglobin C Disease

In the homozygous condition, there is almost 100% hemoglobin C present in the red blood cells. In some patients, there may also be an increased concentration of hemoglobin F. *Homozygous hemoglobin C disease* is characterized by a mild to moderate normocytic-normochromic, hemolytic anemia with splenomegaly. The stained blood smear shows 40 to 90% target cells, a few spherocytes, and slight polychromatophilia. The reticulocyte count is slightly increased. In some instances, rod-shaped crystals (termed *hemoglobin C crystals*) may be seen within the red blood cell in the Wright-stained blood smear, or the crystals may be demonstrated by incubating the red blood cells at 37°C in 3% (w/v) sodium chloride. Hemoglobin electrophoresis shows almost 100% hemoglobin C and less than 7% hemoglobin F. Most patients with hemoglobin C disease live a normal life span.

Sickle Cell Anemia

A person homozygous for hemoglobin S is said to have *sickle cell anemia*. In this disorder, which is confined to blacks, the red blood cells contain 90 to 100% hemoglobin S, with the remainder being hemoglobin F. The symptoms of sickle cell anemia rarely occur prior to about 6 months of age, because hemoglobin F predominates at birth and for a short time thereafter. This disease is usually fatal by the age of 30. The physical properties of the red blood cells have much to do with the clinical manifestations of the disease. Under decreased oxygen tension, hemoglobin S is much less soluble than hemoglobin A. This forces the red blood cell into a rigid sickle-shaped cell when the oxygen concentration is reduced. As a result, clinical crises occur. There is severe abdominal, bone, and joint pain thought to be due, possibly, to plugging up of some of the small blood vessels by masses of the sickled red blood cells. This, in turn, causes infarcts in different organs of the body. The spleen, enlarged during infancy, eventually shrivels up and becomes fibrotic in the adult (autosplenectomy) because of these numerous infarcts. The sickled red blood cells also have an increased mechanical fragility that results in a decreased survival time. There is severe marrow hyperplasia, and changes are produced in the bones.

On a stained blood smear, the red blood cells appear normocytic and normochromic. Some sickle cells are generally present. Target cells, Howell-Jolly bodies, and nucleated red blood cells are usually seen. Polychromatophilia is generally increased, and an elevated reticulocyte count is found. The platelets are usually increased, and there may be moderate neutrophilia. The osmotic fragility test is decreased, and the erythrocyte sedimentation rate is low. Sickle-cell preparations are quickly and strongly positive. Hemoglobin electrophoresis shows a single abnormal band, hemoglobin S, which migrates more slowly than hemoglobin A. The bone marrow is hypercellular due to an increase in the erythroid cells. Cell maturation and morphology in the bone marrow are normal.

Sickle Cell Trait

The *sickle cell trait* is found in approximately 10% of American blacks. In this condition, the patient is heterozygous for hemoglobin S. The red blood cells contain 20 to 40% hemoglobin S and 60 to 80% hemoglobin A. Under normal conditions, sickling of the red blood cells does not occur, there are no clinical symptoms of the disease, and the patient lives a normal life span. There is no anemia present, and the red blood cell morphology is normal. An occasional target cell may be found, but no sickle cells are demonstrable in the stained blood smear. The reticulocyte count is normal, and there is no polychromatophilia on the stained blood smear. The sickle cell preparation is always positive, and hemoglobin electrophoresis shows a band of hemoglobin S. Over 50% of the patients with sickle cell trait do not have the ability to concentrate urine *(hyposthenuria)*.

Under certain conditions, such as a respiratory infection, administration of anesthesia, or airplane flight in a nonpressurized cabin, there may be some sickling of the red blood cells with accompanying clinical manifestations.

Thalassemia

Thalassemia is an hereditary disease found in people of Mediterranean, Asian, and African ancestry. It is caused by impaired production of one of the polypeptide chains of the hemoglobin molecule. The structural formation of the chains is normal, but the rate of formation is de-

creased. Impaired synthesis of the beta chain is the most common, and the term applied to this abnormality is *beta thalassemia*. Decreased production of alpha chains and delta chains may also be found.

THALASSEMIA MAJOR

Thalassemia major, or *Cooley's anemia*, is a homozygous beta thalassemia. This disease generally has its onset during infancy. The most common physical findings are marked pallor and moderate to marked splenomegaly. Enlargement of the liver is also frequently present. Most of these patients exhibit retarded growth, and their facial features show a mongoloid appearance. Patients with Cooley's anemia rarely live beyond the second decade.

There is severe hemolytic anemia present. The peripheral blood smear shows microcytic, hypochromic red blood cells, probably due to the decreased synthesis of globin. There is marked anisocytosis and poikilocytosis. Basophilic stippling, increased polychromatophilia, numerous target cells, Howell-Jolly bodies, and siderocytes are commonly found in the blood smear. Nucleated red blood cells are present in the peripheral blood and may be as numerous as 200 or more per 100 white blood cells. The reticulocyte count is increased. The white blood cell count may be slightly increased, with occasional immature granulocytes present. A slight increase in platelets may also be found. The osmotic fragility test is decreased. The bone marrow shows an erythroid hyperplasia, and storage iron is increased. The plasma haptoglobin level is generally markedly decreased to absent. Hemoglobin electrophoresis most often shows 40 to 60% hemoglobin F. In some cases, hemoglobin A_2 is also increased.

THALASSEMIA MINOR

Thalassemia minor is a heterozygous beta thalassemia that is also known as *Cooley's trait*. This condition is characterized by slight splenomegaly and mild anemia. Patients with this trait generally live a normal life span.

The peripheral blood usually shows a hemoglobin of 10 to 11 g per dl. Microcytic, hypochromic red blood cells are found on the blood smear. Target cells, increased polychromatophilia, basophilic stippling, and an occasional nucleated red blood cell are found on the Wright-stained smear. The reticulocyte count is slightly elevated. The white blood cell count is normal. The bone marrow shows slight erythroid hyperplasia and increased storage iron. Hemoglobin electrophoresis shows 2 to 6% hemoglobin F and 3 to 7% hemoglobin A_2, with the remainder being hemoglobin A.

Acquired Hemolytic Anemias

A hemolytic anemia may develop as a result of exposure to various physical agents such as heat. A substantial amount of third-degree burns to the body will damage red blood cells. The blood smear in these cases will show schistocytes, spherocytes, and irregularly contracted red blood cells. The red blood cells will also show increased osmotic fragility. In cardiac valve disease where the diseased valve has been surgically replaced, mechanical damage to the red blood cells may occur.

Infectious agents, such as *Clostridium perfringens, Bartonella bacilliformis,* and some staphylococcal and other bacterial infections, have been known to produce a hemolytic anemia.

Some chemicals and drugs are capable of denaturing hemoglobin or causing a hemolytic response. Venom from some spiders and snakes may also cause hemolysis of the red blood cells.

ISOIMMUNE HEMOLYTIC ANEMIA

Isoantibodies are antibodies formed by a person who lacks any antigen that would react with this antibody. An example of this would occur if an Rh-negative person were transfused with Rh-positive blood. *Isoimmune hemolytic anemia* will occur as a result of hemolytic transfusion reactions and will also be found in hemolytic disease of the newborn.

HEMOLYTIC DISEASE OF THE NEWBORN

Hemolytic disease of the newborn, or *erythroblastosis fetalis,* is a disorder found in the fetus that manifests itself in the infant during the first several days of life. This disease is usually found in cases of Rh incompatibility where the mother is Rh negative, and the newborn is Rh positive. It is found, with more frequency and less severity, when there is incompatibility within the mother and child's ABO groups. This disorder may also be caused by other blood group systems such as Kell and Duffy. Whenever the infant's blood contains an antigen not present in the mother's blood, a corresponding antibody may be developed by the mother that then acts to destroy the baby's red blood cells.

In hemolytic disease of the newborn, the infant's peripheral blood shows a large increase in nucleated red blood cells, usually present in all stages of development. There is very little anisocytosis; however, a marked polychromatophilia is present. The reticulocyte count is increased and may even be as high as 60%. The red blood cells are usually normochromic and macrocytic. When the hemolytic anemia is due to an ABO incompatibility, there may be marked spherocytosis (accompanied by an increase in the osmotic fragility of the red blood cells). The hemoglobin level at birth is generally slightly lower than normal, decreasing rapidly as the disease progresses. At the same time, the nucleated red blood cells decrease in number and may disappear from the peripheral blood. The white blood cell count is generally elevated, and immature forms of the granulocyte cells are usually present. Platelets are normal to decreased in number. If decreased, there may be a prolonged bleeding time, poor clot retraction, and petechiae. The serum bilirubin level of umbilical cord blood will be above 3 mg per dl. After birth, the bilirubin level rises rapidly and may reach 40 to 50 mg per dl by the third day in cases where no treatment has been given. This rise in bilirubin is due to the indirect fraction of bilirubin. The direct Coombs' test on the baby's red blood cells is positive in all cases except in ABO incompatibility, where the direct Coombs' test is generally negative or weakly positive, becoming negative within 12 hours after birth. The infant with this disorder has an enlarged spleen and liver.

The most common treatment for hemolytic disease of the newborn is the exchange transfusion. If the cord blood bilirubin level at birth is above 4.5 mg per dl, an exchange transfusion is usually carried out immediately. During the first few days of life, the bilirubin level is allowed to rise to 20 mg per dl before an exchange transfusion is performed. More than one exchange transfusion may or may not be required, depending on the severity of the disease.

AUTOIMMUNE HEMOLYTIC ANEMIA

Autoantibodies are antibodies produced by an individual that react with specific antigens within that individual. Therefore, in *autoimmune hemolytic anemia*, the antibodies are produced by the patient's immune system. These anemias may be classified as (1) warm-reactive, (2) cold-reactive, or (3) drug-induced.

Autoimmune hemolytic anemia caused by warm-reactive antibodies may occur without any obvious cause or may be secondary to or associated with various disease states such as viral infections, malignant tumors, systemic lupus erythematosus, and other autoimmune disorders. The clinical symptoms will include weakness and dizziness. Fever may be present, and jaundice is a fairly common finding. This anemia may be variable in its severity, ranging from very mild to very severe. The blood smear generally shows anisocytosis, polychromatophilia, spherocytosis, and some macrocytosis, and nucleated red blood cells may also be present. The reticulocyte count is variable and may show a marked increase. Siderocytes will be increased. The white blood cell count may be increased during the acute phase of the disease. Generally, the platelet count is normal. The autohemolysis test is increased, and the osmotic fragility will be increased during the acute phase but may be normal during periods of remission. The direct antiglobulin test is generally positive but may be negative in cases of weak red blood cell sensitization. Several methods of treatment are used for this disorder. If the hemolytic anemia is secondary to another disorder, treatment of the primary condition may alleviate the hemolytic anemia. In addition, blood transfusions are used to treat the decreased hemoglobin, although steroids are the therapy of choice. When steroid therapy is ineffective, a splenectomy may be performed. Cytotoxic drugs have also been utilized.

Autoimmune hemolytic anemia due to cold-reactive antibodies is caused by antibodies most reactive at temperatures below 32°C. This disease occurs most often in people over 50 years of age and may occur in association with infection, malignancy, or autoimmune disorders. It is most commonly found as a complication of *Mycoplasma pneumoniae*. The two most common cold agglutinins are anti-I and anti-i. A stained blood film generally shows polychromatophilia, possibly some spherocytosis, and agglutination of the red blood cells (unless measures were taken to maintain the blood and equipment at 37°C during smear preparation). The white blood cell count may or may not be elevated. The direct antiglobulin test will be positive if the reagents used contain anticomplement activity. The cold agglutinin titer is increased. Treatment of the patient includes keeping the body temperature above the temperature at which the antibody reacts. Plasmapheresis has been used for the acutely ill patient. Also, treatment of the primary illness may lessen the hemolytic disorder.

Drug-induced autoimmune hemolytic anemia may result from penicillin, stilophen, or an alpha-methyldopa type of drug.

PAROXYSMAL COLD HEMOGLOBINURIA

Paroxysmal cold hemoglobinuria is a rare disorder caused by an antibody described by Donath and Landsteiner, which has thus been named the *Donath-Landsteiner antibody*. It has classically been found secondary to syphilis but has also been seen in viral infections and with no apparent cause.

This disorder manifests itself following exposure to cold, and the patient will exhibit fever, chills, and back and leg pain, along with hemoglobinuria. The patient generally recovers from the attack quickly and may have no symptoms in between attacks.

Laboratory tests show an anemia, the severity of which depends on the severity of the attacks. The reticulocyte count is usually increased. During attacks, the plasma shows marked hemolysis and will contain methemalbumin. The urine contains hemoglobin and methemoglobin, and the serum bilirubin level is elevated. Treatment consists of improving the primary infection, when present, or having the patient avoid cold temperatures.

DISORDERS CAUSING FRAGMENTATION OF THE RED BLOOD CELLS

There are numerous circumstances during which the red blood cells are subjected to physical trauma causing fragmentation and lysis.

Replacement of cardiac valves by prosthetic devices may result in enough damage and destruction to the red blood cell to cause anemia of varying severity. In this situation, the stained blood smear characteristically shows schistocytes. Poly-

chromatophilia and some macrocytosis may also be present. The reticulocyte count will be increased. The bilirubin and plasma hemoglobin may be elevated, depending on the severity of the anemia. Cases where the anemia is severe may indicate a malfunction of the replaced valve, and repeat surgery may be necessary.

Microangiopathic hemolytic anemia is generally a result of fibrin deposits within the small blood vessels, as found in association with thrombotic thrombocytopenia purpura and intravascular coagulation. It is also present in malignant hypertension, disseminated carcinoma, and hemolytic-uremic syndrome in children. The common denominator in these diseases is the presence of small blood vessel disease or pathologic lesions of the small blood vessels. In this anemia, red blood cell fragmentation (schistocytes) and irregular contraction of the red blood cells are very characteristic findings on the blood smear. Microspherocytes may also be present. The reticulocyte count is generally elevated, and the white blood cell count may be slightly to moderately increased. The platelet count may be normal or decreased, largely depending on the primary disorder. The bone marrow usually shows increased red blood cell hyperplasia and megakaryocyte hyperplasia. The plasma hemoglobin is generally increased, urine hemoglobin is present, and hemosiderin can most often be demonstrated in the urine. Therapy usually consists of treating the primary disease. Blood transfusions have been used to treat the anemia when necessary.

PAROXYSMAL NOCTURNAL HEMOGLOBINURIA

Paroxysmal nocturnal hemoglobinuria is a rare, acquired, hemolytic disease. The exact cause of this disorder is unknown. There appears to be an acquired intrinsic defect in the red blood cells that makes the cell sensitive to heat-labile serum factors (complement). The severity of the disorder varies from patient to patient and from time to time in the same patient.

This disorder is characterized by intravascular hemolysis and hemoglobinuria during and following sleep. The peripheral blood shows normocytic-normochromic anemia. The platelet and white blood cell counts are usually decreased. The bone marrow may be hypercellular with erythroid hyperplasia, or, as occurs in some patients, it may be hypocellular. The leukocyte alkaline phosphatase is decreased, and the direct Coombs' test is negative. Diagnosis of this condition may be confirmed by the acid-serum test and the sugar-water test.

POLYCYTHEMIA

Polycythemia is a term used to signify an above-normal hemoglobin, hematocrit, and red blood cell count. It may also be referred to as *erythrocytosis*. This condition is classified as absolute or relative. Absolute polycythemia is further subdivided into secondary and primary polycythemia (polycythemia vera).

Relative Polycythemia

Relative polycythemia is caused by a decrease in the fluid (plasma) portion of the blood. Therefore, the actual number of red blood cells in the blood is not increased, but the number of cells per unit volume of blood is increased.

Relative polycythemia is found in dehydration and in certain cases attributed to nervous stress. The latter condition is termed *stress polycythemia* and is found most often in hard-working, hyperactive, middle-aged males.

The peripheral blood smear shows normocytic, normochromic red blood cells and normal white blood cell, red blood cell, and platelet morphology. The hemoglobin, hematocrit, and red blood cell count are elevated. The white blood cell count may be normal or, in dehydration, slightly elevated. The whole blood volume is decreased, whereas the total red blood cell volume is normal. A normal bone marrow is found in this condition, and the leukocyte alkaline phosphatase is also normal.

Absolute Polycythemia

SECONDARY POLYCYTHEMIA

Secondary polycythemia is caused by an increased level of erythropoietin in the blood, attributable to one of two conditions:

1. Any disorder or circumstance that decreases the arterial oxygen saturation of the blood or decreases the capacity of the hemoglobin molecule to carry oxygen. Specific causes include: residence at high altitudes, chronic pulmonary disease, chronic congestive heart failure, and certain abnormal hemoglobins such as hemoglobin Chesapeake.
2. Certain tumors of the liver, brain, and pituitary gland, renal carcinoma, and occasionally in Cushing's syndrome. In this type of secondary polycythemia, the erythropoietin level is elevated, but the arterial oxygen saturation of the blood is normal and no conditions of hypoxia are present.

The peripheral blood smear shows normocytic, normochromic red blood cells, and normal white blood cell, red blood cell, and platelet morphology. The hemoglobin, hematocrit, and red blood cell count are elevated. The white blood cell count is normal. The whole blood volume is increased as a result of the increased total red blood cell mass. The bone marrow shows erythroid hyperplasia, and the leukocyte alkaline phosphatase is normal.

PRIMARY POLYCYTHEMIA (POLYCYTHEMIA VERA)

Polycythemia vera is a chronic disease of unknown origin that is found most often in patients over 60 years of age. At onset, this disease is characterized by an absolute increase in red blood cells, white blood cells, and platelets. This gives rise to an increased blood volume that may measure two to three times normal. The plasma volume shows little or no change. Because of the increased red blood cell concentration, the viscosity of the blood becomes increased, and the patient shows increased skin coloration. The blood pressure is usually elevated. Increased platelets, along with the increased blood viscosity, may cause the formation of intravascular thrombi. Splenomegaly is a relatively common finding, and an enlarged liver is found in many cases. The arterial oxygen saturation and erythropoietin level are both normal. There is a marked increase in the incidence of peptic ulcer among patients with this disorder.

The peripheral blood smear shows normocytic, normochromic red blood cells, moderate anisocytosis, and slight polychromatophilia. There may be occasional nucleated red blood cells and immature granulocytes present. Atypical platelets or megakaryocyte fragments may also be seen. The relative and absolute number of eosinophils and basophils may be increased, and neutrophilia is usually present. The red blood cell count, hemoglobin, hematocrit, white blood cell count, and platelet count are increased. The reticulocyte count generally shows a slight elevation, not usually over 4%, however. The erythrocyte sedimentation rate is usually decreased. The bone marrow is hypercellular, showing an increase in the granulocytic, erythroid, and megakaryocytic cells. The distribution, morphology, and maturation of the marrow cells are normal. The leukocyte alkaline phosphatase is usually increased, which aids in distinguishing polycythemia vera from other types of erythrocytosis.

Methods of treatment for polycythemia vera include phlebotomies at regular intervals, radioactive phosphorus, and alkylating agents, as used for treatment in leukemia. If the patient does not die from complications of the disease, the bone marrow may become fibrotic until it reaches an aplastic stage. A mild anemia develops, which later becomes marked. Hemorrhagic problems may develop due to platelets that are decreased or abnormal. Hematopoiesis may begin to occur in the liver and spleen. Nucleated red blood cells, myelocytes, and sometimes even myeloblasts may be found in the peripheral blood. Some cases terminate in acute or chronic myelogenous leukemia or myelofibrosis with myeloid metaplasia.

METHEMOGLOBINEMIA

Methemoglobinemia may be inherited as an autosomal recessive trait caused by a deficiency in NADH-methemoglobin reductase, it may be acquired as a result of exposure to various chemical compounds, or it may be caused by one of five hemoglobin M variants. Methemoglobin is different from normal oxyhemoglobin in that the iron in the heme molecule is in the ferric state rather than the ferrous state, and the O_2 is replaced by $-OH$. Normally, less than 1% of the hemoglobin is methemoglobin. One of the main characteristics of these disorders is cyanosis, which gives a bluish color to the skin and mucous membranes.

In *hereditary methemoglobinemia*, infants are cyanotic at birth. Mental retardation may be present, but otherwise the disease is usually benign. A mild polycythemia may sometimes be present. The cyanosis is generally only of importance cosmetically. This disease may be treated with methylene blue taken orally to maintain the methemoglobin concentration below 10%. Ascorbic acid is also used in treatment.

Acquired methemoglobinemia is the most common type of this disorder and is usually due to the toxic effect of such drugs as aniline dyes and derivatives, sulfonamides, nitrates, and nitrites, chlorates, nitroglycerin, and some benzenes, among others. The concentration of methemoglobin in the blood will depend on the degree of exposure to the drug. Cyanosis generally appears when the methemoglobin reaches a level of 15%. Levels exceeding 60 to 70% are generally associated with coma and even death. Treatment consists of withdrawal of the offending drug, and, when symptoms are present, methylene blue or ascorbic acid may be given.

Hemoglobin M disease is characterized by an amino acid substitution in the alpha or beta globin chain. Cyanosis is the only clinical symptom present and is generally not apparent until the infant is 3 to 6 months of age. These individuals lead normal lives and do not respond to methylene blue or ascorbic acid therapy.

SULFHEMOGLOBINEMIA

Sulfhemoglobinemia, when present, is generally the result of exposure to sulfonamides, acetanilid, or phenacetin but may accompany methemoglobinemia. Sulfhemoglobin, once formed, is very stable and remains for the life of the red blood cell. Sulfhemoglobinemia is generally a benign disorder, and about the only symptom it causes is cyanosis. Treatment consists of removing the offending drug.

THE PORPHYRIAS

The *porphyrias* are a group of disorders caused by specific enzyme defects necessary for the synthesis of the heme molecule (Fig. 152). These disorders are characterized by an increased production and excretion of the porphyrins and/or their precursors. The porphyrias will cause cutaneous photosensitivity and/or neurologic abnormalities, depending on the specific defect.

Congenital erythropoietic porphyria causes cutaneous photosensitivity and is one of the rarer types of porphyria. It is inherited as an autosomal recessive trait. In this disorder, there is decreased production of uroporphyrinogen III cosynthetase, which then results in an overproduction of uroporphyrinogen I and, to a

lesser extent, an overproduction of coproporphyrinogen I. These excess porphyrins are then excreted. Exposure to sunlight causes lesions, which heal slowly and eventually lead to scarring and disfigurement. There is generally a mild normocytic-normochromic anemia resulting from red blood cell hemolysis, and there is also ineffective erythropoiesis. Most characteristic is an increased excretion of uroporphyrinogen I in the urine, which may be pink to deep burgundy in color. Splenectomy may improve the anemia, but the primary concern is to protect the patient from exposure to sunlight.

Porphyria cutanea tarda is inherited as an autosomal dominant trait and is caused by a decreased production of uroporphyrinogen decarboxylase. It is manifested clinically by a skin sensitivity to light and to minor trauma. This disease may only manifest itself in the presence of a liver disorder. The urine is generally reddish or brownish in color and contains increased amounts of uroporphyrin I. Improved liver function may effectively decrease the symptoms of the disease. Phlebotomy has also been used to remove iron stores from the liver. An acquired form of porphyria cutanea tarda has been found that is caused by exposure to halogenated aromatic hydrocarbons.

Erythropoietic protoporphyria is inherited as an autosomal dominant trait. It is caused by a decreased activity of heme synthetase, resulting in increased concentrations of protoporphyrin IX in the feces. The red blood cells also contain a marked increase in protoporphyrin IX and will show fluorescent cytoplasm. There is generally no anemia present. This disorder is clinically manifested by a mild sensitivity to sunlight but with minimal lesions and scar formation. Several drugs, including beta-carotene beadlets, and cholestyramine have been used effectively for treatment.

Acute intermittent porphyria causes neurologic abnormalities and is inherited

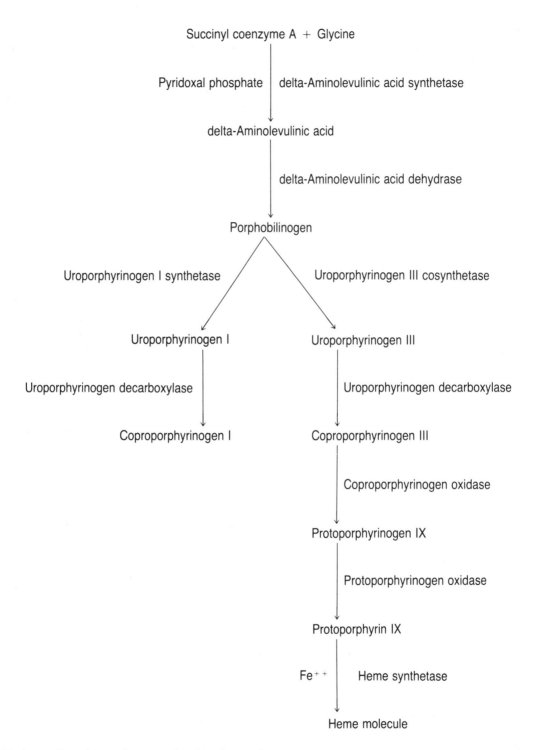

Fig. 152. Heme biosynthesis as related to the porphyrias.

as an autosomal dominant trait. It is caused by a deficiency in uroporphyrinogen I synthetase. The symptoms of this disorder are intermittent and may occur as frequently as several times in 1 year or as rarely as two or three times in the patient's entire life. During the active, or acute, phase, there is usually abdominal pain. Psychologic disturbances and neurologic symptoms may occur. During the active phase, the white blood cell count is usually elevated, and the urine will contain increased amounts of delta-aminolevulinic acid and porphobilinogen. The acute attacks of this disorder have been successfully treated with large amounts of glucose, hematin, and sodium benzoate.

Hereditary coproporphyria resembles acute intermittent porphyria in its clinical picture. It is caused by a decrease in coproporphyrinogen oxidase, which results in increased amounts of coproporphyrin III in the urine and feces. Acute attacks of this disease have been successfully treated with hematin.

Variegate porphyria is inherited as an autosomal dominant trait. The clinical symptoms are very similar to acute intermittent porphyria, except that these patients also show a sensitivity to sunlight. Acute attacks of this disorder are generally precipitated by exposure to such drugs as sulfonamides, barbiturates, anesthetics, and alcohol. This disease is thought to be caused by a deficiency in protoporphyringoen oxidase. The feces contain large amounts of protoporphyrin and coproporphyrin. During acute attacks, the urine will contain increased amounts of porphobilinogen and delta-aminolevulinic acid. This disorder is generally treated in the same way as acute intermittent porphyria.

MALARIA

Parasites that cause malaria in man and other animals belong to the class Sporozoa, suborder Haemosporidia, genus *Plasmodium*. The four species most commonly found in man are *Plasmodium vivax, malariae, falciparum,* and *ovale*.

Malaria is mainly transmitted from person to person through the bite of the female *Anopheles* mosquito. Other means of transmission are through the use of contaminated needles, by congenital means, and through blood transfusions.

The life cycle of the malaria parasite requires two types of hosts: the invertebrate (female *Anopheles* mosquito), where the parasite reaches maturity and the sexual cycle occurs (sporogony), and the vertebrate (e.g., the human), where the immature stages occur and asexual multiplication takes place (schizogony). When the infected *Anopheles* mosquito bites a human, sporozoites are injected into the peripheral blood of the individual. The sporozoites then invade the parenchymal cells of the liver, where preerythrocytic development takes place, ending with the schizont phase. At this time, the parasites rupture the cell, and the merozoites from the schizont penetrate the red blood cells or continue the exoerythrocytic phase by penetrating other liver cells and repeating the cycle, again developing into schizonts.

When the red blood cell has been penetrated by the merozoite, the parasite develops into the trophozoite form and thence to a mature schizont. This process takes 48 to 72 hours and is called *schizogony*. The merozoites rupture from the mature schizonts and penetrate other red blood cells. Fever and chills are associated with the rupture of the red blood cells. The merozoites entering the red blood cell then repeat the process of schizogony, forming mature schizonts from which more merozoites emerge. When several of the preceding asexual cycles have occurred, some of the merozoites enter red blood cells and become sexually differentiated into the male microgametocyte or the female macrogametocyte. In this circumstance, the gametocyte remains in the red blood cell as long as the red blood cell lives and does not influence the patient's symptoms.

The gametocyte is the only form of the parasite that is now infective to the *Anopheles* mosquito. When the mosquito bites the infected person, the gametocytes enter the mosquito and mature in its stomach. The zygote is formed when the microgamete exflagellates and fertilizes the macrogamete. The zygote matures, becoming actively motile, to form an ookinete, which penetrates the stomach wall of the mosquito. It moves to the outside of the stomach wall and becomes an oocyst. The oocyst matures to a sporocyst, which ruptures and gives rise to sporozoites. These sporozoites migrate to the salivary glands of the female *Anopheles* mosquito, where they remain until a person is bitten by this mosquito. At this time, the sporozoites enter the peripheral blood and the cycle is repeated (Fig. 153).

It is important, when diagnosing malaria, to be able to identify the infecting species. This may be accomplished by microscopic examination of thick and thin blood smears stained with Giemsa stain.

Malaria may occur in the chronic, recurrent, or acute form. The patient has sudden onsets of severe chills, along with fever and weakness. Generally, mild anemia is present as a result of shortened red blood cell life span due to the parasite invading the red blood cell. The osmotic fragility of the red blood cells is increased, and due to the hemolysis present, the haptoglobin is decreased to absent. Blackwater fever, although rarely seen, may occur in *P. falciparum* infections. This condition is characterized by acute intravascular hemolysis, chills, weakness, fever, and vomiting. It has sometimes been found in patients who have been treated for malaria with quinine.

PELGER-HUËT ANOMALY

The *Pelger-Huët anomaly* is inherited as an autosomal dominant trait and is characterized by decreased segmentation of the granulocytes, and coarseness and condensation of the nuclear chromatin in the granulocytes, lymphocytes, and monocytes. These changes are most evident in the neutrophil, where the nuclei will appear round, dumbbell-shaped, or peanut-shaped. In the homozygous state, all of the neutrophil nuclei are round or oval. This anomaly, however, is most frequently seen in the heterozygous state, where less than 40% of the neutrophils will contain only a single-lobed nucleus, and the majority of neutrophils contain a bilobed nucleus. In this state, there will be fewer than 10% three-lobed nuclei. These cells appear to function normally.

Acquired or *pseudo-Pelger-Huët* anomaly is most often seen in chronic myelogenous leukemia and myeloid metaplasia but may also be seen in many other diseased states.

CHÉDIAK-HIGASHI ANOMALY

Chédiak-Higashi anomaly is inherited as an autosomal recessive trait and is a lysosomal disorder. There appears to be an abnormality present that prevents normal fusion during the formation of granules in all cells of the body that contain granules. There may be fewer granules, and the granules may be defective. The affected patient generally shows albinism, photophobia, and poor resistance to infection. The disorder is generally fatal by early childhood. The stained blood smear is very striking in that the granulocytes contain large, peroxidase-positive granules in the cytoplasm. There are often multiple granules in the same cell. The lymphocytes and, less often, the monocytes may also contain these granules.

MAY-HEGGLIN ANOMALY

The *May-Hegglin anomaly* is inherited as an autosomal dominant trait. It is characterized by the presence of blue-staining cytoplasmic inclusions (resembling Döhle bodies) in the cytoplasm of the neutrophilic granulocytes and a thrombocytopenia with giant and abnormal-appearing platelets. The inclusion bodies appear to

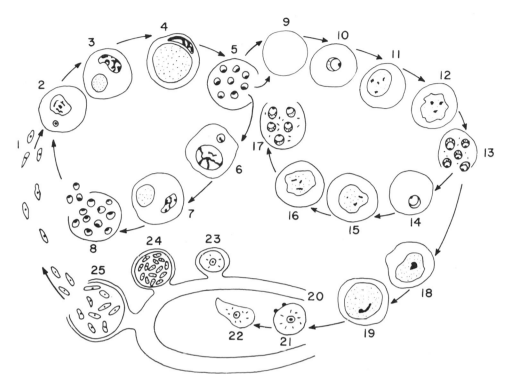

Fig. 153. Life cycle of the malaria parasite. 1, Sporozoites from mosquito. 2, 3, 4, Primary exoerythrocytic parasite in liver cells. 5, Merozoites being released from the ruptured exoerythrocytic schizont. 6, 7, Merozoite of the secondary exoerythrocytic cycle in liver cells. 8, Second generation of merozoites being released from the exoerythrocytic schizont. 9, Red blood cell in peripheral blood. 10, 11, 12, Erythrocytic schizogony in peripheral blood. 13, Erythrocytic merozoites and gametocytes being released from the ruptured erythrocytic schizont. 14, 15, 16, 17, Erythrocytic schizogony. 18, 19, Development of female gametocyte (macrogametocyte) in peripheral blood. 20, Stomach wall of mosquito. 21, Macrogamete. 22, Ookinete. 23, Oocyst. 24, Development of oocyst and production of sporozoites. 25, Sporozoites leaving the ruptured oocyst.

consist of RNA. This anomaly appears to be benign, except that some abnormal bleeding may result from the decreased platelet count. The platelets appear to have a decreased survival time.

ALDER-REILLY ANOMALY

Alder-Reilly anomaly is inherited as a recessive trait and is characterized by the presence of dark staining granules in the neutrophils. These granules are similar to those seen in toxic granulation, but they are slightly larger. The granules may also be seen in the monocytes and lymphocytes. These granules are most often seen in conjunction with Hurler's or Hunter's syndromes, which describe "gargoylism." The basic defect in these diseases appears to be concerned with mucopolysaccharides.

STORAGE DISEASES

The *storage diseases* outlined here represent a group of disorders in which there is an accumulation or overloading of lipid (ceramide) in the cells of the monocyte-macrophage system. This is thought most likely to be due to deficiencies in the enzymes responsible for catabolizing the lipids.

Gaucher's Disease

Gaucher's disease is a rare, chronic disorder caused by a deficiency in the enzyme, beta-glucocerebrosidase. As a result, there is an accumulation of glucose-ceramide within the cells. Patients with this disorder generally have splenomegaly, hepatomegaly, some skin pigmentation, and a hypochromic anemia. The white blood cell count and platelet count are generally decreased. When this disease is found in infants, it is generally characterized by retarded development and neurologic signs. The diagnostic cell, termed the *Gaucher cell*, will be present in the bone marrow and in aspirates from the liver, spleen, and lymph nodes. The Gaucher cell is large, 20 to 80 μm, with a small, eccentric nucleus. The markedly abundant cytoplasm is filled with lipid, giving it a fibrillar appearance.

Niemann-Pick Disease

Niemann-Pick disease affects primarily infants and is most probably due to a deficiency in sphingomyelinase that causes an accumulation of sphingomyelin. These patients shown enlarged livers and spleens and have severely impaired mental development. Death usually occurs within a few months of diagnosis, and few patients live beyond the age of 20 years, with most patients dying between 2 and 3 years of age. In the stained blood smear, vacuoles may be present in the cytoplasm of the lymphocytes and monocytes. Niemann-Pick cells will be found in the bone marrow and spleen. These cells are similar in size to the Gaucher cell and have an eccentrically placed nucleus. The accumulated sphingomyelin gives the cytoplasm a more globular appearance.

Sea-Blue Histiocytosis

Sea-blue histiocytosis is classified as a storage disease because of the accumulation of lipids. The exact cause, however, is not known. Patients with this disorder generally have an enlarged liver and spleen and a thrombocytopenia. The sea-blue histiocytes are found in the bone marrow and frequently in the liver and spleen. These cells are large (20 to 60 μm in diameter), with an eccentric nucleus containing one nucleolus. The cytoplasm contains varying numbers of granules, which are blue to blue-green in color when stained with Wright's stain.

HISTIOCYTOSIS X

Eosinophilic granuloma of the bone, Letterer-Siwe disease, and *Hand-Schüller-Christian disease* have all been categorized as *histiocytosis X* by some hematologists because they all show an abnormal proliferation of histiocytes. The cause of this abnormal proliferation is unknown but may be due to a lysosomal defect. These histiocytes have been found to contain cholesterol.

Eosinophilic granuloma of the bone is found primarily in older children and young adults. Biopsy of the bone shows many eosinophils and histiocytes.

Letterer-Siwe disease is generally found in young children, and death generally occurs within a few months after the onset of the disease. Proliferation of the histiocytes is found primarily in the lymph nodes, spleen, and bone marrow, and, to a lesser degree, in all tissues and in the peripheral blood. Anemia and thrombocytopenia may also be present.

Hand-Schüller-Christian disease is found in older children and affects primarily the bones, where histiocytes are found in the lesions. This disease is more benign and chronic than Letterer-Siwe disease.

INFECTIOUS MONONUCLEOSIS

Infectious mononucleosis was first described in the 1880s. One of the names ascribed to it at that time was glandular fever, a term no longer in use today. In the early 1900s, several cases of "cured leukemia" were reported. These cases are now felt to have been examples of infectious mononucleosis.

The agent responsible for infectious mononucleosis is thought to be the Epstein-Barr virus. It is predominantly a disease of children and young adults between the ages of 15 and 25 and occurs in all races in all parts of the world. As a rule, the symptoms include tiredness, headache, muscle aches, moderate fever (38.3° to 39.4°C) and some enlargement of the lymph nodes. Some patients may show splenomegaly, hepatomegaly, jaundice, and sore throat or cough.

In patients with infectious mononucleosis, the red blood cell count and platelet count are usually normal. The white blood cell count may be variable but is usually normal to slightly elevated. Generally, the white blood cell count is lowest in the beginning of the disease and increases slowly during the first 2 to 5 days after onset, not usually going over 15,000 per µl. There is a relative and absolute increase in lymphocytes, of which 20 to 90% are atypical. These cells vary in size but are usually equal to or larger than the normal lymphocyte. They are often irregularly shaped and are frequently indented by the surrounding red blood cells. The nucleus of the lymphocyte may be round or oval but is often irregularly shaped. The cytoplasm of the cell is often increased in relative size and appears basophilic. This basophilia may appear throughout the entire cytoplasm but more often appears radially or at the peripheral edge of the cell. It is not uncommon to find a rare to few immature lymphocytes as a result of lymphocyte transformation into the blastlike cells in response to stimulation by the virus. Lymphocytes with foamy or vacuolated cytoplasm may also be present. The three types of lymphocytes as suggested by Downey are found in this disorder. Usually, the number of atypical lymphocytes increases for several days and reaches a maximum by the fifth to tenth day. From then on, the number decreases, becoming normal within the next 3 weeks. In some instances, however, some atypical lymphocytes persist for 3 months or more. A serologic procedure, the heterophile antibody test, is positive in 90% or more of the patients with infectious mononucleo-sis. This test is positive in dilutions of 1:112 and above. Generally, relatively high titers are obtained, reaching a peak in the second or third week of the illness and lasting for 2 to 8 weeks. In some cases, a positive test may persist even longer.

The diagnosis of infectious mononucleosis is generally based on the presence of atypical lymphocytes in the peripheral blood, a positive heterophile test, and the patient's clinical symptoms. Other laboratory findings may include elevations in the alkaline phosphatase, serum lactic dehydrogenase, and serum glutamic oxaloacetic transaminase levels. The thymol turbidity and Bromsulphalein tests may also be abnormal.

CHRONIC GRANULOMATOUS DISEASE

Chronic granulomatous disease is inherited as a sex-linked recessive trait and is caused by a defect in white blood cell function. The disease is seen primarily in males and is generally fatal during early childhood because of recurring infections and the development of granulomas. The white blood cell count (primarily neutrophils) does increase during periods of infection. The nitroblue-tetrazolium test is used to diagnose this disorder.

WISKOTT-ALDRICH SYNDROME

The Wiskott-Aldrich syndrome is an immune-deficiency disease. It is characterized by a moderate to marked thrombocytopenia, eczema, and recurrent infections caused by deficiencies in cellular and humoral immunity. During the progress of the disease, there is a decline in the total number of active T lymphocytes. If the patient does not die from infection or bleeding due to the thrombocytopenia, malignant lesions generally form.

LEUKEMIA

Leukemia is an abnormal, uncontrolled proliferation of one or more of the white blood cell-producing cells. Usually, there are qualitative changes in the affected cells, but this does not always have to be true. It is a disease of the blood-forming tissues. The bone marrow is always involved.

The exact cause of leukemia is unknown. There is a possibility that an hereditary predisposition toward the disease exists. Also, there is an increased incidence of leukemia in radiologists and in people who have undergone large amounts of radiation therapy.

Leukemia occurs at any age. Chronic lymphocytic leukemia, however, is usually found in patients over 50 years of age, whereas acute leukemia is generally found in persons under 20 years of age. Chronic granulocytic leukemia is most often found in the 20- to 50-year age bracket.

The major symptoms of leukemia are fever, weight loss, and increased sweating. Enlargement of the liver, spleen, and lymph nodes may occur. The basal metabolic rate is often elevated, and there may be hemorrhagic tendencies if marked thrombocytopenia is present.

The different types of leukemia may be classified according to the duration of the disease, number of white blood cells present in the peripheral blood, and the type of white blood cell involved. (See following outline and Table 21).

1. Duration of disease.
   A. Acute leukemia: a rapidly progressive disease that lasts several days to 6 months.
   B. Subacute leukemia: 2 to 6 months.
   C. Chronic leukemia: the length of this disease is somewhat variable, depending on the age of the patient and the type of cell involved. Most patients live a minimum of 1 to 2 years or more.
2. Number of white blood cells present in the peripheral blood.
   A. Leukemic leukemia: white blood cell count greater than 15,000 per μl.
   B. Subleukemic leukemia: white blood cell count less than 15,000 per μl with immature or abnormal forms of white blood cell present in the peripheral blood.
   C. Aleukemic leukemia: white blood cell count less than 15,000 per μl with no immature or abnormal white blood cells present in the peripheral blood.

In *acute leukemia,* the onset of the disease is sudden, and almost half of all cases occur in children under 14 years of age. There is generally normocytic-normochromic anemia that increases as the disease progresses. The platelet count is low to markedly decreased. The bleeding time is usually prolonged, and there is poor clot retraction. Occasionally, the clotting time

TABLE 21.   CELL TYPE INVOLVED IN VARIOUS LEUKEMIAS

TYPE OF LEUKEMIA	TYPE OF CELL INVOLVED
Acute lymphocytic	Lymphoblast
Chronic lymphocytic	Lymphocyte (small)
Acute myelogenous	Myeloblast
Acute promyelocytic	Promyelocyte
Chronic myelogenous	Immature neutrophils
Eosinophilic	Eosinophil
Acute monocytic (Schilling)	Immature monocyte
Acute myelomonocytic (Naegeli)	Myeloblast showing monocytoid nucleus
Di Guglielmo's syndrome	Rubriblast (myeloblast)
Plasma cell	Plasma cell
Mast cell	Mast cell
Stem cell	Primitive blast
Leukemic reticuloendotheliosis	"Hairy" cell

is also prolonged. The white blood cell count is variable, usually showing a moderate to marked elevation. White blood cell counts of 50,000 to 100,000 per μl are not uncommon. Frequently, however, the white blood cell count may be normal to decreased. Blast cells are present on the peripheral blood smear and may predominate. The bone marrow is hypercellular, with blast cells usually predominating. Acute leukemia is generally treated by *chemotherapy* (the use of chemicals that damage or destroy the cells). Single drugs or combinations of several different drugs may be utilized. (These drugs may also destroy some normal cells.) The primary goal of chemotherapy is to prolong life by eliminating the leukemic cells. When the patient becomes asymptomatic and has only normal cells in the blood and bone marrow, the patient is said to be in complete remission. A patient in partial remission shows improvement, but some leukemic cells remain. The period of time a patient remains in remission is variable, as is the number of remissions possible. In addition, platelet and white blood cell transfusions, as well as transfusions of packed red blood cells, may also be given as needed. The cause of death in patients with acute leukemia is most often infection and/or hemorrhage.

Subacute leukemias are similar to and are usually treated clinically as acute leukemia. The white blood cell count may show elevations up to 50,000 per μl or in some instances may be normal to decreased. The predominant cell present in the peripheral blood is usually the blast, although there are not as many present as there are in acute leukemia. Thrombocytopenia and normocytic-normochromic anemia are also present.

Chronic leukemia has an insidious onset, frequently being symptomless for a long time. Anemia is not usually present until late in the disease. Hemolytic anemia may develop as the disease progresses. Platelet counts are usually normal and may frequently be increased in myelogenous leukemia. In the late stages of chronic leukemia, however, thrombocytopenia and anemia usually occur. The white blood cell count is most often markedly increased and may be as high as 900,000 per μl. However, it is not too unusual for the white blood cell count to be normal to decreased. Less than 10% blast cells are found in chronic myelogenous leukemia, whereas a rare blast cell (or none) is seen in chronic lymphocytic leukemia. Chronic myelogenous leukemia may be treated with busulfan (Myleran) to bring about a state of remission. Eventually, the majority of these patients go into blast crisis, where they present an acute type of myelogenous leukemia. Chemotherapy may or may not induce a remission, and, as in acute leukemia, the main cause of death is hemorrhage and/or infection. Chronic lymphocytic leukemia (CLL) generally has a much longer life span than the other types of leukemia. Alkylating agents, steroids, and irradiation are methods of treatment in current use. However, complete remission is generally not attained, and treatment may be used only when complications occur. Death is usually caused by infection, or, because this is a disease found in the elderly, the cause of death may be unrelated to CLL.

A relatively new (within the past decade) classification of acute leukemias has been developed and is termed the *French-American-British (FAB)* classification of acute leukemias. It divides the acute leukemias into lymphoblastic or myeloblastic. These two main groups are subdivided according to morphology, cytochemical staining results, and, more recently, T and B lymphocyte marker study results. The lymphoblastic leukemias have been divided into three types (L1, L2, and L3), whereas the myeloblastic leukemias have seen separated into six types (M1, M2, M3, M4, M5, and M6).

Acute Lymphocytic Leukemia

Immunologic cell markers are being used on lymphoblasts in addition to T and

B cell markers, which suggests that *acute lymphocytic leukemia* may be classified into one of several categories. The lymphoblast may be classified based on membrane cell markers: immunoglobulins bound to the cell membrane, receptors present on the cell membrane, and formation of rosettes with untreated sheep red blood cells.

At the time of diagnosis, the white blood cell count is generally elevated, with 60% or more lymphoblasts and immature lymphocytes present. In some cases, the white blood cell count may be normal or decreased, in which case there would be relatively fewer lymphoblasts present. A normocytic-normochromic anemia is present, which is generally quite severe. The reticulocyte count is decreased, and thrombocytopenia is present. The bone marrow shows a predominance of lymphoblasts. The periodic acid-Schiff stain is positive, whereas the leukocyte alkaline phosphatase stain is normal. Corticosteroids, vincristine, and asparaginase have been used to achieve remissions.

Chronic Lymphocytic Leukemia

The majority of cases of *chronic lymphocytic leukemia* appear to involve the B lymphocyte. The T lymphocyte is less often involved. The white blood cell count is usually 20,000 to 200,000 per μl, with the peripheral blood smear showing 60 to 95% lymphocytes. These cells are generally the small type of mature lymphocyte that often show a small cleft or indentation in the shape of the nucleus. Lymphoblasts are generally absent from the peripheral blood, but a rare prolymphocyte may sometimes be found. These lymphocytes are somewhat more fragile than normal, resulting in many of the cells being ruptured during the preparation of the blood smear. Therefore, large numbers of smudge cells are usually seen on the Wright-stained smear. A normocytic, normochromic anemia generally develops as the disease progresses. The platelet count is usually normal or shows only a slight decrease. The bone marrow is hypercellular and contains large numbers of the small mature lymphocytes. An autoimmune hemolytic anemia frequently develops during the course of this disease, and the patient shows a positive direct Coombs' test.

Acute Myelogenous Leukemia

The white blood cell count usually shows moderate to marked elevation, with 60% or more of the cells being myeloblasts. Auer rods may or may not be present in the cytoplasm of these cells. Some cases of this disease show micromyeloblasts, a much smaller myeloblast than normal. A severe normocytic-normochromic anemia develops, along with thrombocytopenia. The platelets that are present may be large and bizarre-looking. The bone marrow shows an increased number of myeloblasts. The granulocytes on the blood smear give the following reactions to cytochemical stains: Sudan black B, positive; peroxidase, positive; ASD chloroacetate, positive; leukocyte alkaline phosphatase, decreased; periodic acid-Schiff, faint diffuse granules.

Acute Promyelocytic Leukemia

In *acute promyelocytic leukemia*, the predominant cell in the bone marrow and blood is the promyelocyte. Often, the nucleus of this cell is more immature than usual, and the cytoplasmic granules may be large and abnormal-appearing. There is also an increased incidence of bleeding disorders in this disease. Disseminated intravascular coagulation may occur, which is thought to be due to the release of thromboplastin-like substances by the abnormal promyelocytes.

Chronic Myelogenous Leukemia

The white blood cell count is usually 100,000 to 300,000 per μl at the time of diagnosis. Less than 10% myeloblasts are present in the peripheral blood, and there are numerous immature granulocytes. Eosinophils and basophils are commonly increased, and the percentage of monocytes may also show an increase. Mild normochromic anemia is generally present. The platelet count is often increased, and large forms of the platelets may be present. The bone marrow is hypercellular and usually shows an increased number of myeloid cells, with a slightly higher percentage of immature granulocytes than is present in the peripheral blood. Leukocyte alkaline phosphatase is decreased in this disorder. One arm of the chromosome in pair number 22 is found to be deleted in 70 to 90% of the cases of this disease. This chromosome with its deletion is termed the *Philadelphia chromosome* and occurs in the erythroid, granulocytic, monocytic, and megakaryocytic cells. Patients with this disorder who are negative for the Philadelphia chromosome usually have a poorer prognosis and do not respond particularly well to chemotherapy. Splenomegaly is a fairly constant finding.

Eosinophilic Leukemia

Eosinophilic leukemia is rare. Anemia and thrombocytopenia may or may not be present. Large numbers of immature eosinophils are present in the blood and bone marrow, and the maturation of these cells may be abnormal.

Acute Monocytic Leukemia of Schilling

The white blood cell count is usually moderately elevated, with a predominant number of immature monocytes present. The nucleus of these cells shows a delicate chromatin pattern, one to five nucleoli, and usually appears convoluted or folded. The cytoplasm is variable in amount, generally has few to no visible granules, and may have a serrated border. The bone marrow also shows an increased number of these cells. Anemia and thrombocytopenia are usually present. The monocytic cells stain positively in the nonspecific esterase stain. In this disease, however, the

staining is inhibited by the addition of fluoride.

Acute Myelomonocytic Leukemia of Naegeli

At diagnosis, the white blood cell count usually shows moderate to marked elevation. Anemia is commonly found, and thrombocytopenia may also be present. The most common type of abnormal cell found in this disorder has been described as myelomonocytic, because the cell has characteristics of both the myeloblast and the monocyte. The nucleus is monocytoid, with a fine chromatin pattern, and appears convoluted or folded. The cytoplasm is usually more abundant than that of the myeloblast, and the granules present show characteristics of the granulocytic line of cells. These cells are present in the bone marrow and peripheral blood in all stages of development, from the blast stage to the mature monocyte. Auer rods may be present in the blast cell. Some immature granulocytes are also present in the peripheral blood. In the nonspecific esterase stain, the blasts are negative to weakly positive, whereas the mature monocytoid cells stain positively.

Di Guglielmo's Syndrome

Di Guglielmo's syndrome has been referred to as *erythroleukemia* and *erythremic myelosis* and may occur in the acute or, less commonly, in the chronic form. The white blood cell count may be slightly decreased to moderately elevated, and myeloblasts and immature granulocytic cells are usually found in the peripheral blood. Immature red blood cells may be present in the blood in few to moderate numbers. These cells may appear megaloblastic-like and show bizarre-shaped and multilobed nuclei. Anemia and thrombocytopenia are common findings. The bone marrow is hypercellular and shows a predominance of erythroid cells. The abnormal erythroid cells will show positive staining in the nonspecific esterase stain.

Plasma Cell Leukemia

Plasma cell leukemia is generally found only as a terminal stage in multiple myeloma. The white blood cell count may be slightly to moderately elevated, and the peripheral blood smear shows up to 90% plasma cells.

Mast Cell Leukemia

Mast cell leukemia is extremely rare. Up to 50% of the cells in the peripheral blood may be mature and immature forms of the tissue mast cell, which is difficult to distinguish from the basophil.

Stem Cell Leukemia

In *stem cell leukemia,* the blast cells present are so immature and undifferentiated that they cannot be identified. As the disease progresses, these cells may change and become identifiable. This disorder is rare, found mainly in children, and is generally present in the acute form.

Leukemic Reticuloendotheliosis

Leukemic reticuloendotheliosis is also termed "hairy" cell leukemia and is characterized by the presence of these hairy cells in the blood and bone marrow. These cells are thought to be of lymphocytic origin and show characteristics of B lymphocytes. They are large cells with a diameter of 15 to 30 μm. The nucleus is round to oval in shape and may contain one to five indistinct nucleoli. There is a small to moderate amount of cytoplasm that has hairlike projections around the outer border of the cell. Anemia is a common finding, and the white blood cell count is decreased to elevated, depending on the number of hairy cells present in the peripheral blood. The acid phosphatase stain using L (+) tartaric acid will be positive.

MYELOFIBROSIS

Myelofibrosis, also called *idiopathic myelofibrosis* or *agnogenic myeloid metaplasia,* is a myeloproliferative disorder that is characterized by fibrosis and granulocytic hyperplasia of the bone marrow, with granulocytic proliferation in the liver and spleen. Its basic cause is unknown, and it is generally found in middle-aged or elderly people.

At diagnosis, the patient may show an enlarged liver and spleen, weight loss, a tendency to bruise easily, and a normochromic-normocytic anemia. The anemia becomes more severe as the disease progresses. The stained blood smear characteristically shows teardrop-shaped red blood cells and nucleated red blood cells in numbers out of proportion to the degree of anemia. Polychromatophilia is present, and the reticulocyte count is increased. The white blood cell count is variable but is increased in the majority of patients. Immature granulocytes are generally present on the stained blood smear. Dwarf megakaryocytes or small megakaryoblasts are often present in small numbers in the peripheral blood and, in certain cases, may be present in large numbers. The platelet count is increased in about 50% of cases at diagnosis but decreases below normal as the disease progresses. Large and bizarre forms of the platelets are usually present on the stained blood smear. The leukocyte alkaline phosphatase stain is increased in the majority of cases but may be normal or decreased. The bone marrow is usually hypocellular, and it is often impossible to obtain marrow, except by surgical biopsy. In the early stages of the disease, however, the marrow may be hypercellular and contain an increased number of megakaryocytes, some of which are abnormal. The marrow generally becomes fibrotic, with an abundance of reticulum fibers.

The cause of death is variable and may be due to infection, bleeding, cardiac failure, or a conversion to leukemia. No specific therapy is currently used to treat the basic problem, and patients will generally survive for 1 to 5 years or longer following diagnosis.

MALIGNANT LYMPHOMAS

The term *lymphoma* represents a group of malignant tumors of the lymphoid tissue (excluding lymphocytic leukemia). Various methods for classifying this group of disorders have been suggested. No one classification system, however, has been completely accepted. The lymphomas generally may be divided into two major groups: Hodgkin's disease and the non-Hodgkin's lymphomas.

Non-Hodgkin's Lymphomas

The *non-Hodgkin's lymphomas* may be separated morphologically by cell type into four categories, each of which shows a nodular or a diffuse pattern. (1) In *well-differentiated lymphocytic lymphoma*, the characteristic cell resembles a small lymphocyte. (2) *Poorly differentiated lymphocytic lymphoma* is characterized by lymphocytic cells that may vary in size. The nuclear chromatin is less clumped than in the mature lymphocyte, may contain a visible nucleolus, and may be indented or clefted. There is little cytoplasm. (3) The cells in *histiocytic lymphoma* are relatively large, with fine nuclear chromatin and variable amounts of cytoplasm. The nucleus may be eccentric and may or may not show a nucleolus. (4) *Mixed histiocytic-lymphocytic lymphoma* shows equal proportions of poorly differentiated lymphocytes and histiocytes. (The cells in categories 3 and 4 may not be true histiocytes but may, in fact, be lymphoid.)

At the time of diagnosis, most patients have enlarged lymph nodes, where the disease is primarily located. The white blood cell count is normal, but there may be some abnormal lymphocytes (lymphoma cells) present in the peripheral blood. The hemoglobin level is generally normal in the early stages of the disease. Diagnosis is generally made by examining a lymph node biopsy. The lymphoma cells, however, may also be present in the bone marrow. Chemotherapy and radiotherapy are methods of treatment. In some patients, malignant lymphoma will change into leukemia.

Sézary syndrome, a malignant lymphoma, affects the skin and involves primarily the T lymphocytes. The tumor cells (Sézary cells) are quite characteristic. They resemble a medium-sized lymphocyte with a convoluted nucleus, somewhat resembling the monocyte nucleus. These cells have also been found in patients with mycosis fungoides. Sézary syndrome may be the leukemic phase of mycosis fungoides.

Burkitt's lymphoma is found most often in children in Africa and New Guinea and commonly affects the jaw and facial bones. In American children, a very similar tumor has been found that affects the abdominal and pelvic areas. This lymphoma is very sensitive to chemotherapy, and a complete remission is relatively common.

Hodgkin's Disease

Hodgkin's disease is distinguished from other lymphomas by the presence of Reed-Sternberg cells. This is a large cell, varying in size from 50 to 100 μm or more. There is an abundance of cytoplasm, and the cell usually has irregular margins. The nucleus may be single or multilobed with large nucleoli. These cells are present in the involved tissue.

When a patient is diagnosed as having Hodgkin's disease, his disorder is further classified according to the histologic appearance of the involved tissue: (1) The *lymphocytic predominant* form shows predominantly mature lymphocytes. (2) In the *lymphocyte depleted* form, there are few lymphocytes, but there may be many histiocytes and varying numbers of eosinophils and atypical Reed-Sternberg cells.

(3) The *mixed cellularity* type shows eosinophils, lymphocytes, histiocytes, neutrophils, and plasma cells. (4) In *nodular sclerosis*, bands of collagen are present that divide the tissue into islands. A second classification of the patient's disease can also be done based on the location and extent of the involved tissue. This process is termed *staging*. Prognosis for this disorder depends on both the histologic type and the extent of tissue involvement, as determined by staging.

At diagnosis, the most common finding is an enlarged, painless, cervical lymph node. Recurring fever is also characteristic, and night sweats are a fairly common symptom. A mild normochromic anemia may or may not be present. The white blood cell count may be increased, generally due to a neutrophilia. Increased eosinophils and monocytes may also be present. Reed-Sternberg cells have been found in the blood occasionally. The platelet count is usually normal. The erythrocyte sedimentation rate is commonly elevated.

Generally, the less extensive the disease, the longer the patient will live. Chemotherapy and irradiation are used to treat patients with Hodgkin's disease.

MULTIPLE MYELOMA

The exact cause of *multiple myeloma* is unknown, and there is no evidence that heredity plays a role. This disease is characterized by softening and fractures of the bone. Pain in the bones of the back and, less often, the chest or extremities is common, and multiple bone tumors may be present. Weakness, fever, and weight loss are frequently encountered. Abnormal bleeding may occur. Gastrointestinal symptoms in the form of nausea, diarrhea, and vomiting are also observed in this disease.

The plasma proteins are increased, notably in the globulin portion. On protein electrophoresis, this generally shows up as an increased gamma and less frequently as an increased alpha or beta. The protein types most often found, in order of their frequency, are immunoglobulins G, A, M, and D. The Bence Jones urine test is positive in approximately 50% of cases of multiple myeloma.

Moderate normocytic-normochromic anemia almost always develops in this condition. The peripheral blood smear shows rouleaux formation of the red blood cells. If a red blood cell count is performed and diluted with Hayem's diluting fluid, clumping of the red blood cells occurs due to the abnormal protein. There may be a bluish tinge to the Wright-stained blood smear when it is examined macroscopically. Occasional nucleated red blood cells may be found in the peripheral blood. Polychromatophilia and reticulocytosis may also be present. The white blood cell count is normal to decreased but is seldom increased. A slight increase in eosinophils and lymphocytes may occur, and a few immature granulocytes may be present. Some myeloma cells may also be found in the peripheral blood. The platelet count is generally normal but may be decreased. Some coagulation tests may be abnormal due to interference with some of the coagulation factors by the abnormal plasma protein. The most frequent cause of coagulation defects is the conversion of fibrinogen to fibrin. Increased serum calcium levels may also be present, and bone roentgenographs are abnormal in about 90% of cases of multiple myeloma. The most characteristic finding in the bone marrow is the myeloma cell (a morphologically abnormal plasma cell), which may comprise as much as 95% of all the cells. These cells may be indistinguishable from normal plasma cells but usually show some abnormalities or variations. Generally, the cell is moderately large and contains an eccentric nucleus with one to two nucleoli. The nuclear chromatin is not as fine as in the myeloblast but not as coarse as that found in the plasma cell. The cytoplasm may be basophilic and bright blue or a little lighter in color. Various types of inclusions may be found in the cytoplasm: red-staining crystalline bodies, Russell bodies (eosinophilic globules), and Mott bodies (colorless vacuoles). In certain types of this disease, the cytoplasm will be pink to red in color (flame cell).

HEAVY CHAIN DISEASES

The *heavy chain diseases* are a group of disorders of the lymphoid cells in which there is malignant proliferation of the cells producing immunoglobulins. These cells produce heavy chain fragments without the associated light chains. This may be caused by the deletion of the area in the heavy chain that is responsible for attaching to the light chains. Three types of heavy chain diseases have been found.

Gamma (γ) heavy chain disease resembles lymphoma with atypical lymphocytes and plasma cells present in the peripheral blood. Anemia and leukopenia are generally present, and the platelets are decreased in about 50% of the cases. The bone marrow shows increased plasma cells and lymphocytes. These patients are usually susceptible to infection and have enlarged lymph nodes, spleen, and liver. This disorder is diagnosed by showing the presence of gamma chains in the urine or serum. These chains are reactive on immunoelectrophoresis with antisera to gamma chains but not with antisera to light chains.

Alpha (α) heavy chain disease is the most commonly found form of the heavy chain diseases; it is present as an abdominal lymphoma. The involved areas are generally part of the small intestine and the abdominal lymph nodes, which are infiltrated with lymphocytes and plasma cells. These patients have malabsorption and diarrhea. Small amounts of the alpha chain may be detected by immunoelectrophoresis.

Mu (μ) heavy chain disease is rare and is often found in patients with chronic lymphocytic leukemia. Routine electrophoresis generally shows marked hypogammaglobulinemia. The mu heavy chain is detected by serum immunoelectrophoresis.

WALDENSTRÖM'S MACROGLOBULINEMIA

Waldenström's macroglobulinemia is a disease of the elderly, most often occurring between the ages of 60 and 70. It is characterized by the presence of monoclonal macroglobulins as a result of a proliferation of lymphocytes (and plasma cells). Because of the increased macroglobulins, the blood shows hyperviscosity that may cause neurologic symptoms, visual impairment, and renal problems. Bleeding may occur due to the macroglobulins forming complexes with some of the coagulation factors. The platelets may also become coated with the macroglobulins, thus causing reduced platelet function.

The blood generally shows normocytic-normochromic anemia that may become severe. The white blood cell count is usually normal. In the terminal stages of the disorder, the peripheral blood may contain large numbers of abnormal lymphocytes. Thrombocytopenia is present in about 50% of these patients. Marked rouleaux of the red blood cells is seen on the Wright-stained smear, and the erythrocyte sedimentation rate is elevated. The serum viscosity test is also elevated. The bone marrow usually contains increased numbers of lymphocytes, plasmacytoid lymphocytes, and plasma cells. The periodic acid-Schiff stain is positive and often shows positive inclusions in the cytoplasm and nucleus of the lymphoid cells.

Alkylating agents such as chlorambucil have been used to treat this disorder. The hyperviscosity responds to plasmapheresis. The average life span of patients diagnosed with this disorder is 2 to 4 years.

PLATELET DISORDERS

Thrombocytopenia

Thrombocytopenia is the most common cause of abnormal bleeding and is generally attributed to either decreased platelet production or increased platelet destruction. A third cause of thrombocytopenia is increased platelet sequestration by the spleen; however, this is not very common. Platelets may also be decreased by multiple blood transfusions.

DECREASED PLATELET PRODUCTION

Congenital hypoplasia of the megakaryocytes in the bone marrow is found in a number of clinical conditions: (1) Fanconi's syndrome, where there is pancytopenia and bone marrow hypoplasia, along with various congenital abnormalities. (2) In the newborn, where there is renal, cardiac, and skeletal malformation. (3) In the newborn infected with a virus such as rubella. (4) When the fetus has been exposed to certain drugs such as diuretics in the maternal circulation.

Acquired hypoplasia of the megakaryocytes is generally not caused by replacement of the bone marrow cells by abnormal cells but is, instead, a result of the action of chemicals, toxic drugs, or other physical agents. Exposure to radiation, alkylating agents, cytotoxic drugs, and antimetabolites will cause bone marrow hypoplasia. Usually, the megakaryocytes are the last cell type to return to normal following bone marrow recovery. Occasionally, they do not return to normal, and the thrombocytopenia may persist indefinitely. Some drugs, such as certain thiazides, an estrogen hormone (diethylstilbestrol), and ethanol, selectively decrease megakaryocyte production.

Ineffective thrombopoiesis is found in patients with megaloblastic hematopoiesis due to vitamin B_{12} or folic acid deficiency. In this disorder, the bone marrow generally contains an increased number of megakaryocytes despite the decrease in platelet production. This is thought to be because there is impaired DNA synthesis and, therefore, limited nuclear endoreduplication. The normal increase in cytoplasmic volume does not occur as the megakaryocyte matures. In the bone marrow, the megakaryocytes often appear hyperlobulated, and stained smears will show large platelets. The platelets may have a decreased survival time and may also show abnormal function. This condition is also seen in Di Guglielmo's syndrome, paroxysmal nocturnal hemoglobinuria, preleukemia, and leukemia. It is usually not severe or of clinical significance.

Disorders of the control of thrombopoiesis are not very common and result from an impairment in the mechanisms that control platelet production. Cyclic thrombocytopenia has been described, a condition in which thrombocytopenia and thrombocytosis alternate at regular intervals.

INCREASED PLATELET DESTRUCTION

Increased platelet destruction may occur as a result of immunologic disorders.

Idiopathic thrombocytopenic purpura (ITP) is the most common among the secondary forms of thrombocytopenia and may occur in the chronic, acute, or recurrent form. Acute ITP is found predominantly in children and young adults. It is self-limiting, and spontaneous remissions occur in about 95% of cases. Chronic ITP is found in patients of all ages, but more often occurs in women between the ages of 20 and 40 years. It is felt that people with this disorder have a platelet autoantibody that is responsible for the destruction of the platelets. In this condition, the bone marrow contains abundant megakaryocytes. The platelet count may be markedly decreased to only slightly decreased, and the platelets usually appear large in size and have an abnormal appearance on a stained blood smear. Those laboratory tests requiring normal platelet function will be abnormal: prolonged bleeding time, poor clot retraction, positive capillary fragility, and abnormal prothrombin consumption. Petechiae are present in most patients. The Lee and White clotting time, partial thromboplastin time, and prothrombin time are all characteristically normal. Effective treatment of this disorder usually consists of corticosteroid therapy or splenectomy because the spleen is most responsible for removing the platelets (coated with the antibodies) from the blood. Immunosuppressive drugs occasionally are also utilized.

Drug-induced immunologic thrombocytopenia may be caused by any one of many chemical and physical agents such as antibiotics, hypnotics, analgesics, heavy metals, diuretics, chloroquine, digitoxin, quinine, and tolbutamide, to name a few. Platelet antibodies are the result of a reaction that will occur in only a small number of people exposed to a given drug or chemical. All three factors, the drug, platelets, and the antibody, must be present in the system at the same time for the reaction to occur. Therefore, the treatment of this disorder is to remove the offending chemical or physical agent. Severe thrombocytopenia may occur within 12 hours of ingestion of the drug, or the reaction time may take longer to occur. Bleeding may be severe and begin abruptly. The megakaryocytes in the bone marrow are generally normal in number, whereas those laboratory procedures that depend on platelets will be abnormal. Various serologic tests may be performed to verify the presence of the platelet antibody.

Immunologic thrombocytopenia is associated with a number of other disorders such as autoimmune hemolytic anemias, chronic lymphocytic leukemia, Hodgkin's disease and other lymphomas, systemic lupus erythematosus, and rheumatoid arthritis.

Nonimmunologic thrombocytopenias are varied and are found in disseminated intravascular coagulation, fibrinogenolysis, and other microangiopathic processes. Thrombocytopenia may be present in a number of rickettsial, bacterial, or viral infections as a result of decreased production or increased destruction of platelets. *Thrombotic thrombocytopenic purpura* is a rare disorder, the exact cause of which is unknown. It is characterized by widespread capillary thrombi composed of platelets, hemolytic anemia, changing neurologic symptoms, and abnormal bleeding. The intravascular clotting causes a thrombocytopenia, and the vascular defects also give rise to red blood cell fragments and, occasionally, spherocytes in the peripheral blood. The hemolytic anemia probably occurs as a result of the trauma to the red blood cells. Thrombotic thrombocytopenic purpura affects all ages, although it is most commonly found in the third and fourth decades of life. It is a very serious disease, but at present more than 50% of the patients with this disorder will undergo a long-lasting remission following proper therapy. Treatment consists of the administration of antiplatelet agents and plasma exchange transfusions. In some cases, high doses of steroids are used, and splenectomy may also be helpful.

An abnormal distribution of platelets may also cause thrombocytopenia. The normal spleen sequesters approximately one third of the total platelet mass. In circumstances where the spleen is enlarged (splenomegaly), an increased precentage of the platelets will be found in the spleen, complicating such disorders as Gaucher's disease, Hodgkin's disease, sarcoidosis, and lymphomas.

Massive blood transfusions may also produce a state of thrombocytopenia. The reason for this is that the patient's platelets are lost as a result of hemorrhaging, and bank blood contains few, if any, viable platelets.

Thrombocytosis

A platelet count increased above normal will be found as a result of a variety of circumstances. *Reactive thrombocytosis* describes a moderate increase in the platelet count, which is usually short-lived and asymptomatic. The term *thrombocythemia*, however, refers to a marked increase in the platelet count, which generally persists, and it is considered to be a myeloproliferative disorder.

REACTIVE THROMBOCYTOSIS

Reactive thrombocytosis describes a moderately increased platelet count that generally responds when the underlying disorder is treated. Following splenectomy, the platelet count will generally show an increase above normal on the first to tenth day following the surgery. It will usually peak at 1 to 3 weeks, and begin to decrease in the next 2 to 3 months. In some instances, however, the platelet count may not reach normal levels for a year or more. The platelet count may also show an increase on the third to tenth day following major surgery. In these cases, there may be thrombocytopenia present immediately after surgery. The platelet count generally decreases to normal levels within about 2 weeks following surgery. Within about a day and a half following acute blood loss, a reactive thrombocytosis may also occur. Other conditions showing an increased platelet count are (1) iron-deficiency anemia of short duration, (2) accompanying some malignant diseases such as carcinoma and Hodgkin's disease, (3) following drug-induced thrombocytopenia, (4) in association with increased hematopoiesis, as in patients with hemolytic anemia or secondary polycythemia, (5) during pregnancy, and, (6) in association with various acute and chronic inflammatory and infectious conditions.

THROMBOCYTHEMIA

Thrombocythemia is found most often in mid-adult life and is characterized by a marked increase in the platelet count. Patients with this disorder may have periods of bleeding or thrombosis followed by long periods with no symptoms. Recurring gastrointestinal hemorrhage is the most commonly found bleeding disorder. Thrombosis of both the veins and arteries may develop, with pulmonary embolism as a frequent complication. Splenomegaly is a frequent finding. The most common cause of death is from thromboembolic disorders. The platelet count is usually greater than 1 million per μl and may be as high as 14 million per μl. Platelet production may be as high as 15 times normal. Because of the extremely high number of platelets, it is frequently difficult to obtain an accurate platelet count, and determination of the packed platelet volume is useful. The stained blood smear shows the platelets to be clumped, forming large masses. They also usually show abnormal size, shape, and structure. Platelet life span is generally normal. Megakaryocyte fragments are also frequently present. The red blood cells are normal or may be microcytic and hypochromic due to an iron-deficiency anemia from blood loss. The white blood cell count is usually increased and may be as high as 40,000 per μl. The differential will usually show a neutrophilia with a shift to the left. The bone marrow shows a marked increase in the size, volume, and number of megakaryocytes. The blood coagulation tests are usually normal. In the mild form of this disorder, where the platelet count may not be above 1 million per μl, treatment is not required. Where the platelet count is markedly elevated, however, alkylating agents and thrombocytopheresis are used. Anticoagulants are also employed to prevent thromboembolic complications.

Hereditary Qualitative or Functional Platelet Disorders

Functional platelet disorders may be grouped into one of two classifications: hereditary or acquired. Depending on the disorder, the platelet count may or may not be normal.

GLANZMANN'S THROMBASTHENIA

Glanzmann's thrombasthenia is inherited as an autosomal recessive trait. People who are heterozygous for this trait are asymptomatic. In this disorder, bleeding can be spontaneous and quite severe and will usually begin at an early age. As the patient becomes older, the severity of the bleeding will decrease somewhat. Laboratory studies show deficient in vivo platelet aggregation and deficient platelet aggregation in the presence of collagen, epinephrine, serotonin, ADP, and thrombin. The platelets are reversibly aggregated by ristocetin. The platelet count is generally normal but may occasionally be slightly decreased. Clot retraction is decreased to absent, and the bleeding time is prolonged. When viewed on a Wright-stained blood smear, the platelets appear morphologically normal. The platelets also seem to have a normal release mechanism, and they show a normal shape change in the presence of aggregating agents. The platelets do appear to have less contractile surface protein than normal. Few treatment options are currently available for this disorder, except for transfusion of platelet concentrates.

STORAGE POOL DISEASE

Storage pool disease was previously classified as a thrombopathy. Its inheritance pattern is not yet known. In this disorder, there is a mild to moderate bleeding tendency, and easy bruising is common. The concentration of platelet ADP is reduced, as is platelet factor 3. The acid hydrolases and platelet factor 4 are present in normal amounts, but they are not released normally from the platelet. The release of substances from the alpha granule is below the normal level. There is a decrease in the number of dense bodies in the platelets, and they may also be quantitatively abnormal. The levels of serotonin and calcium in the platelet are also decreased. The platelets will show normal aggregation by high concentrations of ADP but not by collagen. Also, the secondary phase of platelet aggregation will not occur with epinephrine. There is decreased platelet retention using the glass bead column. Storage pool disease may also be found associated with the Chédiak-Higashi syndrome. At present, there is no specific treatment for this disorder.

BERNARD-SOULIER SYNDROME

The Bernard-Soulier syndrome is inherited as an autosomal recessive trait. It is characterized by bruising and moderate to severe bleeding. One of the most striking characteristics of this disorder is the presence of giant platelets, which range in size up to 8 μm in diameter. The platelets also show morphologic abnormalities and have very dense granulomeres. The platelet count is generally mildly decreased. The megakaryocytes in the bone marrow are normal to slightly increased in number and appear morphologically normal. It has been suggested that the platelets have a membrane abnormality. Two types of membrane glycoprotein are lacking in the platelet. In addition, platelets do not bind coagulation factors V and XI normally and bind a decreased amount of thrombin. The platelets also have a decreased ability to adhere to the subendothelium. The bleeding time is prolonged, but clot retraction is normal. Platelet factor 3 concentration is normal. Platelet aggregation by ADP, epinephrine, and collagen is normal, but there is deficient aggregation by ristocetin and thrombin. There is a decreased retention of platelets in the glass bead column procedure. There is no known treatment for this disorder; however, platelet transfusions have been utilized and may be of some aid in stopping bleeding.

WISKOTT-ALDRICH SYNDROME

The *Wiskott-Aldrich syndrome* is inherited as a sex-linked recessive trait. It is characterized by a thrombocytopenia and functional abnormalities of the platelets. Recurring pyogenic infections and eczema are also found in this disorder, secondary to dysfunctions of the B and T lymphocytes. The platelets in this syndrome have been found to have a shortened survival time. In addition, the platelets are characteristically smaller than normal and have a decreased number of granules and dense bodies. Patients with this disorder have been found to respond favorably to splenectomy.

THROMBOPATHY

Thrombopathy is the term used to describe deficient platelet factor 3 activity. This disorder is rare and has been found in patients heterozygous for G-6-PD deficiency. Platelet aggregation has been found to be normal in these cases.

MAY-HEGGLIN ANOMALY

The *May-Hegglin anomaly* is inherited as an autosomal dominant pattern. It is characterized by giant platelets and Döhle inclusion bodies in the neutrophils of the peripheral blood and bone marrow. Thrombocytopenia is usually present but will vary in its degree. Bleeding may or may not be significant, and many patients with this disorder are asymptomatic.

VARIOUS HEREDITARY FORMS OF PLATELET DYSFUNCTION

Some inherited connective tissue disorders and mucopolysaccharide disorders may also show abnormally large platelets and abnormalities in the release of ADP. Patients with *hereditary afibrinogenemia* also show abnormal platelet function studies. There is usually a prolonged bleeding time, a decreased platelet aggregation with low concentrations of ADP, and abnormalities in platelet factor 3 activity. Patients with factor VIII or IX deficiency have also been found to have platelet release abnormalities.

Acquired Qualitative Platelet Disorders

In uremia, the basic defect in the platelets is in their release reaction. This may be due to metabolites that accumulate in the plasma and affect the platelets. There is impaired platelet aggregation and platelet retention. The bleeding time is prolonged, and platelet factor 3 activity is deficient. In this condition, bleeding may be severe at times. Dialysis is of temporary therapeutic value, and the administration of cryoprecipitates will aid in controlling major bleeding episodes.

Many drugs have been shown to inhibit platelet function. Aspirin inhibits the platelet release reaction, preventing the platelets from releasing normal amounts of ADP, ATP, serotonin, and platelet factor 4. High concentrations of aspirin will cause abnormal platelet factor 3 activity. The effect of the aspirin on the platelet lasts for the life of the platelet. In the presence of aspirin, there is also deficient collagen-induced platelet aggregation, and there is no secondary wave of platelet aggregation with epinephrine. Some antihistamines and antidepressants will also inhibit platelet function. Heparin will normally prolong the bleeding time, as will dextran and other plasma expanders. Ethanol affects the platelet release reaction and ADP-induced primary aggregation.

Bleeding disorders will be present in the various paraproteinemias. In macroglobulinemia, there are various abnormalities of platelet aggregation, reduced platelet retention, and deficient platelet factor 3 activity, which are thought to be due to the coating of the platelet membrane with the abnormal proteins.

In acute myeloblastic leukemia, the megakaryocytes in the bone marrow may be small and somewhat abnormal. The resultant platelets are abnormal, showing deficient platelet aggregation and a defective release mechanism.

Bleeding is characteristically found as a

complication in the myeloproliferative disorders (polycythemia vera, chronic myelogenous leukemia, myelofibrosis, and hemorrhagic thrombocythemia). In myelofibrosis and polycythemia vera, platelet factor 3 activity is decreased, and there may also be deficient platelet aggregation. In thrombocythemia, the platelets appear large and morphologically abnormal. There is deficient platelet factor 3 activity and platelet retention, and there may also be defective platelet release. There is a deficiency in membrane glycoproteins in chronic myelogenous leukemia, which places it in the category of an acquired storage pool disease. Micromegakaryocytes are also found in this disorder.

Fibrinogen degradation products present in increased amounts will inhibit ADP-induced platelet aggregation. Fragment E will inhibit thrombin-induced platelet aggregation.

The autoantibodies in idiopathic thrombocytopenic purpura may also cause functional platelet disorders. These patients may have an acquired type of storage pool disease because of the reaction of the antibody with the platelet membrane.

Abnormal platelet aggregation has been found in the beta-thalassemias and sickle cell anemia. Deficient platelet factor 3 activity and abnormal platelet aggregation have been reported in cyanotic congenital heart disease.

COAGULATION DISORDERS

Coagulation Factor Deficiencies

Coagulation factor deficiencies may be due to a deficiency in the synthesis of the protein (leading to a decreased concentration) or may be due to a defective synthesis of the factor (leading to normal amounts of an inactive or abnormally functioning factor). Immunologic procedures are used to test for the presence of coagulation factors. The results of these tests are expressed as positive (+) or negative (−) for *cross-reacting material (CRM +* or

CRM −). A coagulation disorder that is CRM − indicates that the specific substance (coagulation factor) was not present, and the disorder is considered to be caused by a deficiency of the factor. On the other hand, a coagulation disease that is CRM + is considered to have the substance (coagulation factor) present, but it is thought to be functionally abnormal, and it is, therefore, a qualitative disorder.

Factor I Deficiency

A deficiency in fibrinogen is rare, but when it does occur, severe hemorrhaging may result. Congenital deficiencies of fibrinogen may fall into any of three categories: (1) *afibrinogenemia,* in which there is no measurable fibrinogen except trace amounts when tested immunologically. (2) *Hypofibrinogenemia,* where the plasma levels of fibrinogen are lower than 100 mg per dl. (3) *Dysfibrinogenemia,* where the fibrinogen present is functionally abnormal.

Hereditary afibrinogenemia is inherited as an autosomal recessive trait and appears to be the result of deficient synthesis of fibrinogen. This hemorrhagic disorder is present from birth, and there may be severe bleeding from the umbilical cord. There may be bleeding following only slight trauma, subcutaneous hemorrhages, and wound healing may be defective. These patients may, however, have long periods where they have no bleeding, and the disorder is generally not as debilitating as Hemophilia A. In most cases, the blood will not clot. The PT, APTT, and thrombin time are markedly prolonged, and the bleeding time is abnormal in about 50% of cases. Because of the total absence of fibrinogen, the erythrocyte sedimentation rate is generally 0.

Hereditary hypofibrinogenemia has been found to be inherited as both an autosomal dominant trait and an autosomal recessive trait. Generally, the plasma fibrinogen levels are 20 to 100 mg per dl, and little bleeding is seen in infancy. The laboratory test results are similar to those described for hereditary afibrinogenemia but are not as markedly abnormal.

Hereditary dysfibrinogenemia is usually inherited as an incompletely dominant autosomal trait. More than 55 different qualitative abnormal fibrinogens have now been found, and they appear to involve all three aspects of the thrombin-fibrinogen reaction (the enzymatic function, polymerization of the fibrin monomers, and stabilization of the fibrin clot). Most patients with this disorder show few symptoms other than a mild hemorrhagic tendency and some problems with wound healing. The PT and thrombin time generally show variably prolonged results, and the APTT may be normal or prolonged. Chemical or immunologic tests for fibrinogen are generally normal. Procedures testing for clottable fibrinogen (those procedures using a thrombin reagent), however, are abnormal.

Cryoprecipitate and purified fibrinogen may be used to treat the inherited fibrinogen deficiencies.

An *acquired deficiency of fibrinogen* is more commonly found than a congenital deficiency. The acquired deficiency may be caused by impaired fibrinogen production in conditions such as liver disorders. It may occur as a result of excess utilization of fibrinogen, which is caused by widespread blood clotting in vivo, or it may be found as a result of fibrinogen destruction, where rapid fibrinolysis is present in the circulation. It is most commonly found in abnormal obstetric cases and may also occur as a complication of surgery. The fibrinogen titer gives a good picture of the amount of functional fibrinogen present.

Factor II Deficiency

A *congenital deficiency of prothrombin* as a single defect is extremely rare, and it is inherited as an autosomal recessive trait. It is a relatively mild hemorrhagic disorder, and bleeding is most common following trauma. A few cases of dysfunctional prothrombin have also been found. Laboratory tests show both the PT and APTT to be abnormal. The whole blood clotting time may or may not be abnormal, and the Stypven time is abnormal. The most sensitive test for this abnormality is the two-stage prothrombin time, which will show a marked reduction in prothrombin. Stored plasma or a purified prothrombin complex may be administered for treatment.

Prothrombin is produced by the liver and depends on vitamin K for its synthesis. An acquired deficiency in prothrombin is more commonly found in association with a vitamin K deficiency, in which case deficiencies of factors VII, IX, and X are also present. These deficiencies are found in liver dysfunction, obstructive jaundice, in cases in which there is defective absorption or utilization of vitamin K, and in coumarin therapy.

Factor V Deficiency

A *congenital deficiency of proaccelerin* was first described by Owren and was originally designated *parahemophilia*. It is inherited as an autosomal recessive trait and manifests itself clinically in those patients who have inherited the defective gene from both parents. This defect is extremely rare. Clinically, these patients may show varying degrees of mucosal membrane bleeding, easy bruising, gastrointestinal bleeding, and excessive bleeding following dental or surgical procedures. The PT, APTT, and Stypven time are abnormal. The whole blood clotting time and the prothrombin consumption may or may not be abnormal. A factor V assay, based on the prothrombin time, should be performed to determine the extent of the deficiency. Fresh or fresh frozen plasma is used to treat this disorder when necessary.

Acquired deficiencies of factor V have been found in disorders associated with fibrinolysis or intravascular clotting, liver disease, acute leukemia, and hemorrhagic scarlet fever.

Factor VII Deficiency

Congenital factor VII deficiency is a rare disorder and is inherited as an autosomal recessive trait. It produces a severe deficiency in the homozygous patient and a moderate deficiency in heterozygous individuals. Several patients have been found with dysfunctional factor VII. Clinically, these patients generally show mild mucosal bleeding, genitourinary and gastrointestinal bleeding, and significant bleeding following trauma or surgery. The PT is significantly prolonged. The APTT, whole blood clotting time, and Stypven time are normal. A prothrombin time with substitutions may be performed to help identify the factor VII deficiency. An assay for factor VII, based on the prothrombin time, may then be performed to determine the level of factor VII present. This disorder may be treated with stored plasma or a purified prothrombin complex.

Factor VII is vitamin K-dependent and needs a functioning liver for its synthesis. Acquired factor VII deficiency is found in the same conditions that cause acquired deficiency of factor II.

Factor VIII Deficiency

Genetic abnormalities of factor VIII are found in *hemophilia A* (or *classic hemophilia*) and *von Willebrand's disease.* These are the two most common hereditary coagulation disorders. It is currently accepted that several functions can be attributed to factor VIII: (1) Factor VIII:C refers to the coagulant portion of the molecule and represents the ability of the factor VIII molecule to correct coagulation abnormalities associated with hemophilia A. This activity is measured in the APTT and the factor VIII assay procedure. (2) Factor VIII:Ag is the factor VIII-related antigen. (3) Factor VIII:R refers to that part of the molecule which makes possible platelet aggregation in the presence of ristocetin.

(4) Factor VIII:vW is also termed the *von Willebrand factor* and is required for normal platelet adhesion in the hemostatic process.

HEMOPHILIA A

Hemophilia A is inherited as a sex-linked recessive trait and is felt to be the result of a deficiency or dysfunction of the factor VIII:C portion of the factor VIII molecule. Hemophilia A is found most often in persons from northern Europe and their descendents. The condition is transmitted to males by their mothers who have the defective gene on one X chromosome. The female carrier of hemophilia theoretically passes this defect on to half of her sons and half of her daughters. The affected male transmits the defective gene to all of his daughters but to none of his sons because the sons acquire their X chromosome from their mother. Hemophilia has also been found in females, most commonly seen in the heterozygous carrier, where unusually low levels of factor VIII may be seen. Females who are homozygous for hemophilia have been seen in whom the disorder was passed on from the parents (an affected father and a mother carrying the defective gene). In these cases, the disorder resembles that seen in the affected male.

Except in mild deficiencies, this hemorrhagic disorder appears in infancy and remains as a lifelong affliction. Bleeding may occur from the external surfaces of the body, from the gastrointestinal tract, the renal tract, or from the nose or mouth, and may continue for days or weeks if not treated. Bleeding into the tissues can cause serious pressure effects. Hemorrhaging into the joints, causing pain and swelling, may progressively impair joint function and cause crippling.

Patients with classic hemophilia have less than 5% factor VIII activity. The laboratory data are usually characteristic. The platelet count, tourniquet test, PT, and bleeding time are normal. The prothrombin consumption and APTT are abnormal. The Lee and White clotting time is most often abnormal. The thromboplastin generation test or the APTT with substitutions should be performed, followed by a factor VIII assay.

Patients with factor VIII levels of 5 to 10% are considered to have moderate hemophilia. These individuals will also suffer spontaneous bleeding but less frequently than the more severely deficient patients. Mild hemophilia is characterized by factor VIII levels of 10 to 25%. This type is more difficult to diagnose. The patient generally shows a normal Lee and White clotting time and normal prothrombin consumption but may bleed profusely during or following surgery. As a general rule, spontaneous bleeding does not occur unless the factor VIII level falls below 10% of normal. Following surgery or trauma, however, factor VIII levels should be maintained at 30 to 40% of normal.

A few hemophiliac patients develop circulating anticoagulants, usually in the form of antibodies to factor VIII.

Treatment of hemophilia consists of halting any local bleeding by pressure and coagulants and raising the factor VIII level in the blood. There are several therapeutic materials now available for raising the factor VIII level in the blood, including cryoprecipitated fraction of plasma, purified factor VIII, and fresh or fresh frozen citrated plasma. If an anemia is present, fresh whole blood may also be used.

VON WILLEBRAND'S DISEASE

Von Willebrand's disease affects a diverse group of patients and is found more frequently than classic hemophilia. The classic form of this disorder is inherited as an incompletely dominant autosomal trait. There are decreased levels of factor VIII:C, factor VIII:Ag, factor VIII:vW, and factor VIII:R. A more uncommon form of this disorder is inherited as an autosomal recessive trait. This type has very low levels of factor VIII:C and factor VIII:Ag. A

third variety of the disorder shows normal levels of factor VIII:Ag and factor VIII:R and decreased concentrations of factor VIII:C and factor VIII:vW. Other varieties of von Willebrand's disease have also been described.

The clinical manifestations of von Willebrand's disease vary, depending on the severity of the disorder. In classic von Willebrand's disease, abnormal bleeding usually begins in childhood. Easy bruising, bleeding from the gums, gastrointestinal bleeding, and prolonged bleeding following surgery or injury are commonly found. Deep tissue hemorrhages are rare. It has been suggested that the severity of the disease may decrease slightly with advancing age.

A prolonged bleeding time is characteristic of this disorder, and about half of the affected patients show a positive capillary fragility test. Aspirin, which will slightly prolong normal bleeding times, has a marked effect on these patients. The platelet count is normal to slightly elevated, and the platelets appear morphologically normal, although morphologic abnormalities have been reported using electron microscopy. Platelet adhesiveness, as determined by the Salzman method, is reported to be markedly decreased. Platelet aggregation studies show a decreased aggregation in the presence of ristocetin (and normal aggregation with ADP, epinephrine, and collagen). The APTT may be abnormal, depending on the level of factor VIII. The plasma factor VIII activity may range from as low as 1% (rarely) to levels of 30%. The majority of patients show factor VIII concentrations of 5 to 15%. The PT is normal in this disorder, and the Lee and White clotting time is generally abnormal but may be normal in some cases. The prothrombin consumption and clot retraction are generally normal.

Treatment consists of local measures to control bleeding and the administration of fresh or fresh frozen plasma or cryoprecipitate.

Factor IX Deficiency

Congenital deficiency of factor IX is also known as *Christmas disease* and *hemophilia B.* It appears to be inherited as a sex-linked recessive trait in the same manner as classic hemophilia. Inherited factor IX may occur in at least two different forms: CRM− and CRM+. The majority of patients show no detectable factor IX levels by immunologic procedures, whereas a few patients have been shown to have a nonfunctioning factor IX.

This disorder is clinically indistinguishable from classic hemophilia. Both mild and severe forms of the disease have been reported, with the milder forms showing few spontaneous bleeding episodes, but profuse bleeding following surgery or trauma.

The laboratory findings in hereditary factor IX deficiency are similar to those found in classic hemophilia, with the exception of the thromboplastin generation test and the APTT with substitutions. The platelet count, tourniquet test, and PT are normal. The whole blood clotting time, prothrombin consumption, and APTT are abnormal. Before definite diagnosis can be made, a factor IX assay should be performed. In a mildly affected patient, the thromboplastin generation test may not pick up the defect.

Whole blood, plasma, and a purified prothrombin complex are used to treat this disorder. Because factor IX is stable when stored, the plasma or whole blood used does not have to be fresh.

An acquired factor IX deficiency is found in patients receiving coumarin drugs and also in patients with liver disease because factor IX is vitamin K-dependent and requires a functioning liver for its synthesis.

Factor X Deficiency

A *congenital deficiency in factor X* is rare and is inherited as an autosomal recessive trait. Studies have determined that there are both CRM+ (functional or qualitative abnormality) and CRM− (quantitative abnormality) variants of inherited factor X deficiency.

In the heterozygous state, there is no abnormal bleeding. Mild hemorrhagic conditions are manifested in the patient who is homozygous for factor X deficiency.

Because factor X participates in both the intrinsic and extrinsic thromboplastin systems, a deficiency in this factor yields abnormal PT and APTT results. The Stypven time and prothrombin consumption are usually abnormal. The APTT with substitutions, the PT with substitutions, and the factor X assay may be performed for positive identification of this test.

When necessary, this disorder may be treated with stored plasma or with a purified prothrombin complex.

An acquired defect of factor X is found in liver disease, vitamin K deficiency, and patients treated with coumarin drugs. Factor X depends on vitamin K and a functioning liver for its synthesis.

Factor XI Deficiency

Congenital factor XI deficiency is currently thought to be transmitted as an incompletely recessive autosomal trait and is also termed *hemophilia C.*

Bleeding is less severe than in classic hemophilia and spontaneous hemorrhages are rare, although they may occur following surgery or injury.

Laboratory data for factor XI deficiency show a prolonged whole blood clotting time and an abnormal APTT. The thromboplastin generation time is corrected with either serum or adsorbed plasma. The PT is normal. Differentiating factor XI deficiency from factor XII deficiency may be accomplished by substituting known factor XI-deficient plasma and known factor XII-deficient plasma in the APTT substitution test.

When necessary, stored plasma may be used to treat this disorder.

Factor XII Deficiency

Factor XII deficiency, also known as the *Hageman factor deficiency*, is rare and is inherited as an autosomal recessive trait.

It is a unique defect in that there are usually no significant clinical abnormalities. Patients with this disorder show no bleeding or only a minor bleeding tendency, even after trauma or surgery.

The laboratory findings are similar to those found in factor XI deficiency. The whole blood clotting time is prolonged, the APTT is abnormal, and the thromboplastin generation test is corrected by either adsorbed plasma or serum. The PT is normal. A factor XII deficiency may be differentiated from a factor XI deficiency by substituting known factor XII-deficient plasma and known factor XI-deficient plasma in the partial thromboplastin substitution test.

When necessary, stored plasma may be used to treat this disorder.

Factor XIII Deficiency

Factor XIII deficiency has been found to be inherited as an autosomal recessive trait in most instances. Studies have suggested that both a qualitative abnormality and a quantitative abnormality of factor XIII are present.

Clinical symptoms may occur at birth, with bleeding from the umbilical cord. Spontaneous hemorrhage is rare but may occur following surgery or injury, and bleeding into the central nervous system has been found to be more significant in this disorder than in any other hereditary coagulation disorder. Poor wound healing is also characteristic of this factor deficiency.

A simple screening procedure for the fibrin stabilizing factor, employing 5 M urea, is used to diagnose this deficiency in the laboratory. All other routine coagulation screening tests are normal.

When treatment is necessary, administration of plasma is the method of choice.

Prekallikrein Deficiency

Prekallikrein deficiency is thought to be inherited as an autosomal recessive trait. This abnormality has been identified as CRM−, and is, therefore, a quantitative defect.

Like those with a factor XII deficiency, people with prekallikrein deficiency show little to no bleeding tendencies.

Laboratory data shows a normal PT, thrombin time, and bleeding time. The whole blood clotting time and APTT are usually moderately prolonged due to the slow contact activation time caused by the deficiency of prekallikrein.

High Molecular Weight Kininogen Deficiency

High molecular weight kininogen deficiency, or *Fletcher factor deficiency*, is thought to be transmitted as an autosomal recessive trait. Patients with this very rare deficiency are asymptomatic. This disorder is characterized by a prolonged APTT and whole blood clotting time.

Coagulation Disorders Caused by Vitamin K Deficiencies

Factors II, VII, IX, and X are produced in the liver and depend on vitamin K for their synthesis. Therefore, a *vitamin K deficiency* or liver dysfunction may produce coagulation disorders, in addition to coumarin therapy (coumarin impairs the synthesis of the vitamin K-dependent coagulation factors II, VII, IX, and X).

Hemorrhagic disease of the newborn results from vitamin K deficiency. Normally, the newborn has a moderate deficiency of these factors at birth and for the following 2 to 5 days. Routine administration of vitamin K, however, has made this problem relatively rare. This disorder is prevented by administering vitamin K to the mother before delivery and by giving vitamin K_1 to the infant at birth.

Vascular Disorders

Vascular disorders are characterized by bleeding or bruising caused by a defect in the structure or function of the walls of the blood vessels.

In *hereditary hemorrhagic telangiectasia,* there is dilation of the walls of the blood vessels, and they form a very disorganized and tortuous pattern throughout the body. In addition, the walls of the affected blood vessels are very thin. This disorder is inherited as an autosomal dominant trait.

Connective tissue disorders, such as Ehlers-Danlos syndrome, will give rise to abnormal bleeding. Because of abnormalities in collagen and, possibly, elastin, there is vascular fragility, and other coagulation abnormalities are present occasionally that lead to subcutaneous bleeding.

In *scurvy,* the deficiency in vitamin C causes a decreased synthesis of collagen and an intercellular cement substance (between the endothelial cells). This disorder is eliminated by the administration of ascorbic acid.

In vascular disorders, there may be spontaneous bleeding or bleeding as a result of minimal trauma. Petechiae are present, and in some cases, larger superficial hemorrhages may appear secondary to mild trauma. Intramuscular bleeding is rare, but nosebleeds are not uncommon. Generally, the platelet count is normal, as is the blood coagulation mechanism. The bleeding time and tourniquet test are usually abnormal in areas where there is a vascular defect.

Liver Disease

Liver disease may affect all aspects of the hemostatic process, and all of the coagulation factors (except factor VIII) depend on a functioning liver. Factors II, VII, IX, and X need vitamin K for their production. Factors V, XI, and XIII may be deficient in severe liver disease. Factor XII, Fletcher factor, and Fitzgerald factor have also been found to be decreased in liver disease. Quantitative and/or qualitative abnormalities in fibrinogen are also found in most cases of liver disease. For an unknown reason, factor VIII levels are generally increased in disorders of the liver. In the fibrinolytic process, plasminogen activators are generally removed by the liver. In severe liver disease, however, they may not be removed and may continue to circulate, causing activation of the fibrinolytic system.

Patients with chronic liver disease may have severe hemorrhaging. Gastrointestinal bleeding is most common and generally results from an ulcer, esophageal varices, or gastritis.

Laboratory test results will be extremely variable, depending on the severity of the liver disorder and the resultant factor deficiencies. Treatment of the disorder may take the form of administration of vitamin K, factor replacement transfusions, or antifibrinolytic agents, depending on the severity and extent of the disorder and the resultant bleeding.

Disseminated Intravascular Coagulation

Disseminated intravascular coagulation (DIC) has also been termed *defibrination syndrome* or *consumption coagulopathy.* When this disorder does occur, it must be treated as a medical emergency. Thrombin and fibrin are formed in the circulating blood, and the coagulation factors are being constantly utilized. The fibrinolytic system is activated, and large amounts of fibrinogen degradation products are formed. Bleeding, shock, and vascular occlusion develop.

There are numerous causes of DIC: (1) Obstetric problems such as amniotic fluid embolism, a retained fetus syndrome, abruptio placentae, and, less commonly, placenta previa. Amniotic fluid has a clot-promoting activity, and when it enters the circulation, it can initiate the clotting sequence. Necrotic fetal tissue also has a thromboplastic-like effect when it enters the circulation. Placental tissue and enzymes are capable of initiating the clotting mechanism if they enter the maternal circulation. (2) In acute leukemias, some leukemic cells may release thromboplastin-like materials into the circulation. (3) Intravascular hemolysis of various origins. (4) Infections (viral, bacterial, rickettsial, fungal, and protozoal). (5) Massive trauma, burns, or following major surgical procedures where thromboplastic material from the injured tissues enters the circulation and initiates clotting. (6) In tumors, breakdown products from the tumor itself may enter the circulation and show thromboplastic activity. (7) Vascular disorders. (8) Snake venoms from various snakes may contain certain thrombin-like enzymes or substances that may activate factors II or X.

In DIC, when the thromboplastic material enters the circulating blood, intravascular coagulation occurs, with a resultant decrease in fibrinogen, prothrombin, factor V, and factor VIII. Factors VII, IX, and X and other coagulation proteins, namely antithrombin III, alpha-2 antiplasmin, and plasminogen, may also be decreased. The platelet count is generally low because the platelets are used in the coagulation process, and they also tend to adhere to the damaged tissues. An immediate reaction in DIC is the formation of small fibrin strands and microclots. This will cause injury to the red blood cells in the area, and schistocytes and microspherocytes will form. Fibrinolysis is almost always present in DIC and may be activated by the thromboplastic substances responsible for the DIC, activated factor XII, or from plasminogen activators present in the vascular endothelium. The resultant fibrin degradation products formed act as antithrombins and inhibit fibrin polymerization, which may be a major cause of hemorrhage. The reticuloendothelial system is responsible for removing the procoagulants and coagulation products from the system.

The major clinical characteristic of this disorder is significant bleeding, which generally begins quite abruptly. Shock and acute renal failure and thromboembolic manifestations are somewhat common.

In a typical case of DIC, the PT, APTT, and thrombin time are generally prolonged. These tests, however, may be normal for some unknown reason. A normal APTT, however, may reflect the partial coagulation (activated coagulation factors) present in the blood. The platelet count is decreased, as is the fibrinogen titer. (Upon incubation of the tubes from the fibrinogen titer, dissolution of the clots indicates fibrinolysis.) Antithrombin III is usually decreased in this disorder. Tests for fibrinogen degradation products may show increased levels of these substances. It is not unusual, however, to find normal results in these tests because these fragments form a complex with fibrinogen during serum preparation. The euglobulin clot lysis test may be normal due to depletion of plasminogen.

Because DIC occurs secondary to another disorder, the most important aspect of therapy is to treat the primary disorder. To halt the intravascular clotting mechanism, heparin is generally given. Replacement therapy using platelets and/or coagulation factors may sometimes be used if necessary. If the patient is in shock, this must be treated immediately. Whole blood or packed red blood cells are given when indicated.

Circulating Coagulation Inhibitors

Acquired circulating coagulation inhibitors or anticoagulants are relatively rare causes of hemorrhage. They can be divided into two separate classes based on how they affect the coagulation process. (1) Those that act immediately to block the reaction between coagulation factors probably do not destroy the factors. (2) A class of inhibitors that progressively inactivates individual coagulation factors and are primarily immunoglobulins.

A very few acquired antibodies have been found to fibrinogen.

Factor V inhibitors have been found secondary to the administration of streptomycin therapy. The PT and APTT are prolonged in this disorder, and the factor V assay shows decreased levels. Generally, the inhibitors will disappear within several weeks of removing the streptomycin.

Antibodies to factor VIII are the most common inhibitors found and occur in 5 to 20% of the hemophilia A patients. They will also occur in patients with chronic inflammatory diseases such as systemic lupus erythematosus and rheumatoid arthritis, in some women within a few months of giving birth, and in association with drug reactions. Most of these antibodies are of the IgG type. The clinical manifestations of this disorder are very similar to those found in hemophilia A. Treatment of these patients is very difficult. Replacement therapy with factor VIII may produce an increased antibody titer. Spontaneous remissions may occur in some patients.

Factor IX inhibitors occur in about 5% of the patients with this factor deficiency and will also be seen in patients with systemic lupus erythematosus, rheumatic fever, and in some postpartum women. These antibodies appear to act instantly.

Factor XIII inhibitors have been found in patients with this factor deficiency and in some normal individuals following treatment with isoniazid, an antituberculosis drug.

Defects in coagulation have also been found in patients with multiple myeloma, Waldenström's macroglobulinemia, and other protein disorders. The abnormal proteins present may be absorbed by fibrinogen or fibrin, and they will act as inhibitors of fibrin polymerization, causing structurally abnormal clots.

Inhibitors have been found accompanying systemic lupus erythematosus, and a specific lupus anticoagulant has been identified. The lupus anticoagulant causes a prolonged PT and APTT. The bleeding time and thrombin time are normal. It is thought that this anticoagulant affects the prothrombin complex. Other inhibitors found in systemic lupus erythematosus appear to affect factors VIII, IX, XI, XIII, V, and X.

Fibrinolysis

Fibrinolysis, without intravascular coagulation, is most commonly found as a complication of severe liver disease. It is also found as a complication following certain types of surgery (such as lung operations) and in some malignancies and leukemias.

This disorder results from the activation of plasmin within the circulation. The active fibrinolytic system digests factors V and VIII and, in addition, breaks down fibrin and fibrinogen to fibrinogen degradation products. Generally, bleeding is minimal in these patients.

The PT, APTT, and thrombin time are generally prolonged due to the anticoagulant effect of the fibrinogen degradation products. The euglobulin clot lysis time is abnormally short, unless there is depletion of plasminogen. Factors V and VIII are generally decreased. Factor XIII may also be low in some patients. The fibrinogen titer, upon incubation, shows dissolution of the clots.

7

Automation

THE FIBROMETER

The fibrometer offers the hematology technologist a semiautomated procedure for performing coagulation tests.

The complete fibrometer system consists of three separate components: the fibrometer, a thermal prep block, and an automatic pipet, all of which are obtainable from Baltimore Biological Laboratory. The latter two units are not an absolute requirement for use with the fibrometer. When moderate to large numbers of prothrombin times are performed, however, use of the automatic pipet and thermal prep block facilitates the procedure.

COMPONENTS OF THE FIBROMETER SYSTEM

1. *Fibrometer* (see Fig. 154)
    A. The *on-off switch* turns the unit on and off.
    B. The *indicator light* goes on when a temperature of 37°C has been reached.
    C. The *digital readout* gives the clotting time to tenths of a second.
    D. Depressing the *readout reset button* returns the digital readout to 000.0.
    E. There are six *warming wells* in which plasma or reagent may be prewarmed to 37°C.
    F. The *reaction well* holds the plasma mixture that is being tested.
    G. The *probe arm* holds the elec-

trodes. When in operation, it drops down and allows the electrodes to fall in place within the reaction well containing the plasma-thromboplastin mixture.
    H. The *stationary electrode,* located on the probe arm, does not move when the instrument is in operation but functions in conjunction with the moving electrode.
    I. The *moving electrode* is located in front of the stationary electrode on the probe arm. When a coagulation time is being performed, this electrode cycles through the plasma-thromboplastin mixture every half second until a clot forms. This detection system trig-

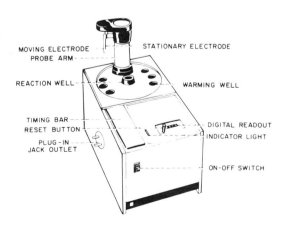

Fig. 154.   Fibrometer.

gers an electronic circuit that stops the timer.

J. The *timing bar* is used to start the timer when the automatic pipet is not used.

K. The *plug-in jack outlet* is used for the attachment of the automatic pipet when it is employed.

2. *Thermal prep block* (Fig. 155)

A. The *on-off switch* is used to turn the heating unit on and off.

B. The *indicator light* goes on and off, depending on the heat demand.

C. The *shallow wells* hold the disposable cups containing the plasma or reagent mixture to allow prewarming to 37°C.

D. The *plastic trays* allow the disposable cups to fit snugly into the shallow wells.

E. The *deep wells* hold test tubes 12 or 13 mm × 75 mm to allow prewarming of the plasma to 37°C.

3. *Disposable coagulation cups*

4. *Fibro-tip:* A disposable pipet tip for use with the automatic pipet.

5. *Automatic pipet* (Fig. 156)

A. The *plug* fits into the plug-in jack outlet of the fibrometer.

B. The *fibro-tip* fits into the hole in the forward end of the automatic pipet.

C. The *plunger*, when depressed, dispenses any liquid in the attached fibro-tip. As the plunger is allowed to retract, the solution in which the fibro-tip rests is drawn up into the pipet tip.

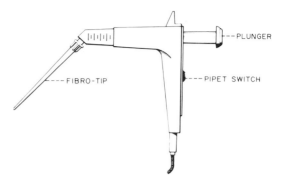

Fig. 156. Automatic pipet.

D. *Alignment indicator*

E. The *0.1 ml calibration mark* is seen as a single notch on the end of the plunger. When this notch is in line with the alignment indicator, exactly 0.1 ml of solution is pipetted.

F. The *0.2 ml calibration mark* is seen as two notches on the end of the plunger. When these two notches are in line with the alignment indicator, 0.2 ml of solution is pipetted. To change from one volume to another, the plunger is merely rotated 180° until it clicks into position.

G. The *pipet switch* is responsible for the activation of the probe arm, electrodes, and timing mechanism. When this switch is in the *on* position and the automatic pipet is plugged into the fibrometer, the aforementioned components become activated as soon as the plunger on the pipet is depressed.

PROCEDURE FOR THE PROTHROMBIN TIME

The prothrombin time procedure (or other coagulation tests) using the fibrometer is basically the same as for the manual method(s) previously described. Therefore, the procedure as outlined here describes the various techniques needed to operate the fibrometer, thermal prep

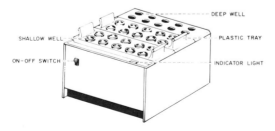

Fig. 155. Thermal prep block.

block, and automatic pipet for the prothrombin time only.

1. Turn the fibrometer and thermal
prep block on and allow the units to
warm to 37°C. This takes about 10
minutes. When the units are at 37°C,
the indicator light on the fibrometer
goes on and remains on as long as the
instrument is at 37°C. The indicator
light on the thermal prep block goes
on and off, depending on the heat
demand.

2. When the indicator light is on, place
the appropriate number of disposable coagulation cups in the plastic
tray over the heating wells in the
thermal prep block.

3. Insert a disposable fibro-tip in the
hole in the forward end of the automatic pipet. Make sure that the pipet
tip fits into the automatic pipet
tightly. (The automatic pipet should
be plugged into the fibrometer and
the pipet switch in the *off* position.)

4. Turn the plunger of the automatic
pipet to the 0.2 ml setting.

5. Completely depress the plunger of
the pipet and place the fibro-tip into
a solution of well-mixed thromboplastin-calcium solution. Allow the
plunger to retract completely.

6. Place the side of the fibro-tip near the
end, on the inside top edge of the
coagulation cup (in the thermal prep
block), so that the tip of the pipet
does not touch the inside wall of the
cup.

7. Depress the plunger, expelling the
0.2 ml of thromboplastin-calcium
mixture into the coagulation cup.

8. Repeat steps 5, 6, and 7 until the appropriate number of coagulation
cups contain 0.2 ml of thromboplastin-calcium mixture and allow to incubate until they have reached 37°C
(2 to 3 minutes).

9. Place the control and patient plasma
in appropriately labeled 12 × 75-mm
test tubes. Allow these test tubes to
prewarm in the deep wells of the
thermal prep block until they reach
37°C (about 3 minutes).

10. Place one of the prewarmed coagulation cups containing 0.2 ml of
thromboplastin-calcium solution
into the reaction well.

11. Turn the plunger of the automatic
pipet to the 0.1 ml setting.

12. Insert a disposable fibro-tip into the
forward end of the automatic pipet.

13. Completely depress the plunger of
the pipet and draw up 0.1 ml of the
prewarmed patient or control
plasma.

14. Change the pipet switch to the *on*
position.

15. Dispense the plasma into the coagulation cup in the reaction well. As
the plunger is depressed the timing
mechanism automatically begins.
Within 1.5 seconds, the probe arm
drops into position, and the electrode action begins. As soon as a clot
forms in the mixture, the electrode
action and timing mechanism stop.

16. Record the prothrombin time, as
shown on the digital readout.

17. Lift the probe arm up to its resting
position, and with a clean, lint-free
cloth, carefully wipe the electrodes.
Depress the reset button to set the
timer at 000.0.

18. All prothrombin times must be performed in duplicate, and the results
should check within 0.5 seconds of
each other. If a prothrombin time is
above 30 seconds, a wider range of
variability is acceptable. If two
fibrometer units are used, it is advisable to run the duplicate prothrombin time on the second unit.

DISCUSSION

1. The electrodes must be kept free of
lint and debris to eliminate falsely
shortened results.

2. If the automatic pipet is not used,
routine 0.2-ml prothrombin pipets

may be utilized. In this circumstance, press the timer bar on the fibrometer when 0.1 ml of plasma is blown into the coagulation cup.

3. The fibro-tips are disposable and should be used only once. When the thromboplastin-calcium solution is pipetted, the same fibro-tip may be used to avoid waste. When pipetting several times, however, the fibro-tip may need to be tightened after every third or fourth use. Loosening of the tip from the pipet causes gross inaccuracies in the amount of solution delivered.

4. If the timing mechanism is started inadvertently, turn the on-off switch on the fibrometer to *off*. Turn the unit back on, replace the probe arm in its resting position, and reset the digital readout.

5. The probe arm on the fibrometer is specifically designed for testing a certain volume of solution. Therefore, when performing a prothrombin time, the 0.3-ml volume probe arm is utilized.

6. When using the automatic pipet, develop the habit of moving the pipet switch to *off* as soon as the plasma has been pipetted and the fibrometer activated.

7. After the plunger on the automatic pipet is depressed, a small amount of solution will remain in the fibro-tip. This is acceptable and has been allowed for in the calibration of the pipet.

MLA ELECTRA 600

The MLA Electra 600 (Fig. 157) is an automated coagulation analyzer designed to detect clot formation by means of a photocell sensing circuit that reads the optical density change when a clot is formed. The plasma specimens to be tested are pipetted into test tubes and placed in the corresponding holes of a circular turntable, where the temperature is maintained

below 10°C. When the instrument is started, the turntable revolves and carries the test samples through a heating zone, where they are warmed to 37°C. When the plasma gets to the test station, the pump dispenses a measured quantity of the reagent (prewarmed to 37°C) into the test tube. A timing circuit is started, and when clot formation occurs, the change in optical density is detected by the photocell, and the timer is halted. The clotting time for that specimen, in seconds, is then printed out on the printer tape. The turntable automatically rotates one space to the next specimen, and the procedure is repeated.

The procedure for the prothrombin time is outlined in this section because this test is most frequently performed on the MLA Electra 600.

COMPONENTS OF THE MLA ELECTRA 600 (Fig. 157)

1. The *turntable* contains numbered spaces for 50 specimens. A refrigeration unit located under the 50 specimen spaces on the turntable maintains the plasmas at a temperature below 10°C.

2. The *pump block assembly* is maintained at 37°C and contains the peristaltic pump, a disposable reservoir cup for the reagent, and a heating zone.

   A. The *pump* is responsible for dispensing an accurately measured amount of the reagent into the plasma sample when the tube reaches the test station (located directly beneath the reservoir nozzle). The reagent is pumped into the test tube forcefully to cause adequate mixing of the plasma and reagent.

   B. The *reservoir* consists of a covered disposable cup with polyvinyl tubing extending from the bottom of the cup. This tubing extends around the pump rotor and

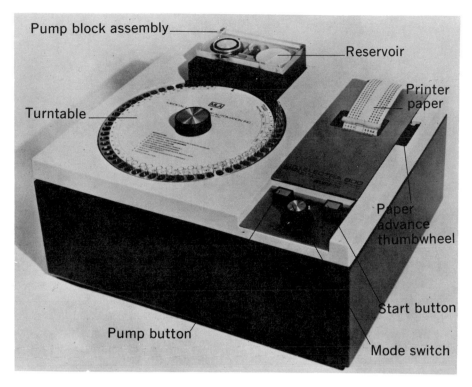

Fig. 157. MLA Electra 600. (Courtesy of Medical Laboratory Automation, Mount Vernon, N.Y.)

ends in a short nozzle in front of the pump block assembly above the test station. When the machine is in the test mode, the reservoir cup is continuously agitated to keep the reagent well mixed.

   C. The *heating zone* heats and maintains the test samples at 37°C prior to and during testing.

3. The *printer timer* prints out the clotting time of the test sample in seconds and tenths of a second. At the same time, a serial number is printed to the left of the clotting time. The *paper advance thumbwheel* is located to the right of the printer paper for manual advancement of the paper.

4. The *control panel area* is located on the right of the instrument and consists of the *mode switch* (test selector), the *pump button*, which is used to prime the pump (fill the polyvinyl tubing with reagent from the reservoir cup), and the *start button* (activates the turntable). The red *pilot light* is lit when the mode switch is on any setting other than the *off* position. Additional controls may be found by lifting the front edge of the printer cover plate. The setting of the *A/B switch* depends on the density of the samples being tested (the anticoagulant and reagents used). Refer to the MLA Electra 600 instruction manual for the proper setting for your laboratory. The *terminal time switch*, when set at 150 seconds, is responsible for printing out a clotting time of 150 seconds when the instrument does not detect a clot in the plasma. The instrument then moves on to the next test sample. The switch may be set at infinity when it is known that the clotting times of the plasma sam-

ples will be greater than 150 seconds. In this setting, the turntable does not automatically advance after a clot has been detected, but advances one station each time the start button is depressed when the printer is not timing. The *alarm switch,* when in the *on* position, causes a buzzer to sound when a clot has not been detected in 150 seconds (only if the terminal time switch is set at 150 seconds). The *reset lever* is located on the left of the printer and resets the serial number to 0001 when pushed forward and released.

5. The *air intake filter* is located in the back of the instrument.
6. The *lamp* for the photo-optical system is located in a recessed pocket in the back of the instrument.

PROCEDURE FOR THE PROTHROMBIN TIME

1. Turn the mode switch to PT and allow a 15-minute warm-up period before using the instrument.
2. Wash the reservoir cup and attached polyvinyl tubing in distilled water.
3. Place a prewarmed quantity of thromboplastin-calcium reagent into the reservoir cup adequate for the number of plasma samples to be tested. An additional 1 ml should be added for priming the pump.
4. Pipet 0.1 ml of the plasma specimens to be tested into 10 × 75-mm glass test tubes and place in the numbered spaces in the turntable beginning with space No. 1. (Do not leave any empty spaces in between samples.) Each plasma sample should be run in duplicate. Allow samples to remain in this position for at least 3 minutes to allow uniform cooling to under 10°C.
5. Place a piece of absorbent material under the nozzle at the test station and prime the pump by depressing the pump switch four times.

6. Push the printer reset lever forward to reset the serial number to 0001.
7. Press the start button to begin testing. The first plasma sample enters the warming zone (37°C), where it remains for 25 seconds. It then moves through the next six warming slots at 25-second intervals until it reaches the test station, where 0.2 ml of thromboplastin is added. The tube remains at the test station until 25 seconds have elapsed or until a clot is formed, whichever occurs last. When a clot forms, the printer types out the clotting time on the printer tape. The next plasma sample then moves into the test station. The serial number to the left of the prothrombin time should coincide with the numbered space the test tube is in (when the serial number is reset at the beginning of each run). The turntable advances each sample to the test station until all samples have been tested and then automatically returns to its home position.
8. Average the duplicate sample readings for each patient and record. Prothrombin times under 20 seconds should have duplicate readings that agree within 0.5 seconds of each other. If there is a wider variation than this, the prothrombin time should be repeated.

DISCUSSION

1. After turning the instrument on each day, inspect the red photo lamp indicator located in the pump block. This lamp should be on. If not, the lamp for the photo-optical system may need to be replaced.
2. Two types of reservoirs are available for use on the MLA Electra 600. The reservoir for the prothrombin time is calibrated to dispense 0.2 ml of reagent. The reservoir for use with the partial thromboplastin time (PTT) is calibrated to deliver 0.1 ml of re-

agent. This cup will either be a different color or have an appropriate marking on the bottom to differentiate it from the 0.2-ml reservoir.

3. The cover of the reservoir cup and the lucite lid of the pump block should be kept on at all times to prevent evaporation and heat loss from the reagent.

4. The pump should be primed whenever new reagent is added to the reservoir. It should be primed prior to depressing the start button. If, however, the start button has been depressed before the pump was primed it may be primed as long as the instrument is not timing a clot.

5. If a clotting time is printed out at the terminal time of 150 seconds, this result should not be reported. Repeat the test on the MLA Electra 600. If similar results are obtained, the test should be done by a manual method. All prothrombin times over 40 seconds should be double-checked using a manual method or the fibrometer.

6. Plasma specimens that are chylous, icteric, or hemolyzed may not show a large enough optical density change with clot formation. In such cases, the test should be performed on the more sensitive special mode, manually, or using the fibrometer.

7. When the mode switch is at the PT setting, or setting No. 1, the print on the tape will be black. At all other settings, the print will be red.

8. When the mode switch is in setting No. 2, the turntable advances at 50-second intervals rather than at 25-second intervals, as when in modes 1, 3, and 4.

9. Maintenance procedures should be performed at regular intervals as outlined below and in the instrument's operations manual.

   A. The air intake filter, located at the back of the instrument, should be cleaned once a month.

   B. The lamp for the photo-optical system generally has to be replaced about once per year. If it begins to darken before this, however, it should be replaced.

   C. The metal, refrigerated trough located under the turntable tends to accumulate moisture and debris. This area should be inspected and cleaned when necessary.

   D. The disposable reservoir cup and associated polyvinyl tubing should be discarded after every 300 test samples or so.

MLA ELECTRA 700

The MLA Electra 700 is similar to but more automated than the MLA Electra 600. The primary operational difference in this instrument is its ability to perform two like or different tests simultaneously due to two photo-optical detection systems and its ability to dispense three different reagents.

COMPONENTS OF THE MLA ELECTRA 700 (Fig. 158)

1. The *turntable* holds up to 60 plasma samples contained in special disposable plastic *cuvettes*. Cooling and heating systems beneath the turntable maintain the plasma specimens at approximately 15°C and warm them to 37°C just prior to and during testing.

2. The *reagent pump system* consists of one pump for each *reagent reservoir* and is responsible for dispensing an accurately measured amount of the reagent into the test samples. A magnetic stirrer is contained in each reagent reservoir.

3. The *pump controls* (three). The *forward* button cycles the pump forward to prime the tubing. The *reverse* button signals the pump to reverse direction and return the reagent in

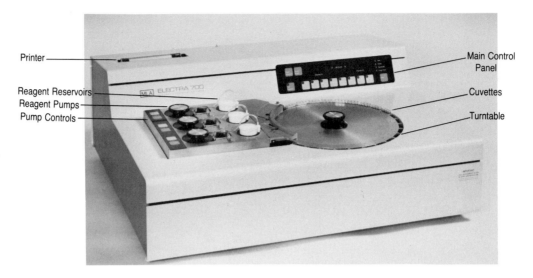

Printer ——
Reagent Reservoirs ——
Reagent Pumps ——
Pump Controls ——
—— Main Control Panel
—— Cuvettes
—— Turntable

Fig. 158. MLA Electra 700. (Courtesy of Medical Laboratory Automation, Mount Vernon, N.Y.)

the tubing to the reagent reservoir. The *pinch valve* closes off the tubing.

4. The *printer* unit first prints out the test name and incubation time and then the clotting time of the test samples, along with the corresponding serial number and position number (on the turntable) for each sample. In addition, the temperatures for the heating trough, reagent incubation and cooling, and specimen cooling are printed out prior to each run of patient samples. The printer will also give the following messages: MISSING TUBE, ILLEGAL TEST, TERMINATED, and NO CLOT.

5. The *auxiliary control panel* is located behind the front panel (pull down to open).

A. The *catch bin* holds the used sample cuvettes as they drop out of the turntable following testing.

B. The *main power* switch turns the instrument off and on.

C. The *turntable release* is used when removing the turntable from the instrument.

D. The *serial number advance* switches (three) for changing the serial number. When reset, the printer will print the next number to be used.

E. The *200/300-second contact activation time* switch is used for two reagent tests (such as the APTT) to set the turntable rotation at specific time intervals.

F. The *automatic/manual* switch sets the instrument to one of these modes. In the manual mode, the incubation times are controlled by the operator, in that the turntable will move only when the operator presses the start button. In the automatic mode, incubation times and testing are automatic.

G. The *normal/long test* switch. In the long position, each patient sample will remain in the test station for a longer period of time. This setting may be desired for samples for which prolonged clotting times are anticipated.

H. The *duplicates/singles* switch allows for test results to be printed in two ways. In the duplicate setting, one serial number is given for the two samples in the same cuvette number, and the results are averaged. In the singles setting, each sample having the same cuvette number is given a different serial number, and the results are not averaged.

I. The *lamp A-B-C* switch allows for one of three different photolamp intensities to be used.

6. The *main control panel.*

A. *Serial number reset.*

B. The *paper advance* advances printer paper.

C. *On/standby.* In the standby mode, the instrument is on, but the cuvette cooling system and reagent stirrers are off. To turn these two systems on, press this botton to the *on* position.

D. The *test mode buttons* are used to select the tests to be performed: *PT* (one or two stage), *APTT, thrombin time, factor assay* (based on the PT and the APTT), and *special test* modes for one or two reagent tests.

E. The *start* button, when pressed, begins the test cycle and provides a printout of the temperatures if the instrument is not in the standby or automatic modes. If pressed two times within 3 seconds, a confidence test is printed. The confidence test indicates any problems present in the optical system, amplifiers, timers, or microprocessors by simulating the change in optical density of a clotting sample.

F. The *catch bin* button indicates a jammed cuvette in the disposal pathway.

G. The *temperature error* indicates a failure in one of the heating or cooling systems.

H. The *automatic* button indicates that the instrument is in the automatic mode.

I. The *long test* button indicates that the instrument is in the long test mode.

J. The *clot time readout* for channel B indicates the verified clotting time for the test sample in channel B.

K. The *clot time readout* for channel A indicates the verified clotting time for the test sample in channel A.

L. The *off scale* indicates that the sample capacity is out of the range of the instrument.

PROCEDURE FOR THE PROTHROMBIN TIME AND ACTIVATED PARTIAL THROMBOPLASTIN TIME PERFORMED SIMULTANEOUSLY

1. Turn the main power switch on.

2. Empty the cuvette catch basin.

3. Press the on/standby button. The button will light when the heating and cooling systems have reached the proper temperature.

4. Set up the pumps with the proper tubing: Pump No. 1, blue tubing, to dispense 0.1 ml of calcium chloride; pump No. 2, red tubing, to dispense thromboplastin (0.2 ml); and pump No. 3, blue tubing, to dispense 0.1 ml of APTT reagent. The tubing nozzles for pump Nos. 1 and 2 should be placed in the test position. Set the tubing for pump No. 3 in the 200/300 nozzle position.

5. Place the reagents into the appropriate reagent cups.

6. Pipet 0.1 ml of the plasma specimens and control specimens to be tested into the plastic disposable MLA cuvettes and place in the numbered spaces in the turntable beginning with space No. 1. (Do not leave any empty spaces in between the samples.) Each plasma sample should be run in duplicate. The plasma samples for the PT test must be placed in red-coded cuvettes, whereas those samples for the APTT test should be placed in blue-coded cuvettes. The instrument detects the color of the cuvette and, in this way, determines

which reagents to add to the test sample.

7. Check the instrument settings: Mode, PT 1/APTT; duplicates/singles for the printer format; 200/300 for the contact activation time; normal/long test (set on normal for routine sample testing); and automatic/manual operation (set on automatic for routine use).

8. Press start two times within 3 seconds if a confidence check is desired.

9. Prime all the pumps. Place an absorbent material such as gauze under each nozzle, and, in turn, press each forward button until the reagent emerges from the nozzle in a steady stream. (As an alternate method place each nozzle into its respective reservoir and prime each pump.)

10. Press start to begin testing.

11. Check the temperature printouts.

12. At the completion of testing, if the instrument will not be used for a while, return the reagents in the tubing to the reagent cup by depressing the reverse pump controls.

13. Empty the catch basin.

DISCUSSION

1. When the instrument's main power is first turned on, it will take approximately 15 minutes for all temperatures to reach their correct values.

2. Reagent cups will hold a maximum of 20 ml of reagent.

3. Additional samples may be added to the turntable as slots become available.

4. The confidence test should be performed at least once per day.

5. Once per month it is advisable to perform the following instrument maintenance: Clean the printer platen, clean the heating and cooling troughs beneath the turntable, clean the cuvette sensor, check temperatures in the four heating and cooling systems, and check the pump volumes.

MLA ELECTRA 750

The MLA Electra 750 is a semiautomated blood coagulation timer (Fig. 159). Clot formation is timed automatically and is detected by means of a photocell that reads the optical density change when the clot is formed. The unit contains a heating block that maintains the reagents and plasma samples at 37°C prior to and during testing. Pipetting of the reagents and plasma samples is done by the technologist, utilizing the disposable-tip, precision pipets included with the instrument. Both oxalated and citrated plasma specimens may be tested with this instrument. An improved sensitivity and optical range allow the instrument to detect the clot on samples that may be chylous, icteric, or hemolyzed (however, hemolyzed specimens should not be used for coagulation testing). There are five mode switches located on the front of the instrument. All routine coagulation testing may be performed on the Electra 750 in addition to thrombin times, fibrinogen assays, factor assays, and saline dilutions.

COAGULYZER II

The Coagulyzer II is an automated unit for performing a variety of coagulation procedures. It detects clot formation photoelectrically. This is accomplished by monitoring the output of a photocell. The plasma test samples are pipetted into cuvettes and placed in the numbered holes of a circular turntable. Sample wells numbered 2 through 60 are cooled at approximately 10°C (±5°C), whereas sample well number 1 is at room temperature. When the instrument is started, the turntable revolves and carries each test sample, in turn, through a heating block, where the plasma specimens are warmed to 37°C. When the first sample gets to the test station, a preset quantity of reagent is automatically pipetted into the cuvette, and

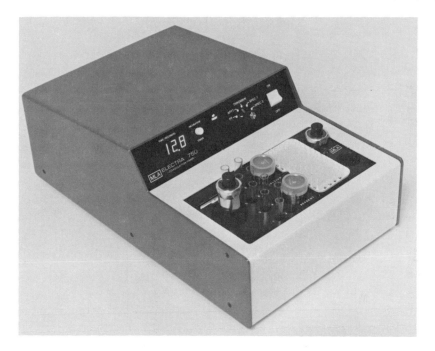

Fig. 159. MLA Electra 750. (Courtesy of Medical Laboratory Automation, Mount Vernon, N.Y.)

the timing mechanism is started. As fibrin formation occurs, this change in optical density is detected by the photoelectric cell, and the timing mechanism is halted. The clotting time, to the tenths of a second, is printed out on the printer tape. The turntable then automatically rotates one space to the next specimen, and the procedure is repeated. In the event that two reagents must be added to the plasma sample, the first reagent is automatically pipetted into the cuvette when it gets to the No. 2 pipet station.

COMPONENTS OF THE COAGULYZER (Fig. 160)

1. The *mode selector switch* may be set at PT-1 (for single reagent PT), *PT-2* (used for the PT when adding calcium chloride and thromboplastin separately), *APTT, APTT (C.A.T.)* (for performing prolonged APTT tests using a constant activation time), and *manual* (for manual operation of the pipettors and timing mechanism).

2. The *on/off* switch turns the instrument on and off.

3. *Manual controls.* When the instrument is in the manual mode, *pipettor #1* and *pipettor #2* operate pipets No. 1 and 2, respectively. The *start* pushbutton moves the turntable to the next position. The *clock start*, when depressed, begins the timing cycle.

4. The *pyrometer* indicates the temperature in the reservoirs and incubation block. The *pyrometer switch* can be rotated between the reservoir and incubation block, depending on which temperature is desired.

5. The *turntable* contains numbered spaces for 60 specimens.

6. The *volume selectors #1* and *#2* are used to set *automatic pipettors #1* and *#2* volumes to 0.1 and 0.2 ml, respectively.

7. The *reagent reservoirs*, left and right, are capable of continuous magnetic stirring. The left reservoir is warmed to 37.5°C.

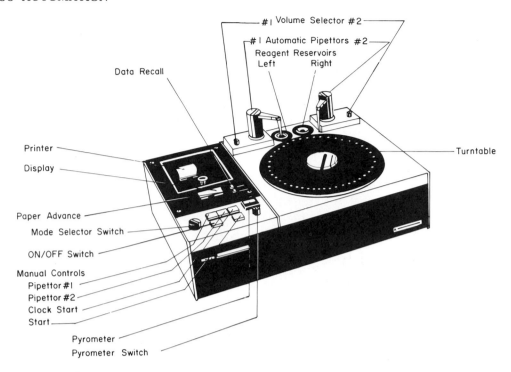

Fig. 160. Coagulyzer II.

8. *Display* indicates the sample number and elapsed time as the sample is being tested.

9. The *data recall* button may be utilized at the completion of the run to display each sample number and clotting time for every sample in the run just completed.

10. The *printer* records the sample number and clotting time for each specimen tested. The *paper advance* button allows manual advance of the printer paper.

The activated partial thromboplastin time (APTT) is outlined in this section because it is a frequently performed procedure and is a two-reagent test.

PROCEDURE FOR THE ACTIVATED PARTIAL THROMBOPLASTIN TIME

1. Depress the power switch, turning the instrument on, and allow 10 minutes for warm-up. Set the mode switch to APTT (or APTT, C.A.T. for a constant activation time). Set both pipets (Nos. 1 and 2) to deliver 0.1 ml of reagents.

2. Place an adequate amount of calcium chloride in the pipet No. 1 well. Add a clean magnetic stirring bar to the reservoir and cover with the lid. Allow a 10-minute warm-up period.

3. Place a sufficient amount of activated platelet substitute in the pipet No. 2 well. Add a clean magnetic stirring bar and cover with the lid. This reagent remains at room temperature.

4. Pipet 0.1 ml of plasma to be tested into the disposable cuvettes and sequentially place them in the turntable beginning with slot No. 1.

5. Depress the start switch to begin testing. The turntable moves counterclockwise one station. The first cuvette is directly below pipet No. 2, where 0.1 ml of activated platelet substitute is automatically added to cuvette No. 1. The turntable remains at this station for 50 seconds (APTT

mode) or 150 seconds (APTT, C.A.T. mode). At the end of 50 seconds (APTT mode) or 150 seconds (APTT, C.A.T. mode), the turntable will move one station forward. When the first cuvette reaches the test station, 0.1 ml of calcium chloride is forcefully pipetted into the sample cuvette, and the timing mechanism is started. When clot formation is detected by the photocell, the timer is halted, and the time is registered on the printer paper. The minimum incubation time per station in the APTT mode is 50 seconds. If the clotting has not occurred within that time, the sample will remain in the test station for a maximum time of 90 seconds or until the sample clots, whichever occurs first. In the APTT, C.A.T. mode, the incubation time per test station is consistently 150 seconds.

6. Average the duplicate sample readings for each patient and record. The duplicate results should agree within ±1.5 seconds of each other.

DISCUSSION

1. The two-reagent test (other than the APTT) may also be performed in the PT-2 mode. Some factor assays are done at this setting. The reader is referred to the Coagulyzer instruction manual for the exact setting to be used in each procedure.
2. It is advisable to keep the reservoir covers on at all times to minimize reagent evaporation.
3. The following procedures may be performed on the Coagulyzer: PT, APTT, prothrombin consumption, PT and APTT substitution tests, factor assays, the thromboplastin generation test, and the Reptilase-R.
4. For coagulation testing performed on the Coagulyzer, use only sodium citrate-anticoagulated blood when plasma is required (serum is utilized

in the prothrombin consumption procedure).

COAGULYZER JR. III

The Coagulyzer Jr. III is a semiautomated coagulation timer (Fig. 161). Clot formation is automatically timed and is detected by means of a photoelectric cell. This unit contains 15 heated *test tube wells* for incubating test plasmas. There are two heated *reservoirs* for reagents, one of which contains a magnetic stirrer. The instrument is turned on by depressing the *on/off* switch. The tube containing the patient plasma is placed in the *reaction well*, and the *start* switch, activating the timing mechanism, is depressed at the same time that the reagent is added to the test sample. If an automatic pipettor is plugged into the *bi-pettor jack*, the timing mechanism is automatically activated as the reagent is pipetted into the test sample. The clotting time is registered on the *digital display* and returns to zero each time the start switch is activated. Only citrated plasma specimens should be used on this instrument. The PT, APTT, factor assays, PT and APTT substitution tests, prothrombin consumption, thromboplastin generation time, and Reptilase-R may be performed on this instrument.

COAG-A-MATE DUAL CHANNEL ANALYZER

The Coag-A-Mate dual channel automated coagulation analyzer detects clot formation by means of a photocell sensing circuit that reads the optical density change when a clot is formed. This instrument automatically pipets all reagents necessary for testing and is capable of performing two like or different test procedures simultaneously. Plasma specimens to be tested are pipetted into small cuvettes in a circular test tray and placed on the instrument in the incubation test plate, which cools the samples prior to testing. When the instrument is activated, the test plate revolves, carrying the test samples

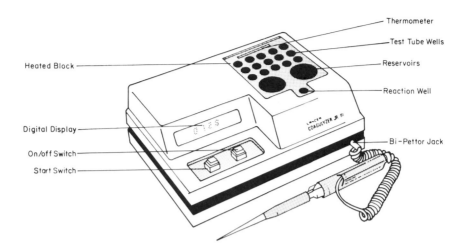

Fig. 161. Coagulyzer Jr. III.

through a heating zone, where they are warmed to 37°C prior to testing. When the first two samples get to the test station, a preset quantity of reagent is automatically pipetted into each of two cuvettes, and the timing mechanisms are started. (If two reagents are required for the test, such as in the APTT, the first reagent is added to each cuvette prior to its arrival at the test station.) When fibrin formation occurs, the photoelectric cell detects the sudden change in optical density, and the timing mechanism is automatically stopped. The clotting time is then printed out on the printer tape to the closest tenth of a second. When both test samples have clotted, the test tray is ready to rotate to the next two test samples. The time elapsed between clot formation and the beginning of the next two tests depends on the cycle time mode that has been selected by the operator.

The Coag-A-Mate dual channel analyzer is capable of performing the majority of coagulation procedures, most notably the PT, APTT, and factor assays. The procedure for performing PTs and APTTs simultaneously is described on the following pages.

COMPONENTS OF THE COAG-A-MATE DUAL CHANNEL ANALYZER (See Fig. 162)

1. *Reagent storage wells* (two) provide reagent storage at room temperature.
2. *Stir cool wells* (two) provide low-temperature reagent storage and magnetic stirrers for constant mixing of the reagents.
3. The *reagent tubing assembly* is color-coded, delivers the reagents from the reagent vials to the test cuvette through inert tubing, and has pick-up and delivery tips.
4. The precision *reagent dispenser pump* is responsible for delivering the exact amount of reagent to the test cuvette.
5. The *reagent incubation arm* warms the reagents (contained in the tubing) to 37°C prior to being delivered into the test cuvette.
6. The *incubation test plate* has a blue area where the plasma samples are cooled and a red area through which the plasma samples are warmed to 37°C.
7. The *circular test tray* is a disposable plastic tray that sits on the incubation test plate. It is capable of holding 48 plasma samples in which incubation and testing occur.

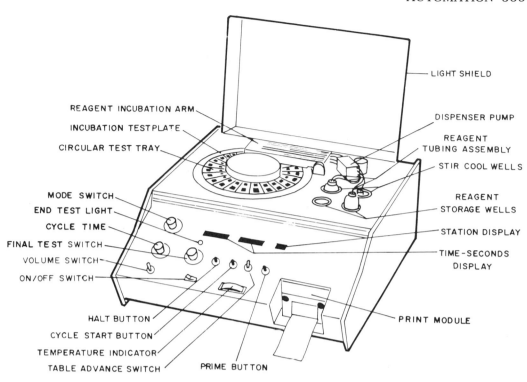

Fig. 162. Coag-A-Mate dual channel analyzer.

8. The *mode switch* is utilized for selecting the test procedure desired: PT, APTT, or PT and APTT. The mode setting also determines the delay time that begins when the reagent is added to the test cuvette. During this period, the instrument does not respond to optical density changes, in case bubbles were briefly formed when the reagent was added to the test cuvette. The delay time in the PT mode is 8 seconds, whereas in the APTT mode it is 20 seconds.

9. The *end test light* is lit, and an audible beep is given at the completion of the final test.

10. The *cycle time* allows the operator to choose the amount of time between tests. In those settings of 50, 110, 150, 240, or 300 seconds, the instrument automatically moves forward to the next test sample at the time set, irrespective of clot formation. In the demand setting in the PT mode, the instrument will automatically index to the next sample in 30 to 150 seconds, depending on clot formation. In the APTT mode, indexing to the next sample occurs between 110 and 300 seconds, again depending on the time of clot formation of the sample in the test station.

11. The *final test switch* should be set at the test station that contains the last sample to be tested.

12. The *volume toggle switch* determines the volume of reagent to be dispensed by the pump.

13. The *on-off switch* turns the instrument on and off.

14. The *halt button,* when pressed, terminates the test cycle and returns the timers to 000.0.

15. The *cycle start button* reactivates the test cycle when it has been stopped.

16. The *table advance toggle switch* advances the circular test tray automatically (when the switch is *up)* or

manually one station at a time (when the switch is *down* and released).

17. The *temperature indicator* shows the temperature in the test station by indirect measurement.

18. The *prime button* activates the pump for priming (filling) the reagent tubing.

19. The *print module records* the test cuvette number, the test, and the clotting time for each test sample.

20. The *time-seconds displays* (two) show the elapsed time to the tenths of a second for the inner and outer test samples.

21. The *station display* indicates the cuvette number currently in the test station.

22. The *decimal point temperature indicator* in the time-seconds display, when lit, indicates that the red area of the incubation test plate is at the proper operating temperature.

23. The *light shield* should be in the *down* position during testing to decrease interfering light, dust, and air circulation.

24. Located on the rear of the instrument are fans, jacks for connecting a chart recorder and a pump, the fuse, and the circuit board cover panel.

PROCEDURE FOR THE PROTHROMBIN TIME AND ACTIVATED PARTIAL THROMBOPLASTIN TIME AS PERFORMED SIMULTANEOUSLY

1. Turn the power on and allow approximately a 15-minute warm-up period, until the red decimal point temperature indicator illuminates.

2. Set the test mode to PT-APTT and the cycle time to either 110 for a 4-minute activation period or 150 for a 5-minute activation period. This activation time represents the time that elapses between the time the partial thromboplastin is added to the plasma and the time that the calcium chloride is added when the test cycle is begun. The volume control should be set at 0.1 and the station display at 23.

3. Place a vial of thromboplastin and a vial of partial thromboplastin in each of the stir cool wells. (Each vial should contain a stir bar.) Place the vial of calcium chloride in the reagent storage well. Cap each vial with the three-hole stopper and connect the reagent tubing assembly into the reagents (red tubing to the thromboplastin, blue tubing to the partial thromboplastin, and white tubing to the calcium chloride).

4. Place a container under the delivery tips in the reagent incubation arm and prime the reagent lines by pressing the prime button. Continue this until the lines are completely filled with reagent.

5. Pipet 0.1 ml of the plasma specimens to be tested into each of the inner (PT) and outer (APTT) cuvettes of the circular test tray beginning with cuvette No. 1 and ending with cuvette No. 22. Cuvettes No. 23 and No. 24 collect excess reagent. Each plasma sample and control should be run in duplicate.

6. Place the test tray on the incubation test plate, being careful to match the notch in the test tray with the notch in the hub.

7. Lower the reagent incubation arm.

8. Set the final test switch to the last cuvette containing plasma to be tested.

9. Close the light shield.

10. Press the cycle button to begin testing. The first plasma samples (one in the inner cuvette and one in the outer cuvette) enter the first of two incubation stations. At the first incubation station, 0.1 ml of partial thromboplastin is added to the outer cuvette for the APTT. At the end of 110 or 150 seconds (depending on the cycle time chosen), the test tray advances the cuvettes one station

until the final test has been completed. When the plasma samples reach the test station, 0.2 ml of thromboplastin (two lines each delivering 0.1 ml) is added to the plasma for the prothrombin time, and the timer is started. At the same time, 0.1 ml of calcium chloride is added to the plasma in the outer cuvette for the APTT. Similarly, the second timer is started. When a clot forms, the timer stops and the clotting time is typed on the printer tape. If a clot does not form within the 110 (or 150) seconds, 000.0 is printed on the tape. In this circumstance, results should be reported as greater than 110 (or 150) seconds.

11. When the last pair of tests has been completed, raise the light shield. Lift up the reagent incubation arm and remove the circular test tray. Discard.

12. Average the duplicate sample readings for each patient and record. Prothrombin time duplicate results should agree within ±0.5 seconds, whereas APTT results should agree within ±1.5 seconds. Samples showing abnormally prolonged results may show a greater difference between duplicate samples.

DISCUSSION

1. Inability of the instrument to detect a clot is generally caused by a burned-out light source.

2. Erratic results may be due to one of several causes: (a) reagents, (b) improper collection or handling of patient specimen, (c) dirty, twisted, or improperly seated reagent tubing, (d) jerky pump operation (pump tubing may need lubrication), (e) delivery tip dirty or in wrong position, or (f) mode switch in wrong position.

3. If the instrument does not become activated when it is turned on, the fuse may need to be replaced.

4. Reagent should not remain in the re-agent tubing for more than 30 minutes after testing has been completed. Remove the reagent and clean the tubing by alternately drawing distilled water and air through the lines using the prime button. Remove the tubing assembly from the pump if the instrument is not to be used right away. See the instrument's operations manual for directions on removing and replacing the tubing.

5. Depending on the usage, the rotor should be removed from the pump and cleaned with isopropanol on a scheduled basis. Instructions for this procedure may be found in the operations manual.

6. The reaction temperatures should be checked routinely. This may be done with a thermistor. The reagent delivery volume should also be checked on a scheduled basis using a calibrated capillary pipet. Instructions for these procedures and the necessary adjustments are clearly outlined in the operations manual.

COAG-A-MATE · X2

The Coag-A-Mate · X2 coagulation instrument detects clot formation by means of a photocell sensing circuit that reads the optical density change when a clot is formed. The instrument automatically pipets all necessary reagents for testing and will perform four tests simultaneously: two different tests in duplicate or four like tests. The plasma samples to be tested are pipetted into small cuvettes in a circular test tray (having a capacity of 48 cuvettes) and placed on the instrument in the incubation test plate, which cools the patient samples prior to testing. When the instrument is activated, the test plate revolves, carrying the test samples through a heating zone, where they are warmed to 37°C for a preset time period prior to and during testing. When the first four samples arrive at the test station, the correct amount of reagent is automatically pipetted into each of the four cuvettes, and the timing mechanisms are started. (If two reagents are required for the test, as in the APTT, the first reagent is added to each cuvette at a set time interval prior to its arrival at the test station.) When fibrin formation occurs, the photoelectric cell detects the sudden change in optical density, and the timing mechanism is automatically stopped. The clotting time is then printed out on the printer tape to the closest tenth of a second. After a preset period of time, the test tray rotates to the next four plasma samples. The circular test tray, carrying the patient samples, is rotated on the incubation test plate at a set rate and is not affected by the clotting time of the patient samples. This timing mechanism is alterable by the operator.

The Coag-A-Mate · X2 is capable of performing the majority of coagulation procedures. The procedure for simultaneously performing PTs and APTTs in duplicate is described under Procedure for the Simultaneous Performance of the PT and APTT.

COMPONENTS OF THE COAG-A-MATE · X2 (see Fig. 163)

1. The *light shield,* placed in the *down* position (at all times except when adding reagents or test samples or when performing maintenance work), decreases interfering light, dust, and air circulation.
2. The *circular test tray* is a disposable plastic tray that sits on the incubation test plate and is capable of holding 48 plasma samples to be incubated and tested.
3. The *incubation test plate* contains a cooled zone for storage of samples prior to testing and a heated zone in the test area that warms the plasma samples to 37°C.
4. The *on-off* switch turns the instrument on or off.
5. The *paper advance keypad* is used to advance the paper tape.

6. The *print module* records on the paper tape the maximum and minimum incubation times, the blank time (time period at the beginning of the test where no clot is detected), the reagent volume, instrument sensitivity, temperature of the testing area, date, cuvette number of sample, name of test, clotting time, and the last cuvette for testing that has been selected by the operator.
7. The *stir cool wells* (four) provide low-temperature reagent storage and magnetic stirrers for constant mixing of the reagents.
8. The *reagent tubing assemblies* are color-coded, inert tubing that have pick-up and delivery tips for transporting the reagent from the reagent vials to the test cuvette.
9. The *reagent dispenser pumps* (two) deliver the exact amount of reagent to the test cuvet.
10. The *reagent incubation arm* warms the reagents (contained in the tubing) to 37°C prior to being delivered into the test cuvette.
11. *Lighted displays*
    A. The *reaction zone temperature indicator* displays the temperature in the testing area. It should be 37°C (±0.5°C). When the instrument is first turned on, the words NOT READY will be displayed until the instrument reaches 37°C (±0.5°C), at which time the word READY will be displayed. During testing, the word BUSY will be illuminated.
    B. The *station number indicator,* during testing, displays the two cuvette numbers that are in the test station by alternating back and forth between the two numbers. When the end test key (see No. 12 below, Touch Entry Panel) is pressed, the words END TEST are displayed. This is automatically set at station 24 unless

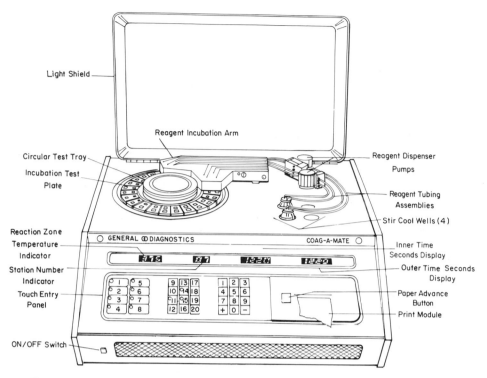

Fig. 163. Coag-A-Mate • X2.

changed by the operator. The *sensitivity* of the clot detection system, which may be set from 1 to 9 as required, may also be displayed on this indicator. The *date* (month/day/year) is displayed when entered into the instrument.

C. The *inner time seconds display* indicates the elapsed time during testing for the two samples in the inner channel on the circular test tray. The display switches back and forth between the two samples. This indicator is also used to display the *volumes* delivered by both reagent dispenser pumps. *Power* is displayed along side of the inner channel when the instrument is on.

D. The *outer time seconds display* indicates the elapsed time during testing for the two samples in the outer channel on the circular test

tray. The display moves back and forth between the two samples. This display also indicates the *blank time,* at the end of which the instrument will begin to monitor clot formation. *Minimum* and *maximum* times will be displayed here, indicating the shortest and longest times the optical sensor will monitor the clot before moving to the next test station.

12. The *touch entry panel* keys are activated by gently pressing them.
   A. *PT* (1) selects the prothrombin time mode.
   B. *APTT* (2) selects the activated partial thromboplastin time mode.
   C. *PT/APTT* (3) allows the operator to run PTs in the inner channel and APTTs in the outer channel simultaneously.
   D. *Fibrinogen* (4) selects the quantitative fibrinogen mode.

E. *TT* (5) selects the thrombin time mode (not yet available for use).

F. *Two-Stage FA* (6) is for a two-stage factor assay mode, which is not yet available.

G. *Special* (7) mode is for custom programming of individual systems.

H. *Modify test* (8) is used to change the standard parameters of test modes.

I. *Prime 1* (9) and *Prime 2* (10) are used to fill the reagent tubing associated with the respective reagent pump.

J. When pressed, *deprime* (11) results in the reagents in the reagent lines being returned to the reagent vials. To return reagents to reagent vial as soon as the last reagent has been dispensed, press enter (22), deprime, and enter. To deprime the reagent tubing in 0.005-ml increments during calibration, pressing deprime will cause the pump that was last primed to deprime 0.005 ml at a time. To return all reagents to reagent vials, press *cancel* (18) and then deprime.

K. *Sensitivity* (12) is used to adjust the sensitivity of the photo-optical system.

L. *End Test* (13) indicates the last cuvette sample that will be tested by the instrument. This is preset at cuvette 24 unless otherwise set before each instrument run.

M. *Pause* (14) may be depressed to momentarily interrupt the test cycle. All tests to which reagents have been added, however, will continue until completion before the instrument stops. When the instrument pauses, an audible beep will sound at intervals until *start* has been pressed.

N. *Recall* (15) may be used to obtain reprints of the previous test run,

as long as the instrument has not been turned off or another test cycle started.

O. *Date* (16) is used to enter the month, day, and year.

P. *Start* (17) is pressed to begin the test cycle.

Q. *Cancel* (18) is used to halt the instrument immediately. Any tests in progress will be lost.

R. *Index* (19) advances the circular test tray one station at a time.

S. *Enter* (20) enters all program changes into the microprocessor.

T. *Numbers* 1 through 9 (right side of the touch entry panel) to enter information into the computer.

U. *+, −* are used in conjunction with the *modify test* (used for sensitivity or volume change) key or the *sensitivity* key to add or subtract.

13. Located on the rear of the instrument are the circuit board cover and a circuit breaker.

PROCEDURE FOR THE SIMULTANEOUS PERFORMANCE OF THE PROTHROMBIN TIME AND ACTIVATED PARTIAL THROMBOPLASTIN TIME

1. Press the rocker switch to turn the instrument on. The words NOT READY will be displayed, indicating that the instrument temperature has not reached 37°C (±0.5°C). When the proper temperature has been reached (37°C, ±0.5°C), the word READY will be displayed. (The instrument cannot be used for testing as long as the words NOT READY are displayed.)

2. Press the PT/APTT key on the touch entry panel (the light on the key should illuminate). To remove the reagents from the reagent lines at the end of every test cycle, press deprime and then enter (deprime should remain lit). Enter the date: Press date, press a two digit number for the

month, the day, and the year, pressing enter after each entry.

3. Place the reagent vials in the stir cool wells: One bottle each of thromboplastin, activated partial thromboplastin, and 0.025 M calcium chloride. Add a clean magnetic stir bar to the thromboplastin and the partial thromboplastin (if recommended by manufacturer). On each vial, place a cap containing an appropriate opening for the reagent lines.

4. Install reagent lines if not in place, using the information given in Table 21.

  A. Insert the appropriate delivery tip into the corresponding hole on the reagent incubation arm, pushing the delivery tip well into the hole until it extends $\frac{1}{16}$ inch below the opening. Without stretching the tubing, firmly press each piece into the appropriate groove of the arm, working from the delivery tip to the base of the arm.

  B. Lightly lubricate each piece of tubing between the collars. Using both hands, grasp both collars on the piece of tubing and stretch tubing around the front of the pump rotor. Slide the tubing into the slot on either side of the stator and position the tubing in the appropriate notch. Both collars should fit firmly on either side of the pump area. Depress the appropriate prime (1 or 2) button to ensure proper seating of the tube around the pump.

  C. Install the pick-up tips into the appropriate reagent vials, making

certain they are inserted to the bottoms of the reagent vials.

5. Prime the pumps to fill the reagent lines. Carefully lift the reagent incubation arm to a 45° angle. Hold a petri dish under lines D, E, and F. Depress and hold prime 2 button on the touch entry panel until all three reagents are expelled from the lines in a steady stream. Repeat, priming line B using the prime 1 button.

6. Pipet 0.1 ml of patient plasma or control plasma into the appropriate cuvettes. Each sample should be run in duplicate. Plasma samples for APTT must be placed into the cuvettes in the outer channel of the test plate. PT test samples should be added to the inner channel of cuvettes.

7. Carefully position the tray on the incubation test plate, matching the notch in the tray with the notch in the hub. Lower the reagent incubation arm so that it is as far down as possible (in a horizontal position).

8. Lower the light shield, making certain that all tubing is completely under the shield. The light shield must be down at all times while the instrument is testing (the busy light will be displayed).

9. Make certain the station number, as indicated on the control panel, corresponds to the cuvette number containing the first sample to be tested. If a different number appears in the station number window, press and hold the index key until the station number corresponds to the first sample.

10. Set the end test station (last cuvette containing a test sample). Press end

Table 21. **PLACEMENT OF REAGENT TUBING FOR THE COAG-A-MATE · X2 (FOR THE PROTHROMBIN TIME AND ACTIVATED PARTIAL THROMBOPLASTIN TIME**

INCUBATION ARM SLOT	TUBING	REAGENT	PUMP NO.	PUMP SLOT NO.
D and E	Red collar (two)	Thromboplastin	2	6 and 7
F	Clear collar	Calcium chloride	2	8
B	Blue collar	Partial thromboplastin	1	3

test, press the two-digit number of the last cuvette, and press enter.

11. Press start to begin testing. Check the printout that is given at this time for the following information: End test station, reaction zone temperature, sensitivity, pumps No. 1 and 2 volumes, blank time (PT and APTT), and minimum and maximum times.

12. During testing, the control panel will show the following: Busy light illuminated, the station number display will shift back and forth between the two cuvette numbers currently at the test stations, the inner channel seconds display will shift back and forth showing the time elapsed or clotting times of the PTs being tested or just completed, and the outer channel seconds display shows the same information on the APTTs.

13. At the completion of testing, the instrument will beep, the busy light will go out, and the word READY will be illuminated. The station display will show the next cuvette number the instrument will begin on. At the completion of testing, raise the light shield and the reagent incubation arm. Carefully remove the test tray. If the outer and inner channels still have empty cuvettes, the tray may be used again.

DISCUSSION

1. During the test cycle, only the on/off, pause, and cancel buttons may be activated.

2. To add more test samples during a run, press the pause key. All tests that have begun will be completed before the instrument will stop. Therefore, once the pause key is pressed, there will be a wait of 6 to 8 minutes before the instrument halts testing (APTT reagent is added to plasma about 5 minutes prior to testing). When the instrument stops, it will beep at intervals, signaling that the light shield may be raised and test samples added. After adding more test samples (a) prime pumps #1 and #2 (if necessary), (b) lower the light shield, (c) set the end test station, (d) press start, and (e) check the printer tape statistics. The instrument will automatically index to the next test station.

3. To stop instrument testing immediately, press the cancel button. When this is done, the duplicate PT and APTT samples being tested will be lost, along with the next two duplicate samples for both tests. Prior to beginning another test cycle (a) prime pumps No. 1 and 2 (if necessary), (b) lower the light shield, (c) index the incubation test plate to the desired cuvette number, (d) set the end test station, (e) press start, and (f) check the printer tape statistics.

4. To shut down the instrument:
   A. Remove the reagent lines from the reagent vials and place in a vial of distilled water.
   B. Clean reagent from the reagent lines by priming the lines with air and distilled water alternately.
   C. Carefully remove the reagent tubing from the pumps. Allow the tubing to remain in the reagent incubation arm.
   D. Lower the light shield. Turn the instrument off.

5. If the results print out as . , this indicates that no clot has been detected, either because clotting is still in progress, clotting occurred during the blank time, the instrument is unable to detect a clot (plasma grossly lipemic, icteric, or hemolyzed or decreased fibrinogen, for example), or no clot was formed for such reasons as no reagent added to cuvette (reagent QNS).

6. Each position in the two pumps must be individually calibrated according to the pump position and the indi-

vidual tubing. It is, therefore, imperative that the tubing be placed in the pump position as indicated and recalibration procedures followed when new tubing is put on.

7. When priming the reagent lines, make certain there are no air bubbles present in the tubing. If there are air bubbles, repriming is necessary.

8. When adding samples to a test tray that has been partially used, add the first PT sample and the first APTT sample to the first cuvette number that has both inner and outer channels empty.

9. The pump rotors should be cleaned at regular intervals. The reagent tubing must also be replaced regularly, depending on the work volume. Whenever the tubing is removed or replaced or whenever the pump rotors are cleaned, the reagent delivery volumes must be checked and adjusted as necessary. The temperature of the incubation arm should also be checked with a thermistor as part of the scheduled maintenance.

COAG-A-MATE 2001

The Coag-A-Mate 2001 (Fig. 164) is able to perform up to 12 PTs or 12 APTTS simultaneously. A single light source is divided into 12 channels, each of which passes through the sample to its own corresponding sensor. The change in optical density of each sample as it clots is detected by the corresponding sensor, and this information is stored until all test samples have clotted, and the results for that run of tests are then printed out on printer paper.

The Coag-A-Mate 2001 is turned on by means of the *on/off* switch and is ready for testing when the *temperature indicator* reads 37°C (± 1°C). By use of the *mode* switch, either PT or APTT is selected, depending on which test is to be run. The reagent *dispenser pumps* will then be set to deliver the correct reagent volumes. The rear panel of the instrument contains a *PT cycle* switch to select sequential testing or simultaneous testing. Also located in this area is the *APTT activation time switch* for setting the activation time at 180, 240, or 300 seconds. The reagents for either the PT or APTT test are placed in the *reagent storage wells*, and the *tubing assemblies* are placed into the reagent vials, fitted into the *reagent incubation arm*, and the tubing nozzles are put into place. Prime No. 1 and prime No. 2 switches are depressed to activate the left and right *dispenser pumps*, respectively, to fill the tubing with reagent. Plasma samples are pipetted (0.1 ml) into the *circular test tray*, which is then placed onto the *incubation test plate* (beneath the *light shield* containing the incubation arm). The *first sample* and *last sample* switches are set to tell the instrument where to begin and end testing. The light shield is kept closed during testing. The test cycle is begun by depressing the *start* switch, at which point the electronic timing mechanism is activated. As each plasma sample is clotted or maximum time has occurred, the *station number display* indicates the sample number, and the clotting time is displayed on the *time-seconds display*. If maximum time has occurred before clotting, U U . U will be displayed, and the test should be repeated by another method. When all testing is complete, the *cycle button/light* will be lit, and the *print module* will print out the sample results with the corresponding cuvette number. Those samples that did not clot will be indicated by - - . - on the printer tape and may be caused by grossly lipemic, icteric, or hemolyzed plasma or decreased fibrinogen, for example. The circular test tray should then be removed, and the instrument is ready for further testing.

THE HEMAPREP AUTOMATIC BLOOD-SMEARING INSTRUMENT

The Hemaprep automatic smear maker (Fig. 165), manufactured by Geometric

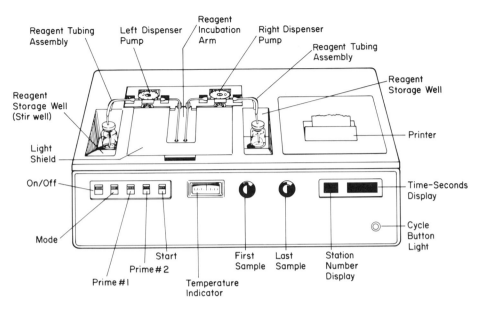

Fig. 164. Coag-A-Mate 2001.

Data Corporation, affords the technologist a fast and simple method for preparing wedge smears of consistently good quality.

PROCEDURE

1. Insert one *spreader* in each *spreader holder* if they are not already in-

stalled. Raise the spreader holder slightly and squeeze gently. Fit the spreader securely in the holder with the notched side facing you.

2. Turn the instrument on by placing the *power swtich* in the up position.

3. Place one (or two) slide(s) in the

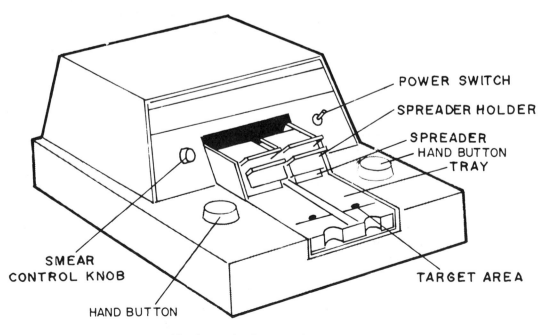

Fig. 165. Hemaprep automatic blood-smearing instrument.

trays(s), making certain the slide(s) is firmly seated.

4. Place a small drop of blood on each *target area*. A capillary pipet, hematocrit tube (nonheparinized), or applicator stick may be used for this step.

5. After the blood has been placed on the slide(s), quickly depress the right or left *hand button* to begin the cycle. When this is done, the slide tray moves back. When the spreader comes in contact with the drop of blood, the slide tray hestitates momentarily, allowing the blood to spread along the edge of the spreader. The slide tray then advances to its original position, pulling the blood into a wedge smear as it moves forward.

DISCUSSION

1. The *smear control knob* alters the speed with which the blood is smeared, allowing the technologist to control the thickness of the blood smear. A setting of 2.5 is generally used for most bloods. If the hematocrit is less than 15%, however, a setting of 3 or 4 is recommended, and, conversely, a setting between positions 1 and 2 should be used on blood specimens with extremely high hematocrit.

2. On the back of the instrument, there is a fuse and a pause control knob that controls the width of the blood smear by allowing the operator to vary the interval of time that the spreader is in contact with the blood before the smear is pulled. When this knob is turned completely clockwise, there is a pause of maximum time, and a full-width smear results.

4. It is necessary to replace the spreaders periodically if they become chipped. They are inexpensive and available from Geometric Data Corporation.

5. If only one smear is prepared on each patient, only one tray (and one spreader) should be routinely used.

6. Reticulocyte smears may also be prepared on this instrument by setting the smear control knob between 3 and 4.

7. Only a small amount of practice is necessary to make blood smears on this instrument. The critical factor is the amount of blood placed on the slide.

8. There may be a small carry-over of cells from one smear to the next. The exact amount has been found to be 0.5% or less. The spreaders should be washed routinely, depending on use, and whenever an excessive amount of blood has been placed on the slide. Clean the spreaders with 0.85% sodium chloride (w/v).

9. A smaller, portable Hemaprep automatic smear maker is also available that does not require electric power and may be used at the patient's bedside.

HEMASPINNER AUTOMATIC BLOOD CELL SPINNER

The Hemaspinner (Fig. 166) is used for preparing a monolayer film of whole blood on a glass slide. A clean glass slide is placed on a platen, and three to four drops of blood are placed in the middle of the slide. When the top of the instrument is closed, the platen spins at high speed for a set amount of time. During this period, excess blood is thrown from the slide into a catch basin, and the resultant slide is completely covered with a thin monolayer of cells. During spinning, a beam of light passes up through the glass slide onto a sensor. When the cells have separated the proper amount, the sensor detects this, and the platen automatically stops spinning. In this way, spreading of the blood is consistent from one smear to the next, regardless of the patient's hematocrit.

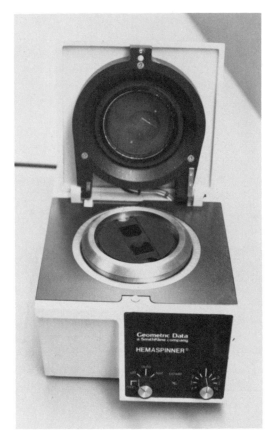

Fig. 166. Hemaspinner.

COMPONENTS OF THE HEMASPINNER

1. The *platen* holds the glass slide in place during the spinning process.
2. The *catch basin* collects the excess blood as it is spun off the slide.
3. The *optical system* automatically stops the spinning process at the point at which the blood cells are beginning to move away from each other but are still close to one another. It consists of a *light source* (located beneath the catch basin) and an *optical sensor* (located on the cover of the instrument).
4. The *mode* switch turns the instrument off, places it in the manual mode (where the spin time is manually set), automatic mode (optical sensing system determines the spin time), or test mode (used to test the optical sensing system).
5. The *power* light, when lit, indicates that the instrument is on.
6. The *spin setting knob* is used to alter the spin time.
7. The *spin* light (not shown) is located on the top of the cover and will be lit while the platen is spinning.

PROCEDURE

1. Lift up the lid on the Hemaspinner. Set the mode switch on auto. The spin setting knob should be on 0.
2. Holding the slide at each end with your fingertips, place the slide in the grooves of the platen. Make certain the slide fits completely within the grooved area of the platen. Failure to do this may result in permanent damage to the instrument.
3. Using a disposable pasteur pipet or plastic straw, place four drops of blood onto the middle of the glass slide. The blood should spread out on the slide to the approximate size of a quarter.
4. Immediately close the top of the Hemaspinner and hold the lid down firmly until the spin light (located on the lid) automatically shuts off.
5. Lift the lid of the Hemaspinner and remove the slide by grasping it at both ends with your fingertips.
6. Allow the slide to air-dry before staining.

DISCUSSION

1. To obtain consistently well-prepared smears, it is necessary to keep the Hemaspinner clean at all times.
   A. After every 25 to 30 slides, the catch basin must be removed and washed and the optical system cleaned.
      1) Remove the platen by grasping the center shaft with the fingers and pulling straight up. (Do not lift the platen by the

outer edges. This will cause the platen to bend, causing the slide to fly off the platen during the spin cycle.)

2) Lift out the catch basin and wash well in running tap water. Dry.

3) Using a piece of water-dampened lens paper, clean the light source (located under the catch basin). Dry with a second piece of lens paper. Repeat this cleaning procedure for the optical density sensor (located on the inside of the lid).

4) Replace the catch basin in the Hemaspinner. Holding the platen by the center shaft, slide it firmly onto the shaft of the Hemaspinner.

B. When making smears, the glass covering of the optical density sensor in the lid may frequently become spattered with blood. Watch for this and clean immediately as outlined above. Any time the glass covering of the light source or sensor becomes dusty or dirty, the spinning time of the Hemaspinner will be affected, and the slides will be incorrectly prepared.

2. The Hemaspinner contains an aerosol removal system. During the spinning process, a positive airflow has been created that travels through a duct in the back of the spin chamber and into a submicron filter.

3. The lid gasket should be changed at least once every 3 months, any time that it appears to be damaged, or when improper sealing occurs.

HEMASTAINER AUTOMATIC SLIDE STAINER

The Hemastainer automatic slide stainer (Fig. 167) is a completely automated slide stainer. In the event of mechanical break-

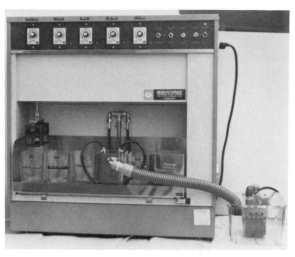

Fig. 167. Hemastainer automatic slide stainer.

down, however, the stainer may be operated manually. The sample slides are placed in a stain rack (slide basket), capable of holding up to 100 slides, and dipped into the staining solutions at timed intervals. Stain station No. 1 contains methanol for fixing the blood smears. The slides are then transferred to station No. 2 containing Wright stain, and from there to station No. 3, which contains a mixture of Wright stain and phosphate buffer (where the major portion of the staining takes place). The slides are then rinsed in running, deionized water, followed by a phosphate buffer rinse. The slides are then dried by forced warm air at the last station. The entire staining process, including drying, takes approximately 12 minutes from start to finish for each batch of slides.

COMPONENTS OF THE HEMASTAINER

1. The *basket hanger* holds the slide basket containing the sample slides.

2. The *slide basket* holds the sample slides. For best results, place the slides in every other slot (maximum load becomes 50 slides).

3. The *stain dishes*, No. 1, No. 2, and No. 3, hold methanol, Wright stain, and Wright stain-phosphate buffer mixture.

4. The *water rinse tray* is station No. 4, where the slides are rinsed.
5. The *water rinse hoses* carry the deionized water to station No. 4.
6. The *drain hose* carries the rinse water back to the recirculating pump tray.
7. *Buffer rinse station.*
8. *Drying station.*
9. *Overflow drain.*
10. The *recirculating pump assembly* pumps the deionized water through the rinse station.
11. The *water inlet hose* carries the water from the pump assembly bath to the water rinse hoses leading into the rinse station.
12. The *pump outlet* supplies electricity to the recirculating pump.
13. The *on/off* switch turns the instrument on and off.
14. The *auto/manual* switch, when set on *auto*, initiates the automatic stain process. When switched to *manual*, the stain basket is removed from the drying station and moves to its position above stain station No. 1.
15. The *right/left* switch moves the stain basket to the right or left.
16. The *swing* switch should be in the *on* position for the automated stain procedure.
17. The *pump switch* controls the recirculating pump and should be in the auto setting for the automated stain procedure.
18. There is one *station timer* for each stain and rinse station. These are used to set the time interval the slides remain in each station.

AUTOMATED STAINING PROCEDURE

1. Prepare stain stations as follows:

Station	Solution
No. 1	500 ml of methanol
No. 2	500 ml of Wright stain (obtain from Geometric Data Corporation)
No. 3	80 ml of Wright stain plus 420 ml of phosphate buffer (obtain from Geometric Data Corporation)
No. 4	Place 1 gallon of deionized water into the pump tank and add 200 ml of phosphate buffer.
No. 5	500 ml of phosphate buffer

2. Set the timers as indicated for each station: No. 1, 10 to 15 seconds; No. 2, 2 minutes; No. 3, 5 minutes; No. 4, 20 seconds; No. 5, 1 minute.
3. Turn the power switch to *on*.
4. Place the freshly prepared blood smears in the staining basket, noting that a small portion of the slide at the top will not be immersed in the stain solution.
5. Attach the slide basket to the basket hanger and tighten the screw.
6. Set the auto/manual switch to *manual*.
7. Set the right/left switch to the *left* position.
8. Set the swing switch to *on*.
9. Set the pump switch to *auto*.
10. Remove the covers from each stain station. Set the auto/manual switch to *auto* to begin the staining process. As soon as the stain basket has reached station No. 3, replace the covers on stations Nos. 1 and 2. These two stain stations should remain covered whenever they are not in use to avoid moisture from the air being absorbed by the methanol.
11. A buzzer will sound at the beginning of the drying station. Wait at least 3 minutes after the buzzer sounds and then set the auto/manual switch to *manual*. The basket will then left out of the drying tube and move auto-

matically to the left and remain above the methanol dish.

12. Loosen the hanger screw and remove the slide basket.

MANUAL STAINING PROCEDURE

1. Prepare the reagents in dishes No. 1, 2, 3, and 4 as outlined above for the automatic method. The water rinse in the metal container is eliminated in this procedure.

2. Place the freshly prepared dry blood smear in the staining basket.

3. Place the rack of blood smears in dish No. 1 for 2 to 3 seconds. Drain the excess methanol back into the dish by holding the rack against the wall of the dish. Replace the lid on the dish.

4. Place the rack of blood smears in dish No. 2 for 2 minutes. Drain the excess stain back into the dish. Replace the lid on the dish.

5. Place the rack of smears in dish No. 3 for 5 minutes. Do not agitate the rack in the stain. Drain the excess stain back into the dish. Do not replace the lid on the stain.

6. Place the rack of smears into dish No. 4 (phosphate buffer) immediately, using a dipping action. Dip the rack about 20 times (1 minute). (If the slides are left in the buffer too long, the stain will fade.)

7. Allow the slides to air-dry.

DISCUSSION

1. For consistently good staining results, it is recommended that the Wright's stain and buffer be purchased from Geometric Data Corporation. Wright's stain may be purchased in the powdered form or in prepared solution.

2. The fixative and staining solutions should be replaced and freshly prepared after approximately 300 slides have been stained or after every 8 to 10 stain baskets have gone through

the Hemastainer, whichever occurs first.

3. The stain and rinse dishes should be cleaned in methanol before adding fresh stain or rinse solutions.

4. If the stain is too intense (nuclei very dark purple), dilute the Wright's stain in station No. 2 with methanol.

HEMATRAK AUTOMATED DIFFERENTIAL SYSTEM

The automated differential system (Fig. 168) is one of the most recent forms of automation to enter the hematology laboratory. Computers have been in use for a much longer period of time and are easily capable of recognizing man-made objects or symbols. In the white blood cell differential count, however, the computer is now being asked to recognize naturally occurring objects, a task made much more difficult by the unlimited variability in cell appearances.

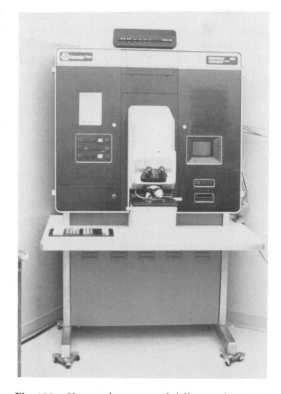

Fig. 168. Hematrak automated differential counter.

In the Hematrak automated differential system, the identification of each cell may be broken down into three steps (1) location of the cell, (2) analysis of the cell, and (3) classification of the cell.

To locate a white blood cell (nucleated cell), a light beam moves back and forth across the microscopic field at intervals of 1 μm until it detects the nucleus of a cell. When the cell nucleus is detected, an electronic window 24 μm × 32 μm is placed at that point by the instrument so that the entire cell should now lie within that window. The spacing between the scanning lines is now decreased to 0.25 μm.

To analyze the cell, special filters are introduced into the light beam of the electronic window, splitting this light beam into three different colors: red, blue, and green. The information obtained from these three different colors passing through the cell goes to the analog section of the instrument, where it is divided into six different density levels (therefore, 18 cell patterns are analyzed). At the lowest density levels, information is obtained about the cytoplasm. The middle density levels give information on the cell nucleus, whereas the highest density levels deal with the darkest portions of the nuclear chromatin. This information is then converted to numeric information and stored in the memory circuits. (The use of these three colors allows the instrument to detect and handle [within limits] differences in the stain intensity that will occur when there is variation in the spreading of the cells, as found in a wedge smear versus a spun blood smear.) Measurements of the cell are made by the microprocessors in the computer by placing lines or patterns of various lengths (from 0.25 μm to 10 μm) and different angles across the cell. These lines are moved across the cell, and the number of times a line falls within the image (of the nucleus, for example) are counted. The shortest lines generally gather information about the texture of the cell, the medium length lines indicate the nuclear shape, and the long lines give information about the volume of the cytoplasm and the shape of the cell itself. All of this information is gathered within milliseconds and totals about 3 million bits of data about the cell. This data is then processed into 96 numbers and is used for cell identification. It includes information on the cell size, nuclear shape and chromatin pattern, ratio of nucleus to cytoplasm, granularity and color of cytoplasm, and presence of nucleoli and vacuoles.

In classifying the cells, the 96 mathematical parameters now in the computer are compared, in a stepwise fashion, with cell data that has been programmed in the computer memory in a "logic-tree" manner. Those cells that do not fit into classification criteria within the computer's memory are remembered by the system and are presented to the operator for identification at the completion of the differential as suspect cells.

After each cell has been analyzed and classified, the instrument again searches for the next cell. This process is carried out by the instrument, field by field, until the preselected number of cells has been obtained by the instrument. Red blood cells and platelets are processed in essentially the same manner as has been described for the white blood cells. The red blood cells are analyzed for size, shape, and hemoglobin density, with the computer analyzing 116 numeric parameters. Platelets are analyzed for nuclear density and size. At the completion of the differential, the cells for review are made available to the operator. It is also possible to store the location of these cells in the instrument's long-term memory. At the completion of the differential and review, the instrument displays a Price-Jones distribution curve (RBC) and a leukocyte profile along with the differential results.

Geometric Data Corporation has manufactured several automated differential systems: Hematraks 360, 450, 450 QP, 480, and 590. The Hematrak 360 is the least automated of the above instruments, whereas the Hematrak 590 is the most sophisticated, having walk-away capabilities, an output of 100 samples per hour, and a bar code method of identifying the patient samples. All models are also programmed to perform reticulocyte counts. All of the Hematrak models are physically very similar (Hematrak 590 is the most different). Therefore, a brief summary will be given below of the Hematrak 360.

COMPONENTS OF THE HEMATRAK 360

1. *System status panel*
   A. The *in calib*(ration) *mode* (1), when lit, indicates that the calibrator thumbwheel is set at a position other than the normal operating position.
   B. The *red cell comments required* (2), when lit, indicates that the operator must enter a platelet estimate and at least one red blood cell comment.
   C. (3) No function.
   D. The *standby* (4) switch turns the microscope light off and on.
   E. *System ready* (5) is lit when the instrument is not in standby.
   F. *A status* (6) indicates a loss of contrast, when lit, and the instrument will not operate.
   G. (7) No function.
   H. *Suspect* (8) will be lit in the stop mode when the instrument locates a suspect cell.
   I. *Out of focus* (9) is lit when the autofocus mechanism limits are exceeded.
   J. *Start* (10) is lit during the scanning and cell counting procedure.
   K. (11) No function.
   L. *Printing not complete* (12), when lit, indicates that the differential has been completed, but the results have not yet been printed.
   M. *Power supply failure* (13), when lit, indicates a power supply failure.
   N. The *power on/off* (14) switch turns the main power to the Hematrak on or off.
   O. *Diff Complete* (15), when lit, indicates that the preselected number of cells has been counted.
2. The *operator panel* contains:
   A. A *calibrator thumbwheel* for use during the instrument calibration check.
   B. *Sample size* selectors to be set according to the number of white blood cells and red blood cells to be analyzed.
   C. *WIN* and *Test 11* toggle switches normally set in the *up* position.
3. The *keyboard* is divided into four functional groups.
   A. Keys to be used for storing cells in the instrument's memory and for use when the Hematrak is interfaced with a central processing computer. These keys are: *Spec, Ident, Comm Code, Opr Ident,* numbers *0* through *9, Delete,* and *Enter.*
   B. Descriptive keys for entering morphology and platelet estimate: *Normal RBC, Aniso, Poik, Micro, Macro, Polychrom, Hypo, Spher, Target Cell, Baso Stip,* blank, *Norm Plate, High Plate, Low Plate, Mark Many, Mod, Slite Few, Toxic Gran, Hyper Seg,* blank, blank, and *RBC Delete.*
   C. Keys for the manual identification of cells, including: *Poly, Band, Lymph, Mono, Eos, Baso, A Lymp, Plasm, Meta, Myelo, Promyelo, Blast, Nucl RBC,* blank (X3), and *WBC Delete.*
   D. Keys for operation of the Hematrak.
      1) *Reset/clear* removes data from the last test sample from the memory circuits.

2) *Suspect* is lit when a suspect cell is located.

3) The *Non-Stop* mode allows the differential to be performed by the Hematrak without stopping and relocates all suspect cells at the end for operator review.

4) The *Video Selec*, when pressed in the non-stop mode, allows the operator to view on the monitor screen the position of the suspect cells in the microscopic field (when reviewing suspect cells). In the non-stop mode, the suspect cell will appear on the monitor screen.

5) *Print*, when pressed, will activate the printer.

6) *Stop* is used to select the Stop mode for performing differentials where the instrument will stop each time a suspect cell is encountered. The instrument will then wait for the operator to enter the identification of the cell before proceeding with the differential.

7) *Halt* will stop the Hematrak counting cycle.

8) *Count Comp* terminates the differential when pressed and reports the differential in percentages.

9) *Transmit* is used to send results to an interfaced computer.

10) *Scan*, when pressed, will begin or continue the Hematrak counting cycle.

4. *Microscope: Eyepieces, 10× objective, 40× objective, stage.*

5. The *manual focus* knob is used to focus the test slide.

6. The *vertical stage position knob* moves the slide vertically.

7. The *horizontal stage position knob* moves the slide horizontally.

8. The *printer* allows the results to be printed on result forms.

9. The *monitor* screen displays the differential results, may display a captured cell, and is used in the calibration of the instrument.

PROCEDURE FOR THE HEMATRAK 360

1. Depress the standby button. The microscope light should come on.

2. Set both eyepieces to the proper focus value. (See the Hematrak system operator's manual for this procedure. The setting for each operator should be ascertained when the instrument is installed in the laboratory. This process is necessary because both the operator and the instrument are using the same objective lens and must be in close focus with each other.)

3. Place a drop of oil on the test slide in the center, about $\frac{1}{3}$ of the distance from the feathered edge.

4. Place the slide on the stage with the feathered edge to the left and the drop of oil over the stage lamp.

5. Place the 40× objective lens into position.

6. Focus the slide and briefly scan from left to right (or right to left). If any of the following are present, the differential should be performed manually:
   A. Numerous immature or atypical cells.
   B. Moderate or marked toxic granulation.
   C. Poorly stained smear.
   D. Excessive dirt, debris, or stain precipitate.

7. If a wedge smear is being used, find a good working area to begin the differential: Approximately 50% of the red blood cells should show no overlapping, with the remainder of the red blood cells overlapping in twos and threes. The white blood cells should be spread well enough to

show the morphology. The field must be centered front to back.

8. Place a normal neutrophil within the large circle of the eyepiece at 11 o'clock. Focus the cell.

9. Press the non-stop button if an uninterrupted differential is desired (suspect cells will be scanned at the end of the differential), or press stop if the operator wishes to review each suspect cell as it is found by the Hematrak.

10. Press reset/clear and then scan. The instrument will now begin to count the preset number of white and red blood cells, and will perform a platelet estimate.

11. If the instrument is in the stop mode, it will stop on each suspect cell, indicating its location in the field on the monitor screen. To display the cell itself on the monitor, press video selec. When the Hematrak stops on a suspect cell, identify the cell and enter it into the differential by using the manual identification keys. Press scan to continue the differential. If the suspect is dirt or debris, press scan to continue the differential, and the suspect will not be included in the differential.

12. When the differential and morphology are complete, the monitor will display the completed differential, red blood cell morphology, a numeric platelet estimate, and the number of red and white blood cells counted. If the instrument was in the non-stop mode, the number of suspect cells will be displayed, and the instrument will be stopped on the first suspect cell. If there are 10 or fewer suspect cells, identify these cells. Press the video selec key to display the location of the cell, identify the cell, and enter it into the differential using the manual identification keys. Press scan. The Hematrak will automatically go to the next suspect cell and indicate the location of the suspect cell on the monitor. Repeat this procedure until all suspect cells have been identified. If a suspect cell should not be included in the differential, press scan.

A. If the Hematrak has detected spherocytes or target cells, it will now go to the first field showing these cells, and the monitor will indicate their location. Examine the cells and then press scan. The Hematrak will show up to five fields displaying these cells before returning to the differential results.

B. To display the Price-Jones distribution curve on the monitor, first display the differential results (press scan if necessary) and then press scan. The leukocyte profile may be displayed on the monitor next by pressing scan. Return the monitor to the differential results by pressing scan.

13. Review the red blood cell morphology and platelet estimate (if necessary). Make any additions or corrections by using the set of descriptive keys for morphology and platelets. If the red blood cell morphology is normal, press the normal RBC key (at least one red blood cell comment and a platelet estimate are necessary before the results can be printed). At the conclusion of this step, the print key should be lit. Place a Hematrak report form in the printer. Press the print key to obtain results on the report form.

DISCUSSION

1. Whenever there is no slide beneath the objective, move the objective to either the right or left of center. Any oil that drops onto the condenser may cause considerable downtime and repair service.

2. Whenever the instrument will not be

used for more than 5 minutes, place it in the standby mode. No warm-up time is necessary when removing the instrument from standby.

3. When using the $40\times$ objective, the area of the large circle, as seen through the microscope, is the area that would be examined using the $100\times$ (high-oil) objective.

4. Each laboratory should have its own criteria for the manual review of abnormal patient results. Such a list may include:

Bands	>5%	Lymphs	0
Monos	>12%	Monos	0
Eos	>9%	Inverse, except in a child	
Basos	>2%		
Atypical lymphs	>5%		
Suspects >10/100 white blood cells			
Red blood cell morphology	—Whenever Pappenheimer bodies or Howell-Jolly bodies are suspected.		
	—Any 2+ red blood cell morphology		
	—Mean corpuscular volume <75 fl, >105 fl		

5. Whenever the reset/clear key is pressed, all values will be erased from the instrument.

6. If you wish to change the call on a previously identified suspect cell after all the suspect cells have been entered, press video selec, press scan until you find the cell, press WBC delete, and enter the correct identification.

7. If you wish to terminate the differential count before completion, obtain the differential in %, press count comp, and continue the routine procedure.

8. The Hematrak system will not make any qualifying statements about anisocytosis, basophilic stippling, target cells, spherocytes, toxic granulation, or hypersegmented neutrophils. When these conditions exist, they must be detected and entered by the operator.

9. If you wish to make a qualifying statement about something that is not listed on the keyboard, first press the blank blue key and then the Sl, mod, or mkd key. Only the qualifying statement will appear in the empty box on the report form. The operator must enter the cell type or condition on the report form.

10. Immersion oil used for Hematrak systems should be a 2:1 mixture of type A and type B immersion oil. Mix two bottles of type A with one bottle of type B.

11. If only a platelet estimate is needed, follow steps 1 to 10 of the Hematrak differential procedure. Approximately 20 seconds after the scan key is pressed, press count comp. Because the instrument bases its platelet estimates on the first 20 fields it views, the estimate will appear on the monitor at this time.

12. If the Hematrak system stops in the middle of a differential, check the front panel. If the out of focus button is lit, look through the microscope:
   A. If the field is out of focus, check that the slide is firmly seated, refocus the field, and press scan.
   B. If there are only a few red blood cells in the field, this may be due to one of two causes:
      1) The end of the smear may have been reached.
      2) There may be "holes" in the smear. If this is the case, press scan and the differential should continue.

HEMA-TEK SLIDE STAINER

The Hema-Tek slide stainer provides a completely automated method for Wright-staining blood smears. The instrument is equipped to hold 25 1-inch × 3-inch glass slides, which are carried by means of a spiral conveyor through the staining procedure, facedown on a platform. These slides are stained at a rate of one per minute, and after staining and rinsing, they are blown dry by a low-velocity blower and then deposited in the slide drawer at one end of the instrument.

The Hema-Tek slide stainer is a self-enclosed unit. The different components making up this instrument will be discussed briefly.

COMPONENTS OF THE HEMA-TEK SLIDE STAINER (Fig. 169)

1. The two *conveyor spirals*, which are turned by a conveyor drive motor, hold the glass slides in place and move the slides through the staining process.

2. The *platen* is a platform that separates the two conveyor spirals. It supports the slides as they are carried through the staining process. It contains three holes through which stain, buffer, and rinse solution are pumped. Grooves located on the platen allow the stain and buffer to mix. A gutter along the sides of the platen allows for drainage of the used solutions.

3. The *conveyor drive motor* (not shown in the illustration) controls the conveyor spirals and the gear asembly and is located on the right, inside the instrument.

4. There are three *volume control knobs*, which are accessible by lifting the lid of the instrument. These black knobs control the amount of solution delivered to each slide. To increase the amount delivered, the knob is turned toward the + (in a clockwise direction), and to decrease the amount of fluid delivered, the knob

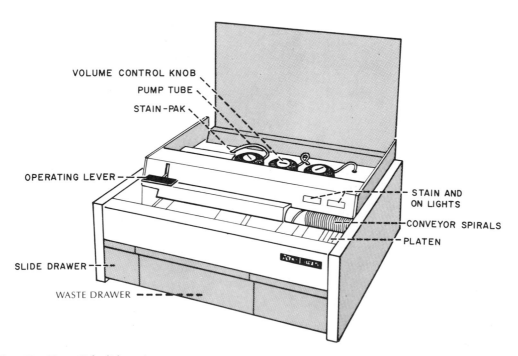

Fig. 169. Hema-Tek slide stainer.

is turned toward the − mark (counterclockwise).

5. There are three *solution pumps* (not shown in the illustration) located in front of the staining pack inside the instrument. They are attached to the volume control knobs.

6. Three *pump tube sets* and *cannulas* are required for transporting the solutions from the reagent bottles, through the reagent pumps, and into the instrument. Each piece of tubing is of a specific length and diameter and contains a cuff situated in such a way that it rests snugly against the pump. The tubing is made of a special type of plastic, and each tube is coded for its purpose. The No. 1 tube is for the stain, the No. 2 tube is for the buffer, and the No. 3 tube is for the rinse solution. (The plastic tubing is available from the Ames Company and their distributors as Hema-Tek Pump Tube Set, No. 4482. The cannulas are obtainable as the Hema-Tek Cannula Set, No. 4483.)

7. There are three *sensing switches* located just above the platen underneath the center enclosed area. Each of these switches is turned on as the slide comes in contact with them while it moves across the platen. When these switches, each attached to one of the three pumps, are on, the pumps become activated and pump the solutions up through the platen onto the slide.

8. The *operating lever* is located on the left, on the enclosed middle section of the instrument. The bottom position of this lever turns the instrument off. When in operation, the lever is in the middle position. The upper position, which must be held in place, is the prime position and allows all three pumps to run continuously.

9. The *stain light* is located on the right, in the middle section of the instru-

ment. When the instrument is on and there is sufficient stain in the *stain pak*, the light is on. When the amount of stain is sufficient to stain only 20 slides (or less) and, therefore, needs replacement, the stain light turns off.

10. The *on light* is located next to the stain light. When the stainer is on or in the prime position, the light will go on.

11. The *fuse* (not shown in the illustration) is located in the right side of the instrument behind the panel.

12. The *dryer fan* (not shown in the illustration) is located behind the right side panel and serves to cool the motors of the instrument and dry the slides.

13. The *slide drawer* is located in the front left of the instrument. It holds up to 100 slides and serves to catch them after staining and drying.

14. The *waste drawer* is located on the right side of the slide drawer, underneath the platen. If an outside waste line is not used, this tank collects all the waste solutions.

15. There is a *circular level* on the top of the instrument underneath the lid. It is important that the bubble be centered and the instrument level when slides are being stained.

16. The *levelers*, for adjusting the instrument to a level position, are located at the bottom front of each end of the stainer.

17. The *drain spout with plug* (not shown in the illustration) is located inside the front of the instrument on the right of the waste tank. It consists of a T-shaped tube and has one plug. If the instrument is to drain into an outside bottle or sink, a piece of tubing is attached to the right side, and the left side is closed with the plug. If the waste drawer is to be used to collect the used solutions, the right side of the tube is closed with the plug, and the solutions are allowed

to drain directly into the waste drawer.

18. The *Hema-Tek stain pak* (No. 4481) is designed for use in the Hema-Tek slide stainer for the routine Wright-staining of blood smears. It consists of prepared stain, buffer, and rinse solutions. It should be placed, in its box, in the back of the stainer, underneath the lid, with the stain on the right side. The appropriate cannulas are then placed in each respective container. The tip of the cannula must be pushed all the way to the bottom of the stain pak.

PROCEDURE FOR THE HEMA-TEK SLIDE STAINER

1. For consistent results, fix the blood smears with methanol and allow them to dry.
2. Place the slide on its side, with the blood smear to the left, into opposing grooves of the conveyor spirals. Make absolutely certain that the slide is placed in the grooves exactly opposite one another. If it is not, the slide will break and may damage the instrument. As the conveyor spirals turn, the slide is moved along toward the platen. When it reaches the platform, the conveyor spirals allow the slide to advance to a facedown position on the platen, and the slide is carried along the platform. The platen is constructed in such a way that there is a very small capillary space between the slide and the platen. As the slide moves along the platform, it triggers the appropriate sensing switch when the slide is over or near the outlet hole. The correct amount of stain then fills the small space between the slide and the platen. The slide, with the stain, then moves along at a specific speed to the sensing switch for the buffer. The buffer emerges, mixes with the stain, and is carried to the end of the platen,

where another switch triggers the rinse solution. The slide is washed, dried by a stream of air, and allowed to drop into the slide drawer. The blood smear is now ready to be examined microscopically.

3. After each use, the platen should be cleaned with methanol. Flood the platen with methanol, and, using soft, clean gauze, wipe the platen from right to left. Care must be taken not to scratch the platen or damage the sensing switches.

PROCEDURE FOR TURNING THE HEMA-TEK SLIDE STAINER ON AT THE BEGINNING OF THE DAY

1. With the stain cannula still in the beaker of clean methanol from the day before, place the operating lever in the *prime* position for about 1 minute. Place the operating lever in the *on* position.
2. Remove the stain cannula from the methanol and place all three cannulas in their respective containers in the stain pak.
3. Place the operating level in the *prime* position until all three solutions emerge through the openings on the platen.
4. Carefully wash the entire platen using methanol and a clean, soft cloth, always wiping the platen from right to left.

PROCEDURE FOR CLOSING DOWN THE HEMA-TEK SLIDE STAINER AT THE END OF THE DAY

1. Remove the cannulas from the rinse, buffer, and stain containers, being careful not to spill any of the solutions on the instrument.
2. Place the cannula from the stain only in a beaker of clean methanol.
3. Place the operating lever in the *prime* position and allow the methanol to aspirate for 2 to 3 minutes. This cleans the stain lines and avoids pre-

cipitated stain, which may build up and block the tubing.

4. Place the operating lever in the *off* position, leaving the stain cannula in the beaker of methanol.

5. Carefully wash the entire platen, or platform area, using methanol and a clean, soft gauze, wiping from right to left to remove precipitated or dried stain and any debris present.

MAINTENANCE

1. It is necessary, at all times, to keep the platen clean and free from any debris. If the platen becomes scratched or marred, this interferes with the staining of the smears.

2. The pump tubing should be replaced once per week or after the use of three stain paks, whichever occurs first. The procedure is as follows:

   A. Remove all three cannulas from the stain pak.

   B. Place the operating lever in the *prime* position until all the tubing has been emptied of its respective solution.

   C. Remove the tubing from each cannula and from the three attachments located in front of the volume controls.

   D. Carefully pull each tube out of the pump.

   E. Using tubing No. 1, attach the end containing the number label to the stain cannula.

   F. Replace the stain cannula in the appropriate container in the stain pak. Using the other end of the tubing, thread it into the rollers, beneath the volume control knobs, until the plastic cuff rests snugly against the arm of the pump. If it is difficult to thread the tubing through the pump, place the operating lever in the *prime* position for a few seconds or pull out the arm of the pump slightly. Attach the tubing to the appropriate tube located in front of the volume control knob.

   G. Repeat steps E and F to replace tubing No. 2 and No. 3.

DISCUSSION

1. Once the slide stainer has been turned on in the morning, there is no need to turn it off if it will be used periodically during the day.

2. If the waste drawer is used to collect the used solutions, it should be emptied at the end of each day.

3. Generally, the best staining results may be obtained using a stain to buffer ratio of 1:2. Some laboratories may prefer a 1:2.5 or a 1:3 ratio of stain to buffer. The volume control knobs may be used to make these adjustments. To accurately measure the stain, buffer, and rinse volumes, prime the instrument, remove the waste chamber, and disconnect the tubing from the underside of the platen. Place each piece of tubing (three) into a 10-ml graduated cylinder. Process 10 blank slides through the stainer. Check the final volumes in each cylinder and divide by 10 to determine the amounts of each solution per slide. The rinse solution should be approximately 1 ml per slide. Make adjustments using the volume control knobs, as necessary. Remeasure the volumes, if adjustment is required, until the proper amounts of stain, buffer, and rinse solution have been obtained.

HEMA-TEK II SLIDE STAINER

The Hema-Tek II slide stainer (Fig. 170) is very similar to the previously described Hema-Tek slide stainer. It is more sophisticated, however, and may be used for more specialized Wright-staining techniques, such as bone marrow and lymph node preparations, in addition to blood smears.

To operate the Hema-Tek II slide stainer,

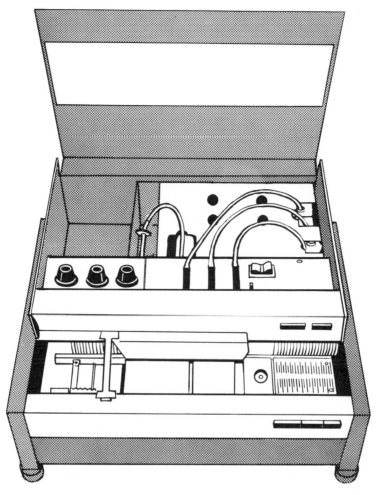

Fig. 170. Hema-Tek II slide stainer.

the *power switch* is turned to the *on* position. The instrument is leveled using the *leveling bubble*. The stain, buffer, and rinse lines are filled with solution from the *Hema-Tek II stain pak* by pressing the *prime* rocker switch. (There are four solution lines: one stain line for fixing the blood smear, one stain line that enters the mixing manifold, one buffer line, and a rinse line.) Slides are placed in the stainer on their sides, with the blood smears to the left, into opposite grooves of the *conveyor spirals*. The first slide is advanced to a facedown position on the *platen*. A *sensing switch* is triggered, and the *stain pump* forces stain from the stain pak

through an opening in the platen to fill the small amount of space under the slide. This step primarily fixes the smear. The slide is then advanced to the next station, at which time the major portion of the stain is removed from the slide, draining into a groove in the platen. A solution of approximately 1:4 stain to buffer mixture is forced through the orifice of the platen to fill the space under the slide. (The buffer and one stain line are connected to a small *mixing manifold* located beneath the platen. These two solutions enter the manifold separately, are mixed, and are then delivered up through the orifice in the platen.) (The stain buffer and rinse volumes may be adjusted using the *volume control knobs.*) When the slide reaches the end of the platen, it advances to a point under the *rinse guard* and is lifted to a vertical position. The slide is then flushed with rinse solution from the *rinse bar* and remains in a vertical position for several minutes, during which time it is dried by a stream of warm air. The slide then drops into the *slide drawer.* During the stain process, all excess and used solutions are drained into the *waste drawer.* There are four *indicator lights: power* (a green light indicates the instrument is on), *prime* (a green light indicates the tubing is being primed), *stain* (a red light indicates the stain pak needs to be replaced), and *waste* (a red light indicates the waste drawer is full).

COULTER ZETAFUGE TM

The zeta sedimentation ratio (ZSR) is determined by use of the Zetafuge TM and is a measurement similar to the Westergren and Wintrobe methods of obtaining erythrocyte sedimentation rates.

Normally, red blood cells are negatively charged and repel each other. In the presence of an increased concentration of fibrinogen and/or gamma globulin, the net negative charge of the erythrocytes decreases, thus permitting an increase in rouleaux formation and a more rapid erythrocyte sedimentation rate.

In the ZSR procedure, a small amount of blood is placed in a capillary tube that is then situated in a vertical position in the Zetafuge. When the Zetafuge is turned on, it revolves at a constant low speed for 45 seconds. During this time, the centrifugal force applied to the tube forces the red blood cells to migrate across the diameter of the tube to the outer wall, where rouleaux formation is speeded up. At the conclusion of the first 45 seconds, the Zetafuge stops and automatically rotates the capillary tube 180°. The Zetafuge restarts, and spins the tube for a second 45-second period. The rouleaux formation (now on

the inner wall) partially disperses, moves across the diameter of the tube, and reforms on the outer wall. The Zetafuge stops and rotates the tubes 180° a second and third time to allow four 45-second centrifuge times. Each time the rouleaux formation moves across the diameter of the tube, it sediments toward the bottom due to the downward force of gravity on the rouleauxed erythrocytes. After centrifugation, the percent of space occupied by the fallen red blood cells is measured. The ZSR, therefore, measures how close the red blood cells approach one another under a specific standardized stress. The packing of the red blood cells depends on their net negative charge, which, in turn, depends on the concentration primarily of fibrinogen and gamma globulin.

The ZSR takes approximately 4 minutes to perform and is unaffected by anemia. The normal range for the ZSR is 40 to 51% and is the same for both males and females. Values of 51 to 54% are considered to be borderline; 55 to 59%, mildly elevated; 60 to 64%, moderately elevated; and greater than 65% markedly elevated.

PROCEDURE

1. Using EDTA-anticoagulated blood, fill one tube three-fourths full for each patient to be tested. (Each tube should be 75 mm long, with an outer diameter of 2.3 mm and an inner diameter of 2.0 mm. These tubes are obtainable from Coulter Diagnostics, Inc.)
2. Plug one end of each tube with clay to a depth of approximately 5 mm.
3. Immediately place the tubes into the sample tube holder (as shown in Figure 171). The tubes must be placed in the Zetafuge so that the instrument is balanced.
4. Push the *power* switch to the *on* position (the switch should light up, indicating that the power is on).
5. Push the *buzzer* switch up to the *on* position (the switch should light up).

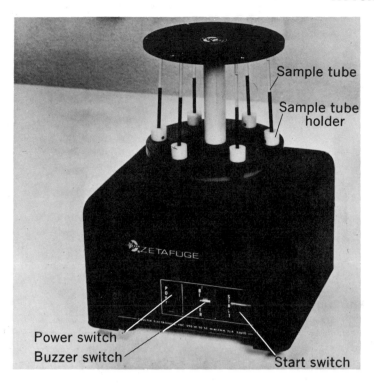

Fig. 171. Coulter Zetafuge. (Courtesy of Coulter Electronics, Inc., Hialeah, Florida.)

(The use of the buzzer is optional, but it warns the operator when the Zetafuge has completed its 3-minute spin cycle.)

6. Depress the *start* switch to begin the spinning cycle. Note the speed indicator, which should move to a horizontal position when the sample holder plate is spinning at full speed.

7. When the buzzer sounds, turn the buzzer switch off.

8. Immediately remove the tubes and read, or place a mark on the tube indicating the level of the sedimented red blood cells. The level to be read is termed the *knee* of the curve (see Figure 172) and indicates the percentage of the blood that is sedimented red blood cells (also termed *Zetacrit %*). An accessory measuring device is available from Coulter Diagnostics, Inc., or, if the level is marked, a hematocrit reader is satisfactory for this reading.

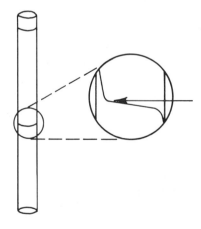

Fig. 172. Sedimented level of red blood cells.

9. Perform a microhematocrit and determine each patient's hematocrit in percent.

10. The zeta sedimentation ratio (ZSR) is then determined by comparing the Zetacrit % to the hematocrit %, as shown on page 336.

$$ZSR\% = \frac{\text{Hematocrit }\%}{\text{Zetacrit }\%} \times 100$$

DISCUSSION

1. At least once a day, check that the mechanism that rotates the tubes 180° is operating satisfactorily. During a complete spin cycle of the instrument, observe the indicator on one of the sample tube holders. This indicator should be pointed alternately in and out during the four spin cycles.

COULTER COUNTER MODEL Fn

The Coulter Counter model Fn is an electronic cell counter used primarily for counting red and white blood cells. It is one of the earlier, basic counters manufactured by Coulter Electronics, Inc. and consists of two units enclosed within one cabinet: the sample stand assembly and the electronic counter. A general description of the instrument follows.

COMPONENTS OF THE COULTER COUNTER MODEL Fn (Figs. 173, 174, and 175)

1. The *numeric readout assembly* consists of numeric glow tubes. The instrument has been calibrated in such a way that the numbers indicated on the glow tubes are the number of cells or particles per μl in the solution being tested.
2. The *dual monitor system* consists of an oscilloscope screen and a micro projection screen.
   A. The *oscilloscope screen* gives an electronic pattern in the form of spikes or pulses for each particle or cell that is counted. The height of each pulse is directly proportional to the volume of the particle.
   B. The *micro projection screen* gives a constant view of the tiny hole (tunnel) in the aperture tube through which the sample passes.

This enables the user to detect any debris that may block the opening during a count.

3. The *sensitivity controls* (three) for the system are set when the instrument is installed and calibrated.
   A. The *attenuation control* determines the overall sensitivity of the electronic amplification. (This is similar to the volume control on a radio.)
   B. The *aperture current control* determines the amount of current that passes between the two electrodes in the sample stand assembly.
   C. The *threshold dial* determines the level above which the pulses of the particles will be counted.
4. The *power switch* turns the instrument on and off.
5. The *sample stand assembly* consists of the beaker platform, the aperture tube, two platinum electrodes, the control piece, and the mercury manometer.
   A. The *beaker platform* holds the sample beaker and should be positioned in such a way that the aperture tube is close to the bottom of the beaker but does not come in contact with it.
   B. The *aperture tube* has a very small hole, or orifice, through which the diluted sample passes. Care should be taken with this tube because the orifice wafer is extremely thin. Aperture tubes may be obtained with various-sized orifices. The 100-μm diameter size is used for red and white blood cell counts.
   C. There are two *platinum electrodes*, one located within the aperture tube (internal) and the second placed outside of the aperture tube (external), immersed in the diluted sample.
   D. The *control piece* connects the

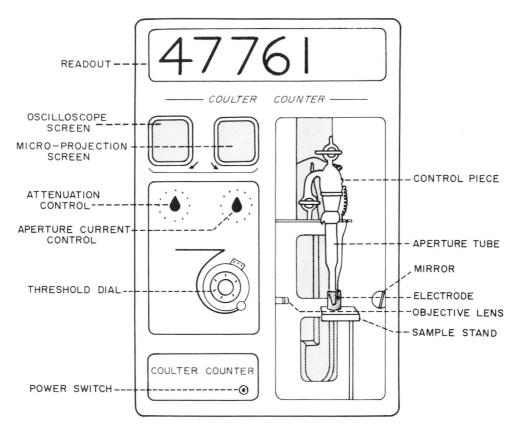

Fig. 173. Coulter Counter Model Fn (front view).

aperture tube to the mercury manometer and contains two stopcocks. Both stopcocks, when closed, are in a horizontal position. To open them, they are turned until they lie in a vertical position. The vacuum control stopcock is used when counting to introduce negative pressure, thus causing the mercury in the manometer to fall. The filling and flushing stopcock, located below and to the left of the vacuum control stopcock, is used in conjunction with the vacuum control stopcock to fill the aperture tube.

E. The *mercury manometer* (Fig. 175) is used to control the exact amount of diluted sample to be counted. The manometer contains three electrodes. One electrode is responsible for starting the particle count and another stops the count as soon as 0.5 ml of diluted sample has been drawn through the orifice of the aperture tube. The third electrode serves as a grounding contact.

6. The *vacuum pump controls* the mercury level in the manometer and is controlled by the vacuum control regulator located above the pump on the same side of the instrument. Attached to the vacuum pump is a piece of tubing pinched off at a predetermined length. This is the *vacuum limit adjustment,* and the length should not have to be changed once it has been set.

7. On the left side of the instrument are four controls for the oscilloscope screen (listed on page 338):

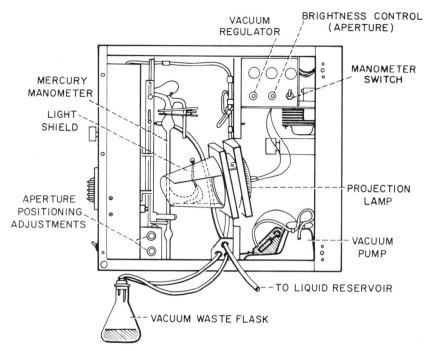

VACUUM
REGULATOR

BRIGHTNESS CONTROL
(APERTURE)

MANOMETER
SWITCH

MERCURY
MANOMETER

LIGHT
SHIELD

APERTURE
POSITIONING
ADJUSTMENTS

PROJECTION
LAMP

VACUUM
PUMP

TO LIQUID RESERVOIR

VACUUM WASTE FLASK

Fig. 174. Coulter Counter Model Fn, side (right) view.

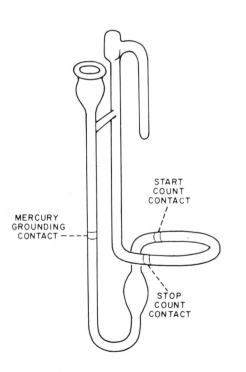

MERCURY
GROUNDING
CONTACT

START
COUNT
CONTACT

STOP
COUNT
CONTACT

Fig. 175. Manometer (Coulter Counter Model Fn).

A. The *intensity control* determines the intensity of the pulses.
B. The *focus control* focuses the pulses.
C. The *horizontal position control* centers the pulses on the oscilloscope screen.
D. The *vertical position control* may be adjusted with a screwdriver and moves the pulses up or down on the screen.

8. On the right side of the instrument near the top, the *vacuum control regulator* is located. Next to this is the light intensity control, which determines the amount of light given off by the *projection lamp* located inside the instrument. The manometer switch is placed to the far right and determines the volume of sample (100 μl or 500 μl) to be aspirated by the instrument. The 500 μl setting is used with the type of mercury manometer described here. On the bottom, near the front of the instrument,

are two *aperture positioning controls* that are used to make corrections in the position of the aperture tube so that it may be seen on the micro projection screen.

9. Located in the front of the Coulter Counter, on a line with the orifice of the aperture tube, is an *objective lens* on the left and a *mirror* on the right. The mirror is adjusted with a screwdriver so that the light source is reflected onto the orifice of the aperture. The objective lens focuses the picture of the orifice onto the micro projection screen.

10. The *vacuum waste flask* is located on the right side of the instrument. It collects the waste as it goes through the instrument.

OPERATING PROCEDURE FOR THE COULTER COUNTER MODEL Fn

1. Turn the power switch to *on*.
2. Preparation of the blood sample.
   A. For a white blood cell count, a 1:500 dilution of whole blood is made.
      1) Add 0.02 ml of well-mixed whole blood to 10.0 ml of 0.85% sodium chloride or Isoton diluent.
      2) Just prior to performing the white blood cell count, add three drops of Zaponin lysing agent or 1% saponin (w/v) (if diluting with 0.85% sodium chloride) or Zap-Isoton lysing agent (if diluting with Isoton diluent) to lyse the red blood cells and platelets.
      3) As soon as the diluted blood sample becomes crystal clear, it is ready to be counted. Once hemolysis is complete, the diluted sample should not sit for more than 10 minutes, otherwise, destruction of the white blood cells will begin to occur.
   B. For a red blood cell count, a

1:50,000 dilution of whole blood is made.
   1) Prepare a 1:500 dilution of whole blood, as outlined for the white blood cell count in the previous section, using 0.85% sodium chloride or Isoton diluent.
   2) Add 0.1 ml of the 1:500 dilution to 10 ml of 0.85% sodium chloride or Isoton diluent. This is now considered to be a 1:50,000 dilution of the whole blood (mathematically, however, it is actually a 1:50,601 dilution).
3. Mix the diluted blood sample well. Avoid foaming. Place the beaker containing the sample on the sample stand, immersing the aperture tube and external electrode in the diluted sample. Move the beaker so that the orifice of the aperture tube (on your left) lies against but not touching the side of the beaker. This ensures a good projection of the orifice onto the micro projection screen.
4. Open the vacuum control stopcock by turning it until it is in a vertical position. This sets up a negative pressure, and the mercury column will fall and come to rest $\frac{1}{4}$ to $\frac{1}{2}$ inch below the horizontal section of the manometer. When the mercury has fallen below the first electrode, a click will be heard. At this time, note that any count lit up on the digital readout asembly is cleared, and the glow tubes read 0.
5. As soon as the click is heard and the glow tubes return to 0, close the stopcock by turning it to the horizontal position. When the stopcock is closed, the mercury begins to rise to its former level in the manometer. As the mercury rises, a corresponding amount of diluted sample is pulled into the aperture tube through the orifice. When the mercury comes in

contact with the first electrode, the count begins. There is a current running through the orifice of the aperture tube between the internal and external electrodes. When a cell or particle passes through the orifice, it produces a voltage pulse that is then registered on the digital readout tubes. All cells contained in the electrolyte that passes through the orifice are counted until the mercury comes in contact with the second electrode on the manometer, at which time the count is stopped. The mercury continues to rise in the manometer a short way, until it reaches a level of equilibrium.

6. While the cells are being counted, watch the oscilloscope and micro projection screens carefully for any irregularities. If dirt or debris partially or completely blocks the orifice of the aperture tube during the count, carefully lower the sample stand containing the beaker and gently wipe the orifice with a small camel's hair brush to remove the debris. Replace the sample beaker and start the count again from step 4.

7. Record the count as shown on the numeric readout assembly, rounding off the count to the nearest hundred. Repeat steps 3, 4, and 5 on the same sample dilution until two counts within 300 cells of each other are obtained. Average these two results.

8. Correction of the counts.
   A. If the count is above 10,000 per μl, it must be corrected for coincidence loss by referring to the coincidence chart obtained with the Coulter Counter instrument. This correction must be made for the small loss in count that occurs when two or more cells enter the aperture at the same time and are registered or counted as only one cell.
   B. When a red blood cell count is performed on the Coulter Counter Model Fn, the result, when corrected for coincidence loss, must be multiplied by 100 before reporting. This is necessary because of the dilution of 1:100 made when the red blood cell count was set up. The Coulter Counter is calibrated to give the direct count using a 1:500 dilution.

DISCUSSION

1. If the cell count exceeds 75,000 per μl, the count should be repeated, using a further dilution. For example, a white blood cell count of 150,000 per μl may be diluted as follows:
   A. Dilute 2.0 ml of the 1:500 dilution with 8.0 ml of 0.85% sodium chloride or Isoton diluent.
   B. The result obtained is multiplied by five after the correction for coincidence loss is made.

2. Before each group of red or white blood cell counts is performed, it is advisable to check what is termed the *background count*. This consists of doing a count on the diluent used for the red and white blood cell counts, to ensure that falsely elevated counts are not being obtained because of contaminated diluent or sample beakers. Background counts of 100 per μl or less are good, and no correction need be made on the cell counts.

3. To avoid interference during the counting procedure, keep all objects, including hands, away from the instrument until the count is completed. Electrical interference may be noted by erratic and sharp pulses seen on the oscilloscope screen.

4. Always make sure that the external electrode is submerged in the diluted sample. For best results, keep it in back of the aperture tube so that it does not interfere with the technol-

ogist's view or block the light so that the orifice cannot be seen on the micro projection screen.

5. Keep the liquid level in the waste flask below the glass tubing at all times. If the level gets too high, it will be drawn into the vacuum pump, which may then become damaged. If the waste does drain into the pump, empty the flask as soon as possible. The pump then generally makes a noise as it pumps. The noise subsides within several hours. If possible pump several milliliters of nondetergent No. 20 engine oil through the pump immediately after the liquid has been removed.

6. On most Coulter Counters, the threshold dial is set at 15 or 20 for white blood cell counts. It is usually necessary to lower this setting when a red blood cell count is done, most often to a threshold setting of 10. This is the only adjustment that needs to be made on the instrument when changing from white blood cell counts to red blood cell counts.

7. There must never be air bubbles or splits in the mercury in the manometer. If these do occur, the vacuum stopcock may be opened and the vacuum regulator adjusted until the mercury falls down into the coalescing bulb. This should bring the mercury back together. Readjust the mercury level and proceed with the count.

8. When the Coulter Counter is not in use, it should be left with either Isoterge (liquid cleaning solution) or electrolyte solution in it, preferably Isoton. To do this, immerse the aperture tube in a sample beaker containing Isoterge or electrolyte solution. Place the free end of the rubber tube (which is attached to the connecting piece on the right of the machine) in a beaker of Isoterge or electrolyte. Ensure that the waste flask is empty. Open both stopcocks on the connecting piece on the front of the instrument. The Isoterge or electrolyte solution then runs from the beaker into the aperture tube, through a connecting tube, and finally out into the waste flask. Leave the stopcocks open for about 10 seconds. Close the stopcocks and leave the instrument as it is. If Isoterge was used, the aperture tube must then be rinsed well with the diluent (electrolyte) just prior to counting.

9. When a series of red or white blood cell counts is being done, it is advisable to rinse the aperture tube with diluent (0.85% sodium chloride or Isoton) after every four of five samples.

10. When the Coulter Counter is to be used periodically throughout the day, it is advisable to keep it turned on. When turning the instrument off at the end of the day, rinse it well with Isoterge, leaving the Isoterge in the counter overnight. To turn if off, merely turn the power switch to *off*.

11. The counting cycle (the amount of time cells are actually being counted by the instrument) should be between 12 and 15 seconds for accurate results. A cycle less than 12 seconds may suggest a broken orifice. Cycles greater than 15 seconds usually indicate a dirty orifice (even though no debris may be seen) or a dirty manometer and mercury. In this case, it is advisable to clean these parts.

12. If it is necessary to alter the vacuum, using the vacuum limit adjustment on the pump itself, this may be accomplished by changing the position of the clamp. To increase the vacuum (lower the mercury level when the vacuum control stopcock is open), move the clamp closer to the pump (that is, shorten the tubing between the pump and the clamp). To decrease the vacuum (raise the mercury level when the vacuum control stop-

cock is open), move the clamp away from the pump (move the clamp toward the free end of the rubber tubing).

MAINTENANCE

1. One of the most important types of maintenance is keeping the instrument clean. Periodically rinsing it with Isoterge during the day helps a great deal.
2. The aperture tube should be removed and cleaned approximately once a week, as outlined in the service manual.
3. If the Coulter Counter is kept clean at all times and the aperture tube is removed and cleaned each week, it should not be necessary to clean the manometer and change the mercury more than once every 6 months. When the manometer needs cleaning, there is a buildup of dirty mercury on the top of the mercury in the mercury reservoir. This will be greater than ⅛ inch. If small bits or drops of mercury are left in the metering section (horizontal U-shaped part of the manometer) when the vacuum stopcock is open, it is time to change the mercury and clean the manometer, as outlined in the service manual.
4. The vacuum pump should be oiled once per week using nondetergent No. 20 engine oil. Place a drop of oil on each of the bearings, the hole in the piston, and in the well next to the barrel.

COULTER THROMBO-FUGE

The Coulter Thrombo-fuge provides a quick (5 minutes) method for obtaining platelet-rich plasma for the semiautomated platelet count.

PRINCIPLE

Whole EDTA-anticoagulated blood is centrifuged in the Thrombo-fuge at a speed of 880 RPM for 20 to 45 seconds. The tube of blood is tilted inward toward the center of the instrument approximately 3° from the vertical. During centrifugation, the blood is forced up inside the outer wall of the tube. The red blood cells, pressed against each other, are forced into rouleaux formation. When centrifugation is complete, the tube of blood is allowed to sit for the remainder of the 5-minute cycle. During this time, due to the rouleaux formation, the red blood cells settle rapidly to the bottom of the tube. At the completion of the 5-minute cycle, platelet-rich plasma is pipetted directly from the tube (supernatant layer), diluted with Isoton, and counted on the Coulter Counter Model Fn. As when using plastic sedimentation tubes, the count obtained is then corrected for coincidence, dilution, and the patient's hematocrit.

COMPONENTS OF THE THROMBO-FUGE (Fig. 176)

1. The *sample plate* contains the *sample tube holders* and *guide plate* and spins during centrifugation.
2. The *sample tubes* fit snugly into the sample tube holder and are kept at the proper angle during the cycle by the sample tube guide plate.
3. The *power switch* turns the Thrombo-fuge on (up) and off (down).
4. The *start switch* initiates the cycle when pressed down.
5. The *buzzer switch* allows for an alarm to sound at the completion of the 5-minute cycle (when in the up position). The buzzer may be turned off by placing the switch in the *down* position. The buzzer also has an automatic cutoff system in that it automatically stops ringing after a short period if it is not manually turned off.
6. The *wait light* remains lit during the entire 5-minute cycle.

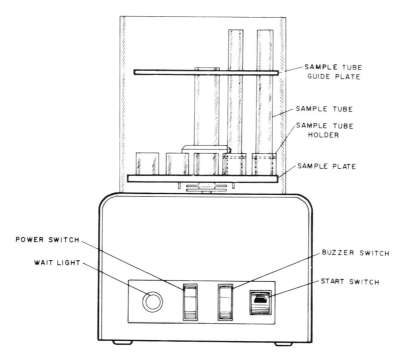

Fig. 176. Coulter Thrombo-fuge.

PROCEDURE

1. Pour 1 ml of well-mixed whole blood into a 10 × 75-mm test tube and place it in the Thrombo-fuge sample plate. If fewer than 10 specimens are to be centrifuged, make certain that the Thrombo-fuge is balanced.

2. Place the splatter shield over the sample plate so it is not touching the sample plate.

3. Turn the Thrombo-fuge on by pushing the power switch up. Place the buzzer switch up and begin the cycle by pushing the start switch down.

4. At the end of the 5-minute cycle, turn off the buzzer and carefully remove the splatter shield without disturbing the sample plate or patient specimens. The tubes must remain undisturbed in the sample plate until testing is complete.

5. Carefully place the pipet tip into the middle of the supernatant plasma layer and withdraw the prescribed amount of plasma for the dilution.

DISCUSSION

1. Extreme care must be taken to avoid red blood cell contamination when pipetting the plasma. For this reason, duplicate dilutions should be made on all specimens, and the counts should agree within 500. If the difference between counts is larger than this, make further dilutions.

2. If more than 1 ml of blood is placed in the test tube, chances are greater that blood will escape from the top of the tube during centrifugation. Therefore, always use the splatter shield.

3. The platelet-rich plasma should be pipetted from the tube within 20 minutes of the completed cycle. If the centrifuged blood sits too long, the platelets will settle out.

4. Occasionally, a sample is encountered that does not yield a large enough plasma layer to allow accurate pipetting. This is generally due to an elevated hematocrit and/or ex-

tremely viscous plasma, in which case an alternative method must be used or a manual platelet count performed.

BIO/DATA PLATELET AGGREGATION PROFILER MODEL PAP-4

Platelet aggregation studies have become important in diagnosing certain platelet disorders. Abnormal platelet aggregation may be drug-induced and may also be found in such conditions as liver disease, uremia, acute leukemia, pernicious anemia, and myeloproliferative disorders.

The Platelet Aggregation Profiler Model PAP-4 employs a photo-optical system for viewing platelet aggregation. In this instrument, there are four independently operated photo-optical systems, or aggregation channels. A sample of the patient's platelet-poor plasma (PPP) is used to set the 100% baseline in each channel. The patient's platelet-rich plasma (PRP) is then placed in each channel to set the 0% baselines. As various aggregating reagents are added to the platelet-rich plasma, the display panel and the printer record the platelet aggregation as it occurs. This information may be stored in the instrument's memory and may be recalled at the end of the test procedure from a single channel or from all four channels. It may then be printed on a single report form or on separate report forms. Multiple copies of the same result may also be printed. The final percent aggregation is determined by the instrument, and a comment section is also available on the printer paper.

This instrument has trace filter switches that make it possible to reduce the oscillations caused by the size of the aggregations. It is also possible to vary the plasma stir speed in each channel. Micro volume samples may be analyzed using a special cuvette adapter. A check of the instrument function can be performed by the operator, using a service diagnostic mode.

COMPONENTS OF THE PLATELET AGGREGATION PROFILER (Fig. 177)

1. The *main power switch* turns the instrument on or off and, when the instrument is turned on, causes the mode switch, paper advance, memory switch, and channel operation switches to light.

2. There are four *channel operation switches*, one for each channel (No. 1 is yellow, No. 2 is green, No. 3 is white, and No. 4 is blue). The first time the button is depressed, a 100% baseline value is read and stored. The second depression of the switch determines the 0% baseline, sets the 0% on the printer paper, and begins the paper transport. Depressing the switch a third time terminates the printing for that particular channel. When all channel switches have been depressed for the third time, the % aggregation and slope for each channel is printed out.

3. The *mode switch* has two settings: (1) When the green light is on, the instrument is ready for testing. If the switch is then depressed, the orange light comes on. (2) The orange light indicates the stir speed position, and the display will indicate the stir speed in each channel. The stir speed may then be changed, using the appropriate *stir speed control* (make certain the test wells are empty).

4. The *temperature indicator* will light when the incubation block reaches 37°C (8 to 10 minutes after the instrument is turned on).

5. The *micro-volume switch* is utilized when micro sample volumes are used. This switch deactivates the magnetic stir bar detector and allows use of the micro stir bar.

6. The *memory switch* is used to initiate the instrument's memory recall. The aggregation patterns generated in each channel will remain in memory

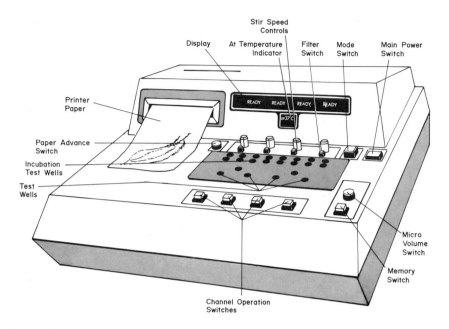

Fig. 177. Bio/Data Platelet Aggregation Profiler Model PAP-4. (Courtesy of Bio/Data Corporation, Hatboro, Pa.)

until another sample is tested in that channel.

7. *Display* will give information concerning the instrument operation, test status, stir speeds, and temperature when the instrument is on.

8. Each channel has its own color-coded *filter switch*. When this switch is activated, the oscillations (a function of the size of the platelet aggregate) generated during platelet aggregation are filtered out. (The platelet aggregations are stored in the memory unfiltered, irrespective of the setting of the filter switch.)

9. The platelet aggregation patterns are printed out on the *printer paper,* which may be manually advanced by depressing the *paper advance switch.*

10. There are four *incubation test wells* maintained at 37°C for each of the four channels.

11. There is one *test well* for each of the four channels, in which the platelet aggregation is tested and monitored.

PROCEDURE

1. For each patient plasma to be tested, obtain a platelet-poor plasma specimen and a platelet-rich plasma specimen. Prepare the aggregating reagents (ADP, epinephrine, collagen, ristocetin, and/or arachidonic acid) according to the manufacturers' directions.

2. Turn the instrument on. When the instrument is first turned on, the display will read INSTRUMENT NOT READY. In 8 to 10 minutes the incubation block will reach 37°C, and the at temperature indicator will light. The display will then read READY for each of the four channels.

3. Pipet 0.5 ml of PPP into a 8.75 × 50-mm aggregometer cuvette. Pipet 0.45 ml of PRP into one to four aggregometer cuvettes, depending on how many channels are to be utilized for testing.

4. Place one or more of the PRP cuvettes into the test wells of the incubation block for approximately 2 minutes.

Place a magnetic stir bar into each cuvette.

5. Set the 100% baseline: Place the PPP cuvette into the test well. Depress the appropriate channel operation switch one time. When the display reads PPP SET, remove the cuvette. Repeat this procedure for the other three channels if they are to be used.

6. Set the 0% baseline: Insert the patient's PRP cuvette into the test well. Depress the appropriate channel operation switch one time. The display should read "0%." If the display reads LO RANGE or HI RANGE, however, this indicates that the difference in the otpical densities of the PRP and PPP are not greater than 5% and less than 95%, respectively. The platelet count on the plasma specimens should be rechecked and/or the specimens prepared once more. Depress the channel operation switch one more time. If the display reads STIR BAR, add the stir bar, depress the appropriate channel operation switch again and repeat steps 5 and 6. Repeat the above procedure for each channel to be utilized, using the appropriate PRP cuvette in each channel.

7. Perform the platelet aggregation test: Add 0.05 ml of the reagent directly into the PRP cuvette in the test well. At the termination of the test, press the appropriate channel operation switch. Repeat this step for each channel being used. When the testing has been terminated in each channel, the printer will print the percent aggregation for each channel. (See Figs. 178 and 179 for examples of normal and abnormal platelet aggregation response.)

DISCUSSION

1. To stop a test before its conclusion, press the channel operation switch. Only that channel will be affected.

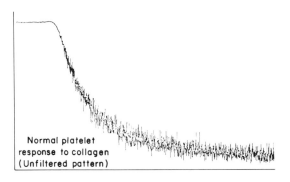

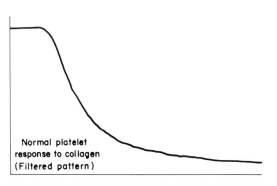

Normal platelet response to collagen (Unfiltered pattern)

Normal platelet response to collagen (Filtered pattern)

Fig. 178. Normal platelet response to collagen as shown on the platelet aggregometer (filtered and unfiltered patterns).

2. For micro-volume testing, 0.2-ml PPP and PRP volumes are used in place of the routine 0.5- and 0.45-ml volumes. The test is performed in the same manner as the platelet aggregation test, except that a micro-volume adapter is used in the test well, 7.5 × 55-mm cuvettes are needed, and a micro magnetic stir bar is used.

3. To recall the previously run results from the instrument's memory, all channels must be in the READY position, as shown on the display. Press the memory switch. NO PRINT should appear on the display in each channel. Press the channel operation switch for each channel to be recalled. PRINT should appear on each channel's display. (If the oscillations

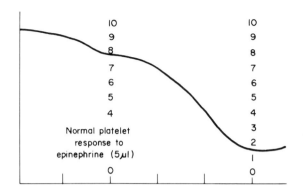

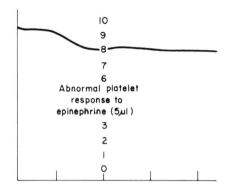

Fig. 179. Normal and abnormal platelet response to epinephrine as shown by the platelet aggregometer.

are to be filtered out, press the trace filter switch for the desired channels at this time.) Press the memory switch a second time. The printer will automatically begin printing and will label the form PRINT FROM MEMORY. The % aggregation and slope will be printed for each channel activated.

4. Each platelet aggregation graph is numbered according to the channel in which it was run. This number is printed on the graph every 30 seconds during operation.

5. This instrument has a diagnostic mode, which is used to determine if the instrument is functioning properly. The procedure for entering this mode and performing the tests is very clearly outlined in the instrument's operations manual.

6. The magnetic stir motor in each channel turns on when PPP SET appears on the display. It shuts off at the end of the aggregation step. If the test is left unattended for a period of time, the stir bar motor will automatically shut off in 2 hours.

7. The blood specimen should be collected carefully, using a plastic syringe and plastic test tubes. Place 9.0 ml of whole blood into a plastic test tube containing 1.0 ml of 0.11 M sodium citrate. Mix gently. There should be no hemolysis present.

8. To prepare platelet-rich plasma, centrifuge the whole blood at 150 × g for 5 minutes. Remove the platelet rich plasma using a plastic pipet. If red blood cells are present, centrifuge the plasma for an additional 5 minutes. Prepare the platelet-poor plasma from an aliquot of the platelet-rich plasma by centrifuging it at 1500 × g for 15 minutes. The platelet-rich plasma should have a platelet count of 250,000/μl (± 50,000 per μl) and may be obtained by adding platelet-poor plasma to the platelet-rich plasma as necessary. The platelet-rich plasma should be capped and allowed to sit at room temperature for a minimum of 30 minutes and a maximum of 3 hours after blood collection.

9. The normal range for each of the platelet aggregation reagents should be established by each laboratory.

10. The platelet aggregation procedure should not be performed on any patient who has ingested aspirin within 8 days prior to the test. Aspirin inhibits platelet aggregation and would, therefore, mask any qualitative platelet defect present. Other compounds that inhibit platelet aggregation are antihistamines, alcohol, cocaine, tricyclic antidepressants, dipyridamole, and

nonsteroidal anti-inflammatory agents.

11. In most cases of von Willebrand's disease, the platelets fail to show aggregation with ristocetin but do aggregate with the other reagents.

COULTER COUNTER MODEL S

The Model S Coulter Counter has made a significant contribution to the busy hematology department. On all blood samples, this instrument reports the white blood cell count, red blood cell count, hemoglobin, hematocrit, MCV, MCH, and MCHC. Results are received on a printed card, and the analysis is completed 40 seconds after the whole blood has been introduced into the instrument. Blood samples may be introduced at a rate of one every 20 seconds.

The Model S Coulter Counter consists of five connected units:

1. The *diluter* aspirates, pipets, dilutes, mixes the blood, lyses the red blood cells, and "senses" (i.e., senses the current changes between electrodes and senses the hemoglobin at the photodevice).
2. In the *analyzer*, the counting, measuring, and computing of the results take place.
3. The *power supply* supplies voltages necessary to run the electronic system.
4. The *printer* receives the digital information from the power supply and prints these results on report cards for the technologist.
5. The *pneumatic power supply* furnishes the diluter with the necessary vacuum and pressure.

These five units may be further subdivided into two separate systems: the electronic system and the pneumatic system.

COMPONENTS OF THE MODEL S COULTER COUNTER

1. *Diluter unit* (Fig. 180).
   A. Aspirators
      1) Whole blood.
      2) Capillary blood (1:224 dilution).
   B. Blood-sampling valve.
   C. Touch control bar.
   D. Aperture baths.
      1) White blood cell bath.
      2) Red blood cell bath.
   E. Hemoglobin sensing (photosensitive) device.
   F. Removable bar in front of the aperture baths contains the bulb for hemoglobin measurement and separate light sources to illuminate the orifices of the aperture tubes for projection onto the aperture projection screens.
   G. Diluent dispenser assembly.
   H. Bubble trap.
   I. Red blood cell count mixing chamber.
   J. Waste chamber.
   K. White blood cell mixing chamber.
   L. Lysing chamber.
   M. Mercury manometer.
   N. Vacuum/isolator chamber.
   O. On the bottom right of the instrument in the front is located a control panel that contains:
      1) Aperture count button.
      2) Aperture clear button applies back pressure to the apertures in case they become blocked with debris.
      3) Bath drain button empties the aperture baths and adjacent chambers ($A_2B_2C_1$) when they are used in conjunction with the pinch valves under these chambers.
      4) Bath rinse button fills the aperture baths with Isoton and is used to prime the Isoton supply into the diluter unit.
      5) Aspirator toggle switch, to be set depending on the blood sample used: whole blood or blood diluted 1:224 with Isoton.

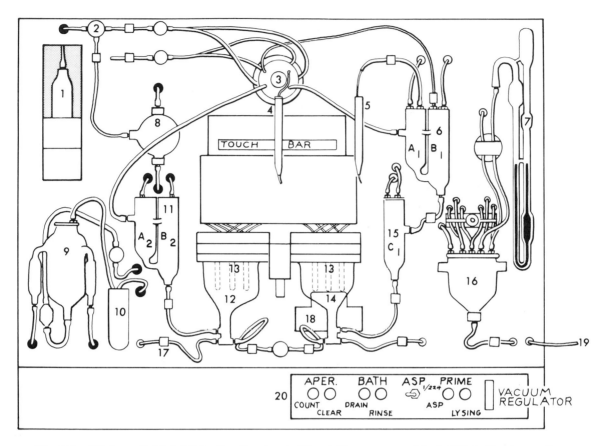

Fig. 180. Diluter unit. Model S Coulter Counter. 1, Diluent dispenser assembly. 2. "T". 3, Blood-sampling valve. 4, Aspirator (whole blood). 5, Aspirator (1:224 dilution). 6, WBC mixing chambers. 7, Manometer. 8, Bubble trap. 9, Waste chamber. 10, Foam trap. 11, RBC mixing chambers. 12, RBC aperture counting bath. 13, Apertures. 14, WBC aperture counting bath. 15, Lysing chamber. 16, Vacuum/isolator chamber. 17, Pinch valve. 18, Hb. device. 19, Lyse supply. 20, Control panel.

6) Aspirator priming button.
7) Lysing fluid priming button.
8) Vacuum regulator wheel.

In the rear of the diluter unit, there is a cable connecting the diluter to the analyzer unit. A tank panel, also located at the back of the diluter unit, receives a vacuum and two pressure lines (25 psi and 5 psi) from the pneumatic supply unit. In addition, a diluent and waste connection are present on this panel. The switch panel is a mechanical timer, contains five switches, and is located in the inside rear of the diluter unit above the tank panel. The cam assembly, or timing mechanism, can be seen by lowering the mid-panel door in the back of the diluter unit. It consists of two timing motors, 16 cams, and associated tubing. Below the drip pan in the front lower section of the diluter unit is the pneumatic junction panel. It receives 25 psi from the cam assembly and 25 psi, 5 psi, and vacuum from the tank panel and distributes these pressures and vacuum to each of six pneumatic cards located inside the left and right panel doors (three cards per side).

A more detailed description of the switch panel, timing mechanism, pneumatic cards, control panel, and blood sampling value follows.

A. The switch panel (mechanical timer) is made up of five switches, each of which has the following functions:

1) Switch No. 1 is activated by the touch control bar and turns motor No. 1 (of the timing mechanism) on.
2) Switch No. 2, activated by cam No. 1 (of the timing mechanism), keeps motor No. 1 on and also turns off the red light and turns on the green light (behind the touch control bar). In dropping, switch No. 2 activates motor No. 2.
3) Switch No. 3 is activated by cam No. 11, keeps motor No. 2 on, and brightens the optic lights.
4) Switch No. 4 is activated by cam No. 12 and commands the timer/hemoglobin card to obtain a hemoglobin reference value.
5) Switch No. 5, activated by cam No. 18, resets the timer/hemoglobin card to begin the counting cycle.

B. The timing mechanism (cam assembly). The timing mechanism consists of two motors and 16 cams. Timer motor No. 1 operates cams 1 through 8 for a period of 20 seconds. Timer motor No. 2 operates cams 11 through 18 for the second 20-second period. When the touch control bar is pushed, motor No. 1 operates for 20 seconds. At the end of this time, motor No. 2 goes on, and motor No. 1 is stopped. If, however, the touch control bar is pushed at the end of 20 seconds (when the light turns from red to green), motor No. 1 is immediately reactivated, and both motors are in operation at the same time. As the cams and switches are activated, the pressure and vacuum from the pneumatic supply unit go through the tank panel to the timing mechanism and the pneumatic junction panel (located inside the front of the diluter unit), where it then goes to the six pneumatic cards.

C. Pneumatic Cards
The filling and emptying of the various chambers in the diluter units are operated by pumps, valves, and cylinders located in the pneumatic cards. These pumps, valves, and cylinders are in turn dependent on and operated by the timing mechanism. There are three pneumatic cards on the right side of the diluter (R-1, R-2, and R-3), and three pneumatic cards on the left side of the diluter (L-1A, L-2, and L-3). The function of each of the pneumatic cards is outlined in the instrument's operations manual.

D. Blood-Sampling Valve
The blood-sampling valve consists of three parts, held together by a long center pin. The front section has four fluid pathways, each of which has respective tub-

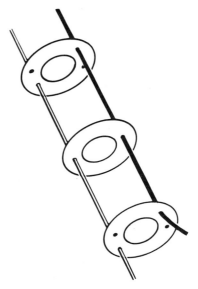

Fig. 181. Blood-sampling valve, position 1.

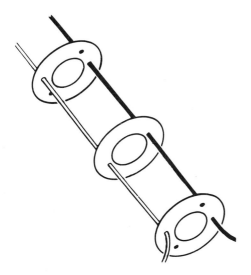

Fig. 182. Blood-sampling valve, position 2.

ing fitted into it. The middle section has two fluid pathways or holes. There are four holes in the rear section connected to respective tubing. The center section is movable and rotates between two positions. In position 1 (Fig. 181, black line), the middle section links up the top hole on the right side of the rear section with the top hole on the corresponding side of the front section. The whole blood is aspirated through this passageway. The center section then rotates to position 2 (Fig. 182, black line), where it links together the bottom right hole on the rear section with the bottom right hole on the front section. At this time, the center section still contains a measured segment of blood (44.7λ). While the center section is in position 2, 10 ml of Isoton is forced through this passageway, mixing with the blood in the center section, and emptying into the white blood cell mixing chambers. The center section remains in position 2 while approximately 1 ml of the first dilution (1:224) is removed from the white blood cell mixing chamber (B_1) and aspirated through the tubing, through the top left passageway of the blood-sampling valve (Fig. 182, white line). The center section rotates to position 1, where 10 ml of Isoton is forced through the lower left passageway (Fig. 181, white line), picking up the measured segment (44.7λ) of diluted blood from the center section. This rediluted sample then empties into the red blood cell mixing chamber. It is extremely important that all parts of the blood-sampling valve be kept clean.

2. *Analyzer unit* (Fig. 183)
   A. Oscilloscope module and system monitors.
      1) Oscilloscope screen.
      2) Aperture projection screen.
      3) Data rejection lights.
   B. Electronic circuit cards, as listed below:
      1) Three pre-amp cards.
      2) MCV card.
      3) Timer-hemoglobin card.
      4) Computer card.
      5) Two voting cards, right (WBC) and left (RBC).

In the rear of the analyzer there are cables connecting the analyzer to the diluter and to the power supply.

3. *Printer* (Fig. 184)
   A. Printout card opening (two printer sleds).
   B. Two "ready" lights (one above each sled).
   C. Digital information window.

A cable connecting the printer to the power supply is located at the back of the printer.

4. *Power supply unit* (Fig. 185)
   A. A/D converter card.
   B. Data selector card.
   C. Timing generator card.
   D. AC input voltage meter.

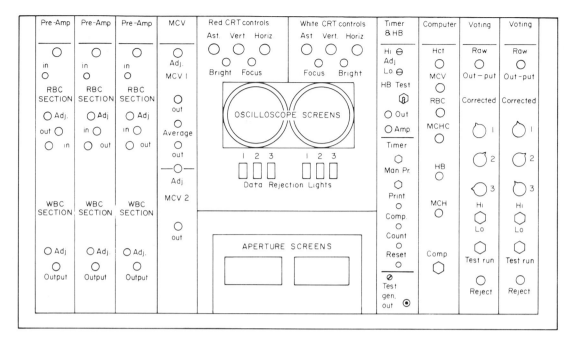

Fig. 183. Analyzer unit, Model S Coulter Counter.

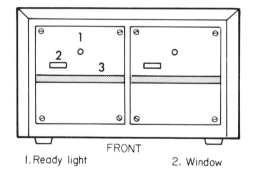

FRONT

1. Ready light   2. Window

3. Card insert (sled)

Fig. 184. Printer unit, Model S Coulter Counter.

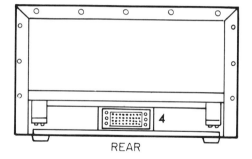

REAR

4. Printer to power

E. Power supply modules.

F. Main power switch.

Cables connecting the power supply to the printer and to the analyzer units are located in the back of the power supply unit, along with the computer interface connector and the AC line cord connector.

5. *Pneumatic power supply unit* (Fig. 186).

    A. High-vacuum gauge.

    B. 5-psi gauge and regulator.

C. 25-psi gauge and regulator.

D. High-pressure gauge.

E. Preset regulator.

F. Power switch.

G. Vacuum trap bottle.

H. 5-psi outlet.

I. High-vacuum outlet.

J. 25-psi outlet.

K. Air filter.

L. Lubricator (oil) container.

The power connector cord and the filter are located on the right side of

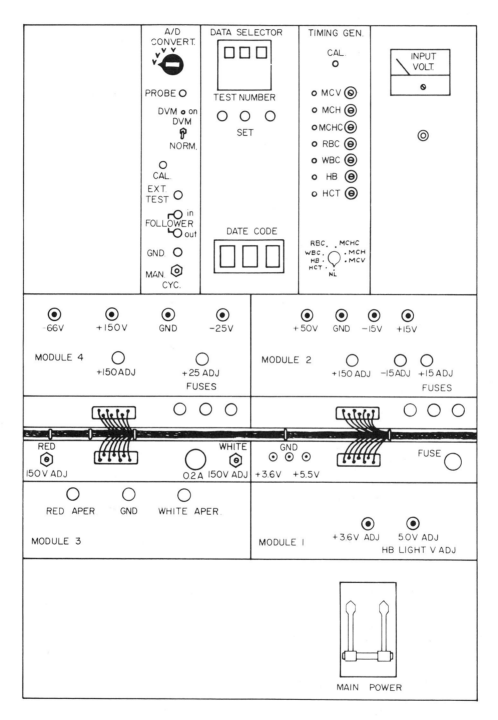

Fig. 185. Power supply unit, Model S Coulter Counter.

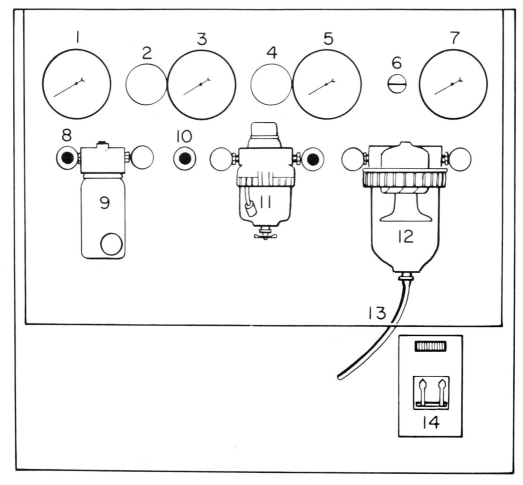

Fig. 186. Pneumatic power supply unit, Model S Coulter Counter. 1, High-vacuum gauge. 2, 5-psi regulator. 3, 5-psi gauge. 4, 25-psi regulator. 5, 25-psi gauge. 6, Preset regulator. 7, High-pressure gauge. 8, High-vacuum outlet. 9, Vacuum trap bottle. 10, 5-psi outlet. 11, Lubricator (oil) container. 12, Air filter. 13, Waste line. 14, Power switch.

the unit. The pneumatic power supply unit supplies and is connected to the diluter unit with two pressure lines and one vacuum line.

PROCEDURE AND OPERATION OF THE MODEL S COULTER COUNTER

1. Collect 5 to 6 ml of whole blood and place immediately into a tube containing EDTA.
2. Whenever the unit has been flushed completely with Isoton (or if the baths have been manually drained and rinsed), prime the instrument by

cycling two samples of normal whole blood.
3. Place the Coulter S recording card in one side of the printer and label with the patient's name and hematology accession number.
4. Mix the tube of blood well and check for clots, using two applicator sticks.
5. Place the well-mixed tube of whole blood under the aspirator, inserting the aspirator at least 1 inch into the blood.
6. Press the touch control bar, and keep the aspirator in the blood until the red light behind the bar lights up. Re-

move the tube of blood, and when the light turns green, wipe the outside of the aspirator clean with a piece of gauze. The aspirator will draw up approximately 1 ml of whole blood (0.9 to 1.1 ml). In the blood sampling valve, a measured portion of this blood (44.7λ) is removed and forced into the white blood cell mixing chamber with 10 ml of Isoton from the diluent dispenser assembly. The blood and Isoton (1:224 dilution) are mixed in these two chambers (A_1B_1). A small portion (1 ml) of this dilution is siphoned off, returned to the blood-sampling valve, and forced into the red blood cell mixing chambers with 10 ml of Isoton, to give a final dilution of 1:50,000 in the red blood cell mixing chambers (A_2B_2). While the blood is being rediluted and mixed in the red blood cell mixing chambers, 9 ml of the original dilution (1:224) of blood is forced from the white blood cell mixing chamber into the lysing chamber below it. Lysing reagent (1 ml) is forced into this chamber and mixes with the diluted blood to give a final dilution of 1:250. The dilution remains in the lysing chamber long enough to cause complete lysis of the red blood cells. During this short period, the previous blood sample is drained from the baths into the waste chamber. Isoton then enters the baths, and a hemoglobin reference reading is made (prior to the hemoglobin reading of the diluted blood sample). From the C_1 chamber the dilution is then forced down into the white blood cell aperture bath (contains three apertures). As in the Model Fn Coulter Counter, each aperture contains an internal electrode. There is one external electrode in the bath. A specific amount of diluted blood is drawn through each orifice of the ap-

erture tubes for a period of 6 seconds. The current between the external and internal electrodes changes each time a cell passes through the orifice of the aperture. This produces a voltage pulse, the magnitude of which is proportional to the size of the cell. In the analyzer unit, the voltage pulses are counted for 4 seconds, amplified, and shown on the oscilloscope screen. Three red blood cell counts are being performed at the same time. An average of the three counts is made and recorded. If debris, dirt, or other malfunction is present in one of the apertures, the corresponding red data rejection light comes on, and that red or white blood cell count will not be used. The two remaining counts are averaged. If two of the counts are rejected, the three data rejection lights come on, and a 0.0 count is recorded. The sample must then be run through the machine again. While the white blood cell count is being performed in the unit, a beam of light from the movable bar in front of the aperture bath passes through the diluted blood sample in the white blood cell count aperture bath onto a photosensitive device. This component measures the amount of light that passes through the solution and converts this into a hemoglobin reading that is recorded. When the white blood cell and hemoglobin dilution is forced into the aperture bath on the right, the red blood cell dilution is forced into the aperture bath on the left. The red blood cells are counted at the same time and in the same way that the white blood cells are counted. In addition, the MCV of the red blood cells is electronically derived and recorded. The hematocrit is then calculated from the values received from the red blood cell count and MCV. The MCH and MCHC are also calculated. The final results for all seven tests are printed out on the special card placed in the printer. It is possible to put two reporting cards in the printer at the same time, one in each sled. The side of the printer that prints the first report is indicated by a red light coming on as soon as the card is placed in the printer unit.

7. If 1 ml of whole blood is not available or if fingertip blood is used, add 44.7λ of whole blood to 10.0 ml of Isoton (1:224 dilution). (Precalibrated 44.7λ pipets are available from Coulter Electronics, Hialeah, Florida.) Before the count is performed, change the aspirator switch to the 1:224 dilution. Mix the diluted sample well, and place it under the capillary blood aspirator. Press the touch control bar, and allow the instrument to aspirate the entire diluted sample. (It is desirable to make up all micro dilutions in duplicate or triplicate and average the results. If, however, there is a large discrepancy between results, new dilutions should be made.) The diluted sample, when it is aspirated by the instrument, flows directly into the white count mixing chambers, omitting the first blood dilution. The procedure then continues as for the undiluted blood sample described in step 5.

ELECTRONIC SYSTEM

The Model S Coulter Counter has been designed in such a way that it becomes important for the technologist to understand some of the electronics involved in this system. For purposes of troubleshooting problems and as a routine periodic check, it is important to know how to test some of these electronic systems. The basic elements in the Model S are the apertures and counting system. The internal electrodes inside the apertures are all connected to an amplifier on one of the three pre-amp cards in the analyzer unit. The input signal received from the internal electrode in the aperture tube is sent to the pre-amp card, where it is amplified. If this pulse is large enough to exceed a preset threshold voltage, the pulse is applied to a circuit that provides output voltage in proportion to the number of input pulses it receives. The outputs for the red and white blood cell counts then appear as vertical pulses on the oscilloscope screen. From the pre-amp cards, the output voltage goes to one of two voting cards. Both voting cards are identical. One card, however, is used for the white blood cells and the second is used for the red blood cells. In the voting card, the three output voltages are received, averaged, and corrected for cell coincidence passage. If one or more of the signals disagrees with the others, however, it is discarded, and the appropriate data rejection light goes on. If only one count is rejected, the other two counts are averaged and used. If all three signals are different, however, all three data rejection lights go on, and the entire count must be repeated using another blood sample, or a recount may be performed. Pre-amp cards two and three also have an output to the MCV card. The two pulses received by the MCV card are corrected for cell coincidence passage and are averaged for the MCV value. For the hemoglobin, the output signal from the photosensing device goes to the timer-hemoglobin card (first for the blank and then for the sample), where it is amplified and converted into an output voltage that can be used as a linear function of the hemoglobin. The timer-hemoglobin card also contains the electronic circuitry for controlling the reset, counting, computing, and printing function. The computer card receives the hemoglobin, MCV, and red count outputs from their respective cards, and computes the hematocrit, MCH, and MCHC.

The A/D converter card (analog to digital converter card) located in the power supply unit converts the information from the analyzer unit into digital information. It also contains a digital voltmeter, which is used to check voltages in the systems of the machine. The data selector card contains the test number unit that determines the number to be printed on the recording card. Once set, this number increases by one each time the machine is cycled. The date may also be selected and printed on the card by using the date code. The four power supply modules supply the proper voltages to be used in the complete system.

The two printers in the printout unit automatically alternate if two printout cards are inserted. If one printer is not working, the second printer continues to operate each time.

MAINTENANCE

Keeping the instrument clean is most important in maintaining accurate results with a minimum number of test rejections. It should also be remembered that when control results are only slightly out of range, there is generally a small malfunction somewhere. Continuing to use the instrument under these circumstances results in increasing the error and sending out invalid reports. When control values do not check, no matter how small the error, time should be taken to ascertain the trouble.

1. Procedure to be followed at the beginning of each day.
   A. Turn on the power supply unit. Allow the instrument to warm up for approximately 30 seconds. Empty the vacuum trap bottle on the pneumatic power supply if it contains any fluid. Check the oil level. Turn the pneumatic power supply on and wait 30 seconds for warm-up.
   B. Drain Isoterge from the aperture baths. Depress the rinse button in the control panel to fill the aperture baths with Isoton. Depress the count button until the printer

begins to print. This drains the waste chamber.
   C. Inspect the following switches to make certain they are in the operating or normal position:
   1) A/D converter card toggle switch.
   2) Card R-1 toggle switch.
   3) Voting card.
   4) Computer card.
   5) Timer/hemoglobin card.
   6) MCV card.
   7) Control panel (aspiration switch).
   D. Make certain that the orifices of the apertures are visible on the aperture screen and that they are free of blockage or debris.
   E. Cycle Isoton through the instrument four or five times, through the whole blood aspirator, using the touch control bar. Make certain that:
   1) Approximately 1 ml of Isoton is being aspirated, that the blood sampling valve changes position correctly, and that there are no air bubbles in the lines from the blood sampling valve.
   2) The bubble rates in the red cell and white cell mixing chambers are correct.
   3) The transfer rates are correct.
   4) The red cell, white cell, and lysing chambers are draining completely.
   5) The outside of the white cell aperture bath is clean.
   6) The vacuum isolator and waste chambers drain completely.
   7) The gauges on the pump are all reading correctly when the unit is at rest.
   8) The setting on the mercury manometer is correct.
   9) The diluent dispenser piston

is making a full stroke with no hesitation.

F. It is necessary to clean the apertures with Clorox after every 400 to 500 blood samples, as described in the operations manual.

G. Clean the blood sampling valve after every 500 counts. Place the toggle switch on pneumatic card R-1 in the *down* position. Unscrew the black knob of the blood sampling valve and remove the center section of the sampling valve. Wash all three parts well with Isoterge and rinse with Isoton. Keeping all inside surfaces wet with Isoton, reinstall the blood-sampling valve. Turn the black knob finger tight. Place the toggle switch on card R-1 in the *up* position.

H. Drain the Isoterge from the aperture baths and rinse two or three times with Isoton.

I. Cycle Isoton through the machine two to three times by way of the whole blood aspirator, using the touch control bar. Place a printout card in the printer on the last cycle of Isoton to check the background counts. The red blood cell counts should register 0.02 or less and the white blood cell count, 0.4 or less.

J. Employ the six-way attenuator for a routine voltage check, as described in the operations manual.

K. Run the appropriate control blood specimens through the instrument. These results should check within the 2 S.D. limits of your laboratory.

2. Daily shut-down procedure.

A. Carefully clean the outside of the unit of any spilled blood.

B. Pull out pneumatic card L-1A from the left side of the diluting unit. Aspirate 50 to 60 ml of Isoterge through the instrument, through the whole blood aspirator, using the aspirator button on the control panel, until the top left cylinder in the pneumatic card is free of blood. It may be necessary to tilt the pneumatic card to facilitate the removal of blood. Periodically, air may be aspirated through the whole blood aspirator in place of the Isoterge. This also aids in the removal of the blood. It is usually not possible to remove all of the blood on the spring in the middle cylinder of the pneumatic tube. Remove as much as possible by this procedure and allow the Isoterge to remain in the system overnight. This generally loosens the small amount of blood, and it will be flushed away in the cleaning process the following day.

C. Cycle Isoterge through the instrument two times, using the touch control bar.

D. Depress the drain button in the control panel to remove the Isoton from the aperture baths. Fill the baths with Isoterge. Drain the vacuum isolator chamber, carefully pulling out the pinch valve. Depress the count button until the liquid entering the vacuum isolator chamber is green. During this procedure, be careful that the Isoterge level in the aperture baths does not fall below the level of the aperture orifices. It is usually necessary to add more Isoterge to the baths once or twice during this process. Drain the vacuum trap by pulling out the pinch valve. The aperture tubes should now be filled with Isoterge.

E. Shut off the power supply and pump units. Place the metal protective shield cover on the diluting unit.

3. Routine maintenance.
   A. Never leave blood in the aspirator or sampling valve for more than 1 or 2 minutes after the results have been obtained.
   B. Whenever the instrument is not going to be used for a while (15 or 20 minutes), drain or rinse the baths with Isoton. Aspirate approximately 10 ml of Isoton or Isoterge through the whole blood aspirator, using the aspirate button on the control panel.
4. Cleaning procedure—after every 1,000 counts.
   A. Turn off the power supply and pump units.
   B. Very carefully remove the white cell double mixing chamber from the associated tubing and stoppers. Clean the chamber with Isoterge and a small laboratory cleaning brush. Rinse well in tap water and then distilled water. Replace the chamber on the instrument and carefully hook up the tubing and stoppers.
   C. Remove the red cell double mixing chamber and clean in the same manner as outlined in step B.
   D. Remove the lysing chamber and clean in the same manner as outlined in step B.
   E. Remove the white cell aperture bath and clean as outlined in step B.
   F. Remove the red cell aperture bath and clean as outlined in step B.
   G. Turn on the power supply and pump units. Fill the aperture baths, using the rinse button in the control panel.
   H. Remove the filter from the right side of the pneumatic pump unit. Wash in warm water and replace.

DISCUSSION

1. When a problem is encountered with the Model S Coulter Counter, it is advisable to proceed with the start-up procedure as outlined previously, making certain all switches are in the proper position, bubble rates and transfer rates are correct, the blood sampling valve is clean and operating correctly, the apertures are clean, the pneumatic power supply gauges are reading correctly, and the diluent dispenser piston is making a full stroke with no hesitation. If the six-way attenuator results are within ±002 of the original reading, the problem is always in the pneumatic system. (There are only a few electronic problems that do not show up on the six-way attenuator printout. In these instances, the malfunction will show up by taking a reading of the reference voltages.) If the six-way attenuator readings vary more than ±002, the problem is in the electronics. This reading is then helpful in isolating the malfunctioning circuit. The next step is to check the appropriate reference voltages for the particular parameter(s) in question. If it is possible to correct an inaccurate voltage reading by adjustment back to the original reference voltage, the six-way attenuator reading should then be within ±002 of the original reference. Refer to the Model S Coulter Counter instruction manual for the procedure to follow when checking the reference voltages.
2. The Model S Coulter Counter should be calibrated only by the Coulter service representative.
3. In cases where the white cell count is above 30,000 per μl, it is advisable to perform the count by another method, such as manually, or on the Coulter Model Fn. In this circumstance, no part of the result reported by the Model S should be used. If the white blood cell count is not too high, the blood may be diluted 1:1 with Isoton, run through the instru-

ment, and all results except the red blood cell indices multiplied by two. On the diluted blood, however, the white blood cell count should still not exceed 30,000 per μl.

4. In cases where the white blood cell count is below 1,500 per μl, a manual white count should be performed. In this case, the results reported by the instrument, except for the white blood cell count, are acceptable and may be reported.

5. Care should be taken to ensure that the white cell aperture bath does not overflow. When this occurs, the fluid dries on the outside of the bath and may interfere with the hemoglobin reading.

6. When using the secondary aspirator for previously diluted blood (1:224 dilution), remove any whole blood in the primary aspirator by first cycling Isoton through the instrument, using the touch control bar. This avoids leaving blood in the line for more than 15 minutes.

7. If the white blood cell count or the red blood cell count and hematocrit continuously give results of 0.0, double-check to make certain the external electrodes are immersed in the solution in the aperture baths.

8. If one or more of the data rejection lamps continuously light up, check the aperture orifices for dirt or debris.

9. After using the secondary aspirator, do not forget to change the switch in the control panel to the left for whole blood aspiration.

COULTER COUNTER MODEL S PLUS

The Model S Plus Coulter Counter is similar to the Model S Coulter Counter. This new model, however, has a more compact and less complicated pneumatic system and is more computerized than the Model S Coulter Counter. In addition, this instrument performs whole blood platelet counts and tests the degree of anisocytosis (RDW) on patient samples, in addition to the seven parameters tested by the Model S Coulter Counter.

The Model S Plus Coulter Counter consists of five connected units:

1. The *power supply unit* furnishes regulated voltages to run the electronic system and also provides the necessary pressures and vacuum to the diluter unit and reagent system.

2. The *diluter unit* aspirates, pipets, dilutes, mixes the blood, lyses the red blood cells, physically moves the blood sample through the unit for testing, and senses the samples in the baths.

3. The *analyzer unit* contains electronic cards that control the sequence of the various operating cycles of the diluter unit. Messages are received from the diluter unit, and the analyzer counts, sizes, measures, and computes this information, which is then sent to the printer unit in the form of test results. Information is also sent from this unit to the X-Y recorder.

4. The *printer unit* gives a printed copy of the test results obtained by the instrument.

5. The *X-Y recorder* provides a graph of the platelet size distribution and also simulated platelet distributions based on test pulses as part of the electronic voltage check.

COMPONENTS OF THE MODEL S PLUS COULTER COUNTER

1. *Power supply unit* (Fig. 187): Numbers in parentheses refer to numbers indicated in the figure and explained in the legend.

   A. Main power switch (13) turns the electronic system on (up position) and off (down position).

   B. Control voltage indicator lamp (12) should be lit when the main power switch is on.

   C. Line voltage meter (14) should in-

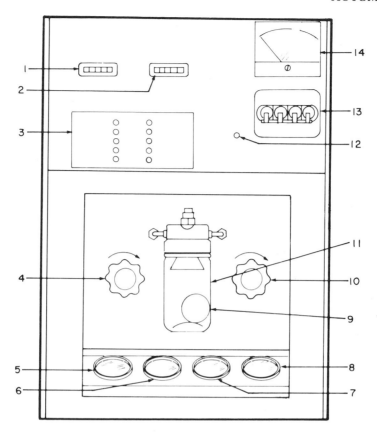

Fig. 187. Power supply unit, Model S Plus Coulter Counter. 1, Compressor run meter. 2, Total hours meter. 3, Monitor. 4, 5-psi pressure regulator. 5, 6, 7, 8, Pneumatic gauges. 9, Ball. 10, 30-psi pressure regulator. 11, Vacuum trap bottle. 12, Control voltage indicator lamp. 13, Main power switch. 14, Line voltage meter.

dicate 105 V to 125 V. The instrument should not be operated if the meter reading is outside these limits.

D. Compressor run meter (1) indicates the number of hours that the pneumatics have been activated.

E. Total hours meter (2) indicates the number of hours the power supply unit has been on.

F. The monitor (3) contains indicator lights. Seven of these lamps indicate voltage problems when lit (such as a blown fuse). When the pneumatic system is at rest (gauges register 0) or not fully activated, this lamp is on. Pneu Temp and Elec Temp are lit if the temperature in the pneumatic system or electronic system becomes too hot.

G. The vacuum trap bottle (11) should be empty. If it contains liquid, there is a leak somewhere in the diluter unit, allowing fluid to enter the vacuum lines.

H. The pneumatic gauges (5, 6, 7, 8) indicate the amount of pressure and vacuum being introduced into the diluter unit. The 5-psi pressure should read exactly 5-psi, the vacuum should be 20 inches Hg $\pm$ 2 inches, the 60-psi pressure should read 60 psi $\pm$ 5-psi, and the 30-psi pressure should be 30 psi $\pm$ 1 psi.

I. The pressure regulators (4, 10) may be used by the operator to adjust the 5-psi pressure and the 30-psi pressure. The vacuum and the 60-psi cannot be adjusted by the operator.

J. The main power pack containing fuses and voltage jacks is located on the right side of the unit, near the front. The control module, also containing fuses and voltage jacks, is on the same side of the unit near the back.

K. Filters (two).

Power cables connecting the power supply unit to the printer, analyzer, and X-Y recorder are located in the back of the unit along with the signal cable and +9 V power cable to the analyzer unit. The pneumatic portion of the unit connects into the back lower right of the diluter unit through the 60-psi, 30-psi, 5-psi, vacuum, and waste lines.

2. *Diluter unit*

A. Front of door (Fig. 188)
   1) Whole blood aspirator tip (14) through which the whole blood sample is drawn.
   2) Whole-blood push button (13) initiates the whole blood cycle.
   3) Diluent dispenser spout (21).
   4) Diluent dispenser push button (22) delivers approximately 10 ml of diluent through the diluent dispenser spout.
   5) Microsample aspirator (15), through which 10 ml of the 1:224 diluted microsample is drawn.
   6) 1:224 dilution push button (16) initiates the microsample cycle.

B. Back of front door
   1) Blood sampling valve cylinder moves the blood-sampling valve between positions 1 and 2.

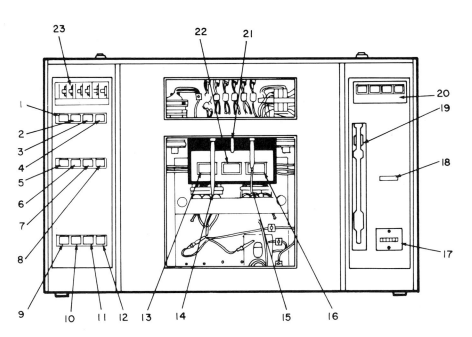

Fig. 188. Diluter unit front, Model S Plus Coulter Counter. 1, Prime button. 2, Drain button. 3, Rinse button. 4, Clear button. 5, Print button. 6, Plot button. 7, Recount button. 8, Continue (cont) button. 9, Power-on button. 10, Power-off button. 11, Start-up button. 12, Shut-down button. 13, Whole blood push button. 14, Whole blood aspirator tip. 15, Microsample aspirator tip. 16, Microsample push button. 17, Test cycle display. 18. Vacuum adjust regulator. 19, Mercury manometer. 20, Liquid level monitors. 21, Diluent dispenser spout. 22, Diluent dispense button. 23, Month/day/year selector.

2) Blood-sampling valve.
3) Rinse cup, through which 4 ml of diluent is pushed during the backwash cycle (cleaning of the whole blood aspirator between samples).
4) Rinse cup cylinder moves the rinse cup into position for the backwash.
5) Knurled nuts holding the aspirator tips in position.

C. Center front of diluter unit (door open) (Fig. 189)
1) RBC diluent dispenser (2) delivers approximately 10 ml of diluent for the RBC dilution.
2) WBC diluent dispenser (24) delivers approximately 10 ml of diluent for the whole-blood WBC dilution. It also dispenses approximately 10 ml of diluent when the diluent dispenser button is pushed.
3) Pinch valves (26).
4) Locking lever (25) (attached to pinch valve) in the up position releases pressure from the tubing to help eliminate pinched tubing.
5) Backwash pump (4) delivers 4 ml of diluent through the blood sampling valve to the whole-blood aspirator into the rinse cup during the backwash cycle.
6) Hemoglobin blank pump (22) delivers 5 ml of diluent to the hemoglobin cuvette to be read as the hemoglobin blank.
7) WBC and RBC sample pumps (23) (red in color) are each 0.5 ml pumps and act to aspirate the blood through the blood sampling valve.
8) Lyse pump (23) is responsible for moving 0.7734 ml of lyse reagent into the WBC aperture bath.
9) RBC vacuum isolator chamber

(7) contains a vacuum of 6 inches Hg during the counting cycle. It is attached to the RBC aperture block through the sweep flow lines. During the count cycle, this vacuum is responsible for drawing the diluted blood sample through the apertures.
10) WBC vacuum isolator chamber (18) operates in the same manner as the RBC vacuum isolator chamber. There are, however, no sweep flow lines coming into the bottom of the WBC aperture housing.
11) Aperture housings (one RBC and one WBC) contain the aperture blocks.
12) Apertures (three RBC apertures and three WBC apertures) (19) are contained in the aperture blocks. The RBC apertures are 50 μm in diameter and the WBC apertures are 100 μm in diameter.
13) Aperture baths (6, 21), two (RBC and WBC), contain the diluted blood samples that are pulled through the apertures and into the vacuum isolator chambers during the counting cycle. The back of each aperture bath contains three openings that are tightly fitted around the front of the corresponding aperture block, creating an air-tight seal.
14) Sweep flow lines (8) (three) are attached to the bottom of the RBC aperture housing. During the count cycle, diluent is pulled up through these lines behind the aperture tube opening (aperture bath is on other side of the aperture) and out through the top of the aperture housing to the vacuum isolator chamber. This steady

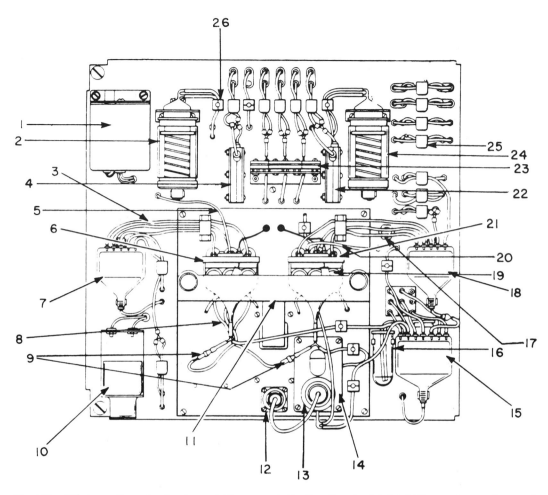

Fig. 189. Diluter unit, center front panel (door open), Coulter Counter Model S Plus. 1, Sweep flow tank. 2, RBC diluent dispenser. 3, Sweep flow lines (3). 4, Backwash pump. 5, Overflow line. 6, RBC aperture bath. 7, RBC vacuum isolator chamber. 8, Sweep flow lines (3). 9, Check valve. 10, Overflow cuvette. 11, Light bar. 12, Hemoglobin lamp plug. 13, Hemoglobin lamp. 14, Hemoglobin cuvette. 15, Waste chamber. 16, Foam trap. 17, Needle valve (microsample aspiration). 18, WBC vacuum isolator chamber. 19, Aperture. 20, Overflow line. 21, WBC aperture bath. 22, Hemoglobin blank pump. 23, WBC and RBC aspiration pumps and lyse pump. 24, WBC diluent dispenser. 25, Locking lever. 26, Pinch valve.

stream of diluent moves the red blood cells out of the sensing area.

15) Sweep flow tank (1), through which sweep flow lines pass prior to entering the RBC aperture blocks.

16) Overflow lines (5, 20), one leading from the WBC aperture bath and one from the RBC aperture bath. If the baths are filled to the top with fluid,

the overflow leaves the aperture baths through these lines and goes to the overflow cuvette.

17) Light bar (11) (removable) contains the lamps necessary to see the apertures in the viewing screens on the analyzer unit.

18) Hemoglobin lamp plug (12).

19) Hemoglobin lamp (13).

20) Hemoglobin cuvette (14),

where the hemoglobin reading is made.

21) Check valve (9), WBC bath, allows air bubbles to flow in only one direction, into the aperture bath.

22) Check valve (9), RBC bath, same function as check valve in WBC bath.

23) Waste chamber (15).

24) Needle valve (17) for adjusting microsample aspiration rate.

D. Left front panel of diluter unit (Fig. 188)

1) Month/date/year selector (23).

2) Prime push button (1) applies vacuum to the apertures and sweep flow lines, turns on the aperture current, and activates the pneumatic system (pressures and vacuum). (The pneumatic system automatically shuts off when the diluter unit has not been cycled for approximately 15 minutes.)

3) Drain push button (2) empties the RBC aperture bath and both vacuum isolator chambers into the waste chamber and empties the WBC aperture bath into the hemoglobin cuvette.

4) Rinse push button (3) fills both aperture baths with approximately 10 ml of diluent, empties the hemoglobin cuvette into the waste chamber, and empties the waste chamber.

5) Clear push button (4) applies 5-psi pressure onto the inside of the aperture block to clear any debris that may be blocking the aperture.

6) Print push button (5), when pressed, produces a printout on the last sample introduced into the instrument.

7) Plot push button (6) produces a graph of the platelet data from the X-Y recorder on the blood sample just previously introduced into the instrument.

8) Recount push button (7) flashes if there is a vote-out during the cycle. When activated, it initiates a recount.

9) Cont push button (8) (along with the recount button) blinks when there has been a vote-out. If a recount is not desired, this button is pushed and the cycle continues.

10) Power-on push button (9) turns on the power (originating from the power supply) to the diluter unit, analyzer unit, and the printer.

11) Power-off push button (10) turns off the power to the diluter unit, analyzer unit, and printer.

12) Start-up push button (11) activates an automatic sequence of five cycles of the diluter unit. This cleans and primes the unit with diluent and lyse reagent.

13) Shut-down push button (12) activates an automatic sequence of five cycles of the diluter unit with cleaning reagent to clean the unit.

E. Right front panel of diluter unit (Fig. 188)

1) Liquid level monitors (20): Low diluent, low cleaner, low lyse, and full waste.

a) 5 psi of pressure is placed on the small line extending into the waste and reagent containers. If a bubble of air escapes from the bottom of this tube in the reagent containers, or, conversely, if no bubble of air escapes from the tube in the waste container, the appropriate push button illuminates when the corresponding reagent supply is low or the waste container is full. An audible beep also sounds when the monitor is on. At this point, five more blood samples (instrument cycles) may be run.

2) Vacuum regulator (18) regulates the amount of vacuum applied to the apertures (applied directly to the vacuum isolator chambers and through the open lines to the apertures).

3) The mercury manometer (19) is a gauge for the aperture vacuum. During the count cycle, the upper level of the blue indicating fluid should be at the point labeled AA and should not vary more than $\frac{1}{4}$ inch. When the instrument is at rest (pneumatic system turned off), the upper level of the blue indicating fluid should be at level BB.

4) Test cycles display (17) indicates the number of times the instrument has been cycled. This counter is not adjustable by the operator and does not advance during the start-up and shut-down cycles of the instrument.

F. Left side of diluter unit
The vacuum and pressure lines enter the diluter unit from the power supply at the back left of the diluter unit.

1) Diluter control card is computer operated and controls the solenoid valves located on the floor of the diluter unit (left side). Each of the solenoids has a color-coded pneu-

matic (pressure or vacuum) line attached to it. The function of each solenoid is printed on the side of the diluter control card. The pressures and vacuums in these pneumatic lines are responsible for the dilution and movement of the sample and reagents through the diluter unit during instrument cycling and diluent dispensing. As each solenoid is activated, the indicator light (located on the front panel of the card) for that particular solenoid is lit. The button next to the indicator light may be used to operate that solenoid manually.

2) Hemoglobin regulator card

G. Right side of diluter unit
Reagent and waste lines are attached to the diluter unit at the back right of the unit.

1) Vacuum isolator chamber receives high vacuum and is connected to the vacuum regulator and the mercury manometer.

3. *Analyzer unit* (Fig. 190)

A. The oscilloscope screen (10) represents the cells as they pass through the apertures and are counted. Each pulse shown on the screen represents a cell. The size of the cell is indicated by the height of each pulse (the larger the cell, the higher the pulse).

B. White and red CRT (cathode ray tube) controls (9) are utilized to adjust manually the pulses on the oscilloscope screens.

C. Voting display matrix (1) corresponds to the different counts performed by the instrument (horizontal axis) and the apertures counting the cells (vertical axis) (the apertures are numbered from left to right). If one of the

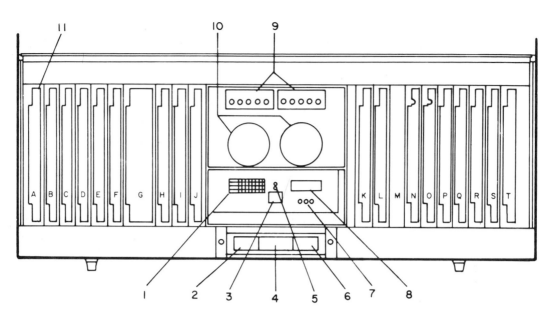

Fig. 190. Analyzer unit, door open, Coulter Counter Model S Plus. 1, Voting display matrix. 2, RBC aperture viewing screen. 3, Error code display. 4, System status indicator. 5, DVM/test number indicators. 6, WBC aperture viewing screens. 7, Set test number buttons. 8, DVM/test number display. 9, CRT controls. 10, Oscilloscope screens. 11, Electronic cards: A, RED PERCentile 2; B, RED PERCentile 1; C, MCV; D, EXTended MEMory; E, MEMory; F, Central processing unit; G, Analog to digital converter/CALibration; H, RED/WHite CounTeR; I, APerture CURrent/SIGnal GENerator; J, Power supply MONitor/BUFFer; K, MEMory; L, PLATelet ADC; M, empty; N, PRE-AMPlifier (red); O, PRE-AMPlifier (white); P, PULSE EDitor (ap 1); Q, PULSE EDitor (ap 2); R, PULSE EDitor (ap 3); S, Particle VELocity; T, PLATelet PROCessor.

three parameters being measured (except hemoglobin) does not agree within four S.D. of the other two measurements, the count votes-out (values will be rejected), the corresponding lamp lights on the voting matrix, and the other two counts are averaged and reported. If two measurements are rejected by the instrument, all data for this parameter will vote-out and all three lamps (for apertures 1, 2, and 3) will be lit.

D. DVM/test number (5) indicators are represented by two lamps. The DVM lamp is lit when the cal/norm switch on the ADC/calibration card is in the cal position, and also at the beginning and end of the cycle when the hemoglobin blank and patient sample, respectively, are read. The test number

lamp should be lit at all other times during normal operation of the instrument.

E. DVM/test number display (8), when the instrument is at rest, displays the test number of the next sample to be cycled through the instrument. When a sample is introduced into the instrument, the hemoglobin blank is immediately read. The voltage reading of the blank is then displayed on the screen in place of the test number. The counting cycle then begins and the number 1 is displayed. This indicates that the first platelet count is being performed. If a second, third, fourth, or fifth platelet count is necessary, the corresponding number is displayed while that count is being performed. At the completion of the counting cycle, the hemoglobin is read, and the voltage reading (indicating how much light passed through the sample) appears on the display. The test number for the next sample then replaces the hemoglobin reading and remains displayed until the next sample is introduced into the instrument.

F. Set test number push buttons (7) (three) are located directly beneath the DVM/test number display and are used to set manually the test number as desired.

G. Error code display (3) indicates a problem or malfunction of the instrument. During normal, problem-free operation of the instrument, 00 is displayed on this indicator. When any number or letters are displayed, the operator should refer to the error code display table in the Coulter S Plus operator's reference manual for an explanation of the code and the action to take. Most of the codes listed indicate electronic problems and customer service must be called. An exception to this is a code 10, which indicates a "no fit" platelet count. If codes 12 or 13 are displayed, the reagent (or waste) liquid levels may need to be replenished (or emptied).

H. RBC and WBC aperture viewing screens (2, 6) show the aperture through which the diluted sample is drawn during the count cycle. These screens should be watched carefully for debris that may block the aperture and cause vote-outs on the counts of MCV.

I. System status indicator (4) is located between the two aperture viewing screens. This display indicates the sequence of events as they are taking place during the test cycle. During a normal, problem-free cycle, the following sequence of events appears on the indicator: INTRO SAMPLE, WIPE, COUNT, ANALYZE, DATA ACCEPT, BACKWASH, READ HGB, READY. READY is displayed when the instrument can accept another sample. NOT READY (as shown during a startup or shut-down cycle) indicates that the instrument cannot accept a sample. SYSTEM FAULT indicates a malfunction in the instrument. DATA REJECT appears when there has been a vote-out.

J. Electronic cards
The electronic cards (11) are responsible for the functions of the analyzer unit as previously described. In addition, voltage checks of the electronics are made and the instrument is calibrated manually by use of these cards.

4. *Printer Unit* (Fig. 191)

A. Printer sleds (1) (two), into which the printout cards are placed.

B. Indicator lights (3) (two) are used to indicate which sled will report the next blood sample. When placing a printout in each sled, the sled with the first printout placed in it will cause the lamp to be lit. If the lamp blinks, the

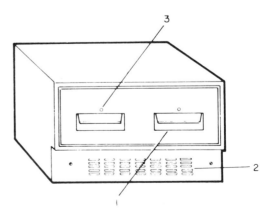

Fig. 191. Printer unit, Coulter Counter Model S Plus. 1, Printer sled (2). 2, Filter. 3, Indicator lights (2).

slip is not seated correctly and the result will not be printed.

C. Filter (2).

D. On/off switch located on the back of the unit.

The printer unit is connected to the power supply through a power cable and to the analyzer unit through the printer signal cable.

5. *X-Y recorder* (Fig. 192)

A. X-axis controls (1, 2) consist of the zero knob, which sets the pen on 0 on the horizontal axis, and the gain control, which adjusts the sensitivity for the horizontal axis.

B. Y-axis controls (5, 6) are the zero knob, which sets the pen at 0 for the vertical axis, and the gain control, which adjusts the sensitivity for the vertical axis.

C. Power on/off push button (4) turns the recorder on and off.

D. Pen up/down push button (3) is not utilized when the recorder is used with this instrument because the pen is automatically

lowered and raised when necessary. Do not touch this button.

PROCEDURE AND OPERATION OF THE MODEL S PLUS COULTER COUNTER

1. Whenever the instrument has not been cycled for approximately 15 minutes, the pneumatic system (pressures and vacuums) automatically turns off. In this case, depress the prime button.

2. As soon as the pressure and vacuum gauges register correctly, check that READY is displayed on the system status indicator.

3. Wipe the aspirator tip in case there is a drop of diluent at the end.

4. Place the tube of blood under the whole blood aspirator tip, inserting the aspirator at least 1 inch into the blood.

5. Press the whole blood push button and keep the aspirator in the blood sample until WIPE is displayed. Remove the blood sample and immediately wipe the aspirator tube with a piece of gauze moistened in dilu-

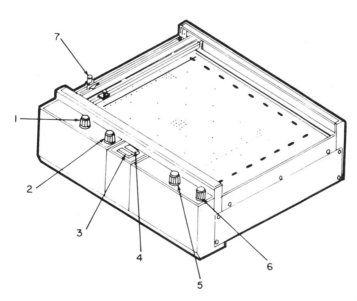

Fig. 192. X-Y recorder, Coulter Counter Model S Plus. 1, Gain control knob (X axis). 2, Zero control knob (X axis). 3, Pen up/down button. 4, Power on/off button. 5, Gain control knob (Y axis). 6, Zero control knob (Y axis). 7, Pen holder.

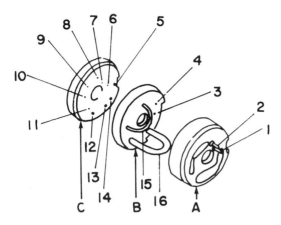

Fig. 193. Blood-sampling valve, Coulter Counter Model S Plus. Whole-blood aspiration. RBC and WBC dilutions are performed simultaneously. RBC dilution, position 1 (as shown above): Whole blood enters line 1 (section A), goes through passage 4 (section B), and out of sampling valve through passage 6 (section C). Center section rotates counterclockwise to position 2: Diluent enters line 2 (A), goes through passage 4 (B) picking up the blood sample, and out passage 7 (C) to RBC aperture bath. [Remaining whole blood aspirated travels through passage 3 (B) and out passage 6 (C).] WBC dilution, position 1: Whole blood enters back of section C through passage 10 into loop 15 (B) and out line 8 (C). Position 2: Diluent enters section C through back of passage 11, through loop 15 (B), picking up blood sample, and out passage 9 (C) to aperture bath. Microsample aspirations: Diluted sample enters back of section C through passage 12, into loop 16 (B), and out passage 14 (C) to the WBC aperture bath. Midway during the aspiration, the middle section rotates to position 2. The dilution continues to enter the back of passage 12 (C), into an etched-out passageway in the back of section B, and out passage 14 (C) to the WBC aperture bath. At the same time, diluent enters the back of passage 5 (C), through loop 16 (B), picks up the diluted blood, and carries it out passage 13 (C) to the RBC aperture bath.

ent. Do not put your hands or any object near the whole blood aspirator tip during the remainder of the cycle. Approximately 1 ml of whole blood is drawn up into the instrument through the blood-sampling valve. This blood sample is split into two pathways prior to reaching the blood sampling valve. One half of the sample enters the back of the blood-sampling valve, where it enters the valve and fills the small metal loop for the WBC dilution. (See Figure 193 for a

diagram of the blood-sampling valve.) The remaining portion of the sample enters the front of the blood-sampling valve for the red blood count dilution. The blood-sampling valve changes to position 2. As soon as this is accomplished, approximately 10 ml of diluent enters the back of the blood-sampling valve, picks up the 42.9λ of whole blood contained in the small loop, and carries it to the WBC aperture bath, where it enters through the bottom left of the bath. At the same time, approximately 10 ml of diluent enters the front of the blood-sampling valve and picks up the 1.6λ of whole blood in the center section. This blood and diluent go directly to the RBC aperture bath, where they enter through the bottom left of the bath. While the blood is being aspirated, the diluent is draining from the RBC aperture bath into the waste chamber, and the WBC aperture bath is draining into the hemoglobin cuvette. As soon as the aperture baths have been drained, the diluted blood samples enter the RBC and WBC aperture baths, respectively, through the tubing at the bottom left of each bath. As the dilution for the WBC is entering the WBC aperture bath, 0.7734 ml of lyse reagent is entering the WBC aperture bath at the bottom right side (1:251 dilution) of the bath. At the same time, 14 bubbles are introduced into each aperture bath through tubing attached at the bottom of each bath. These bubbles (the number may vary between 12 and 16) are utilized to mix completely the diluted blood sample. While the aperture baths are filling, the hemoglobin cuvette is being drained into the waste chamber. As WIPE is displayed, an internal voltage check is automatically performed (voltage patterns are displayed on the oscilloscope screens), and the hemoglobin cuvette is filled with diluent (5 ml) for the hemoglobin blank reading. At this point, the instrument is ready to count. COUNT is displayed, and a 4-second counting cycle takes place. At the beginning of the first 4-second count cycle, the voltage reading for the hemoglobin blank is shown on the DVM/test number display. This number immediately changes to the number 1 to indicate the first counting cycle. As in the Model S Coulter Counter, each of the apertures contains an internal electrode. There is one external electrode in each aperture bath. When the pinch valves between the aperture housing and the vacuum isolator chambers are opened, the vacuum (present in the vacuum isolator chambers) draws the diluted blood sample through each aperture (into the vacuum isolator chamber) for a period of 4 seconds. As the diluted blood sample passes through the aperture, the current between the external and internal electrodes changes each time a cell passes through the aperture. This produces a voltage pulse, the magnitude of which is proportional to the size of the cell. The white blood cells are counted from the WBC aperture bath on the right side. From the RBC aperture bath, the red blood cells and platelets are counted. At the same time that the red blood cells are counted, the MCV is determined from the size of the voltage pulses. As the red blood cells and platelets pass through the RBC apertures, those particles measuring 2 to 20 μm^3 are counted as platelets, whereas all particles above 36 μm^3 are enumerated as red blood cells. All cells between 36 and 360 μm^3 are used to determine the MCV. The red blood cell count, white blood cell count,

platelet count, and MCV are all measured through three apertures. Up to five 4-second platelet counts are performed by the instrument on each cycle, depending on the platelet count of the sample introduced. The instrument automatically counts the platelets for these additional cycles, up to five, until the equivalent of a 190,000 to 250,000 per μl platelet count is attained. As each platelet count is performed by the instrument, the number corresponding to the platelet count being done (2, 3, 4, or 5) appears on the DVM/test number display. During the first count cycle, three platelet counts, red blood cell counts, white blood cell counts, and MCVs are performed simultaneously (one count through each aperture). When the counting cycle(s) has been completed, ANALYZE appears on the system status indicator, and the analyzer unit compares the counts from each aperture. If all three results for each parameter tested (RBC, WBC, platelet count, and RDW) agree with the others within four S.D., DATA ACCEPT appears on the system status indicator, and the three counts are averaged for a final result. If one count does not match the other two, the corresponding data rejection lamp lights on the voting matrix, and the other two counts are averaged for the final result. A total vote-out for a parameter is obtained when none of the counts agree within four S.D. of each other. In such instances, all three data rejection lamps are lit, DATA REJECT appears on the indicator, and the cycle stops. The recount and cont buttons flash for 30 seconds. If a recount is desired on the rejected parameter, push the recount button. If a recount is not wanted, either push the cont button or wait 30 seconds and the cycle will continue. The aperture baths will then empty (RBC bath into the waste chamber and the WBC bath into the hemoglobin cuvette) and refill with diluent. BACK-WASH appears on the system status indicator, and 4 ml of diluent is pushed through the blood-sampling valve and out the aspirator tip into the rinse cup, which has moved into a locked position beneath the aspirator. HGB READ is displayed on the indicator, and the amount of light passing through the diluted hemoglobin sample is read. The voltage reading is displayed on the DVM/test number display. The hematocrit (RBC × MCV), MCH (hemoglobin ÷ RBC) and MCHC (hemoglobin ÷ hematocrit) are calculated in the analyzer unit. Immediately, the printer unit prints the results of the nine parameters.

6. If 1 ml of whole blood is not available or if fingertip blood is used, add 44.7λ of whole blood to one aliquot (approximately 10 ml) of diluent from the diluent dispenser. Mix the diluted sample carefully to avoid bubbles, and place the vial under the microsample aspirator tip. Press the 1:224 dilution push button directly behind the aspirator and allow the instrument to aspirate the entire sample. The diluted sample enters the back of the blood-sampling valve and goes into and completely fills the large loop of the center section. (See Figure 188 for a diagram of the blood-sampling valve.) It continues through the blood-sampling valve and leaves by way of the back of the valve, going directly to the WBC aperture bath. During the aspiration of the microsample, the blood-sampling valve moves to position 2. The large loop is now completely filled with the original microsample dilution (359.55λ). Diluent then enters the blood-sampling valve at the back,

picks up the diluted sample in the large loop for the RBC dilution, and carries it to the RBC aperture bath, where it enters the right bottom side of the bath. While this is occurring, the diluted sample continues to be aspirated through the back of the blood-sampling valve but now enters the trough in the middle section and continues out the back of the blood-sampling valve, where it goes directly to the WBC aperture bath, entering through the line at the top of the bath. The cycle continues as described for the whole blood cycle, with one exception. The microsample aspirator tip is not backwashed with diluent. Instead, a vacuum is applied to the microsample aspirator tip for a short period at the end of the cycle, immediately before the READY light comes on. This is for cleaning purposes.

PLATELET COUNT AS PERFORMED ON THE COULTER COUNTER MODEL S PLUS

During the count cycle, as the platelets and red blood cells pass through the apertures, those particles that are between 2 and 20 μm^3 in size are counted as platelets. In the analyzer unit, as the platelets are counted, they are divided into groups (channels) according to size. This information is then used for plotting the platelet graph. It has been found that normal platelets, when graphed according to size and number, are log-normally distributed and yield a log-normal curve (see Fig. 194). There are platelets smaller than 2 μm^3 and larger than 20 μm^3. If the upper limit was increased to count platelets above 20 μm^3, however, red blood cells might be included in the platelet count. Therefore, a graph is made of the size distribution of the platelets. If the analyzer recognizes this platelet count as having a log-normal distribution, it chooses the peak of the curve and the lowest point on either side of the peak. Using the two low points, the

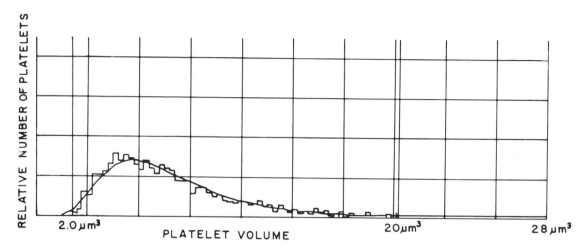

Fig. 194. Graph of normal platelet size distribution, Coulter Counter Model S Plus.

platelet data are fitted to a log-normal curve and extrapolated to read from 0 to 70 μm³; everything within this curve is counted as platelets. The first graph of the platelet count is a graph of the actual count between 2 and 20 μm³. If the platelet count then shows log-normal distribution, a fitted curve is graphed from 0 to 70 μm³ over the original curve, and all platelets contained within the curve are counted and reported as the platelet count. If the platelets do not show log-normal size distribution, this is recognized in the analyzer, and the curve only extends from 2 to 20 μm³ (Fig. 195). The symbol $ appears on the printout form, signifying a "no-fit" platelet count. The platelet count result that is printed may not be valid because it represents only those platelets contained in the curve between the two valleys (not between 2 and 20 μm³). See Figure 195 for a no-fit platelet curve. To have a valid count, a fitted curve must be obtained. The criteria for a fitted curve are a platelet count above 20,000/mm³, log-normal distribution (positive curve), and no platelet count vote-out.

RED CELL DISTRIBUTION WIDTH (RDW)

The RDW is essentially an indication of the degree of anisocytosis. The size of red blood cells shows a normal distribution

curve (Gaussian curve). The RDW is determined and calculated by the analyzer using the MCV and red blood cell count. The point on the curve (the MCV reading) at which 20% of the red blood cells are larger than the rest is recorded as the 20th percentile, and the point at which 80% (the MCV reading) of the red blood cells are larger is noted as the 80th percentile (Fig. 196). The space between these two points represents the RDW. Mathematically, the RDW is determined as follows:

$$RDW = \frac{(20\text{th percentile} - 80\text{th percentile})}{(20\text{th percentile} + 80\text{th percentile})} \times \text{Constant}$$

The constant represents the number that is required to give a normal value of 10 to this test. The normal range for the RDW is 8.5 to 11.5.

START-UP PROCEDURE

The entire start-up procedure should be performed at the beginning of each day or when the instrument has not been used for several work shifts. If there is a malfunction of the instrument that is not identified by an error code or if control results are not within acceptable limits, the start-up procedure should also be performed to help locate the problem.

1. Check the liquid level in the waste, diluent, lyse reagent, and cleaning

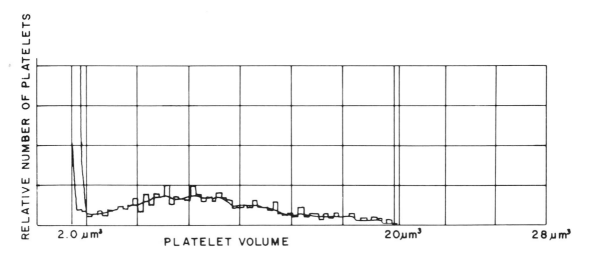

Fig. 195. Graph of no-fit platelet size distribution, Coulter Counter Model S Plus.

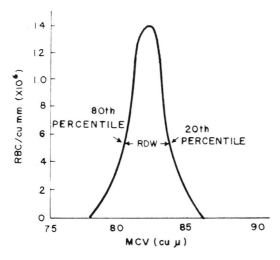

Fig. 196. Normal red blood cell size distribution showing RDW.

reagent containers. Empty or fill these containers as necessary.

2. In the diluter unit, check that the tubing in each pinch valve is not pinched by rolling the tubing between your thumb and forefinger (manually open those pinch valves not containing a lock). Unlock the pinch valves (place the locking lever in the *down* position). Empty the overflow Accuvette.

3. Check the power supply unit. The line voltage meter should read 105 V to 125 V. (Do not operate the instrument outside of these limits.) The control voltage indicator lamp should be on. Check the monitor lamps (the only one that may be lit is the pneumatic lamp unless there is a problem). Inspect the vacuum trap bottle. If liquid is present in the bottle, empty (all pressures must be at 0 and the diluter unit must be turned off).

4. Press the prime button on the diluter unit. The pneumatic light on the power supply unit should go out. Inspect the pneumatic gauges on the power supply unit and ensure that they maintain the proper pressures.

5. Turn the power on in the X-Y recorder. Uncap and place the pen in position.

6. Raise the front cover on the analyzer unit and lock into position. All switches on the electronic cards should be in the down position. Check that the ext mem card has flashing Fs. (If the instrument has not been used for several shifts, it will probably be necessary to set the DISPLAY switch, ext mem card, to on.)

7. Open the door on the left side of the

diluter unit and inspect the Hgb reg card. All switches should be in the *down* position.

8. The error code on the digital display assembly should read 00 or 10.

9. On the diluter unit, set the month/day/year thumbwheel. Inspect the mercury manometer and make certain the upper level of blue indicating fluid is at exactly the AA reference mark. Adjust if necessary. Carefully push the light bar into place, being careful not to pinch any tubing. Inspect the aperture viewing screens. If any debris is present on the apertures, remove this using the clear button before proceeding.

10. Make the necessary adjustments of the baseline images on the oscilloscope screen.

11. Check the operation of the drain, clear, rinse, and prime buttons by operating each one individually and by checking that they function as previously outlined. While depressing the prime button, inspect the sweep flow lines. They should contain no air bubbles.

12. Depress the start-up button. With the front door of the diluter unit open, watch for normal reagent flow and cycling of the instrument. (No bubbles will be introduced into the aperture baths.) Also check the backwash operation on the door of the diluter unit. At the conclusion of the cycle (about 2 minutes), the READY sign should appear, and the baths and tubing should be free of cleaning reagent. Dispense and discard two 10-ml aliquots of diluent from the diluent dispenser.

13. Cycle clean diluent through the whole-blood aspirator at least five times, noting the following (the MCV generally rejects, in which case depress the cont button):
    A. The diluter unit appears to be cycling correctly.

B. Fourteen (12 to 16) bubbles enter each aperture bath (at the rate of about two bubbles per second).

C. The top line of the blue indicating fluid in the mercury manometer should not vary more than $\frac{1}{4}$ inch during the count cycle.

D. The system status indicator shows the proper sequence of messages.

E. While WIPE is displayed, electronic self-test pulses are displayed.

F. Perform a background count on the final diluent cycle. The counts should not exceed the following limits: WBC, 00.2; RBC, 0.01; hemoglobin, 00.1; and platelets, 003. If no results print out for the platelet count, the platelet count is greater than 0 but less than 1,000 per μl.

G. Record the hemoglobin blank voltage as shown on the DVM/test number display, and the hemoglobin read voltage that appears on the display when HGB READ is displayed on the system status indicator. As a general rule, the higher the difference between the two readings, the higher the hemoglobin background count.

14. Dispense 10 ml of diluent into each of two clean vials. Aspirate the first sample of diluent through the microsample aspirator. During the cycle, check that an error code is not displayed. Also check the system status indicator for the correct sequence of messages. Aspirate the second sample of diluent through the microsample aspirator and record the background count. It should not exceed those limits set for the whole blood mode.

15. Perform the electronic voltage checks: The RAM/ROM memory test, ramp-pulse electronic test, and the precision-pulse electronic test.

These should be performed by specially trained technologists. The procedure is outlined in the Coulter Counter Model S Plus reference manual.

16. Prime the instrument by cycling two samples of whole blood through the whole-blood aspirator.

17. Perform quality control procedures as outlined for your laboratory.

SHUT-DOWN PROCEDURE

1. Press the shut-down button on the diluter unit. The instrument cycles cleaning reagent through the diluter unit five times, cleaning the tubing, vacuum isolator chambers, aperture baths, diluent dispensers, and hemoglobin cuvette. This procedure should be done at least once every 24 hours. As soon as this cycle is completed, bleed off the pressures and vacuum by pressing and releasing solenoid No. 17 on the diluter control card until the vacuum and pressures read 0.

2. If the instrument will not be used for one or more work shifts, perform the following:
   A. Turn the bright knob for the oscilloscope screens off (turn the knob fully counterclockwise).
   B. On the ext mem card, set the display switch to off.
   C. Pull the light bar on the diluter unit out (release the bar by pressing the two side buttons) a very short distance until the lights go out.
   D. Lock the pinch valves in the open position (place the locking levers in the up position).
   E. Turn off the X-Y recorder. Remove and cap the pen.

3. If the instrument will not be used for several days, set the battery on/battery off switch (ext mem card) to off, shut off the diluter unit, and the main power circuit breaker on the power supply unit.

CLEANING PROCEDURES AND MAINTENANCE

1. Once per month, remove the five air filters, wash in warm, soapy water, rinse, and dry.

2. After every 1,000 cycles of the instrument (or weekly, whichever occurs first), the blood-sampling valve must be cleaned and the apertures cleaned with Clorox.

3. Once per month and also when the instrument is calibrated, voltage readings for the instrument should be taken and recorded.

These procedures should be performed by specially trained technologists. See the Coulter Counter Model S Plus operator's reference manual for these procedures.

DISCUSSION

1. Refer to the back of the Coulter Counter printout slip for the description of the seven codes and symbols that may appear on the slip when a patient specimen is reported by the instrument. The symbols for a count exceeding the instrument maximum, a vote-out, and an incomplete computation appear in the box corresponding to the problem test. A notation for SA (single aperture) appears in that box (top left, above WBC) and indicates from which aperture the results were printed if the results were not derived from an average of all three apertures. The remaining three symbols (no fit, recount, clear) are noted in the box to the right of the SA box (op codes box).

2. The front door of the analyzer unit must remain closed during normal operation of the instrument. Fans are located in this unit to maintain the necessary cooling of the unit.

3. To obtain a valid platelet count: (a)

the platelet count must be above 20,000, (b) there can be no total platelet vote-out, and (c) a positive curve must be obtained.

4. The test number will only sequence to the next number when a micro-sample or whole-blood sample is introduced into the instrument.

5. If the vacuum-adjust wheel is adjusted manually and the mercury column does not change, there may be a leak in the vacuum system.

6. Reagent and waste-container replacement: Carefully unscrew the pickup tube assembly from the container to be replaced. Pull it straight up and out of the container. With one hand, pull the mouth of the new container upward as far as possible. Hold it in this position and place the pickup assembly straight into the new container and completely screw the assembly into place. Proceed as follows: (a) Waste container replaced: press button No. 19 (dil cont card), press the full waste button, and wait for READY to be displayed. (b) Diluent replaced: Press the start-up button. At the completion of the cycle, press button No. 18 (dil cont card) and hold it depressed until the liquid level in the RBC vacuum isolator chamber is $\frac{1}{4}$ inch from the tips of the white fittings (do not allow the chamber to overflow). Drain the vacuum isolator chambers (drain button). Fill the aperture baths, press the low diluent button, and wait for READY to be displayed. (c) Cleaning reagent replaced: Press the low cleaner button. The shut-down cycle should continue. (d) Lyse reagent replaced: Place the lyse container on the same level as the diluter unit. Drain the aperture baths. On the dil cont card, press and hold in button No. 2 and press button No. 4. Release button No. 2 and then release button No. 4. Keep repeating this procedure until the lyse reagent flows steadily with no air bubbles into the WBC aperture bath. Press solenoid No. 6 to drain the hemoglobin cuvette. Drain the aperture baths and refill with diluent. Press the low lyse button and wait for READY to be displayed.

7. It is advisable to keep a spare cube of diluent adjacent to the instrument. This prevents unnecessary mixing of the diluent and the resultant formation of microscopic air bubbles in the diluent when it is hooked up to the instrument.

8. Aperture baths do not generally have to be removed except in cases where an aperture cannot be unplugged or in the case of a leak around the aperture fitting.

9. Buildup of protein on the orifices of the apertures first causes an increase in the MCV, followed by a decrease in the counts.

10. Whenever a problem is encountered in the diluter unit, it will be due to one or more of four possible problems in the pneumatic lines or fluid lines: (a) a pinched line, (b) a plug, (c) a leak, or (d) a defective component.

11. When filling vials with diluent for microsamples, the microsample dispensing system must be used to obtain accurate dilutions.

12. Microsamples should be run within 1 hour of diluting to obtain an accurate platelet count and within 4 hours for the hemogram.

13. If the aperture baths must be removed, turn off all power to the instrument and unplug the instrument from the wall socket.

14. If two of the same fuses blow within a short time, there may be a problem. Do not replace the fuse until the cause has been located.

15. If a printout on a single aperture is desired, turn the rotary knob on the ap cur/sig gen card to the appropriate

aperture, put a card in the printer, and press the print push button.

16. Erratic red blood cell and white blood cell counts may be caused by a dirty blood-sampling valve.

17. It takes 34 to 50 seconds for each whole-blood sample to cycle through the instrument and for results to be obtained. The variation in time is due to the number of platelet counting cycles that are necessary. Only one sample may be introduced into the instrument at a time.

18. The Model S Plus Coulter Counter has been found to be linear within the following ranges: WBC, 0.5 to 99,900 per μl; hemoglobin, 3.0 to 30.0 g per dl; RBC, 1,000,000 to 7,000,000 per μl; MCV, 50.0 to 200.0 fl; platelet, 30,000 to 700,000 per μl; and RDW, 5.0 to 20.0. The preceding figures are dependent on particle-free diluent. In cases where these values are exceeded, the blood may be diluted 1:2 with diluent and the results (except MCV, MCH, MCHC, and RDW) multiplied by two.

19. In some situations (leukemia), the white blood cells may be more fragile than normal. When the blood is cycled through the instrument, especially through the apertures, these cells may rupture. Consequently, they are not counted and thus yield an invalidly low white blood cell count. In these instances, the white blood cell count should be performed manually.

20. If agglutination of red blood cells is present (patient with a cold agglutinin), the red blood cell count will be invalidly low and the MCV invalidly high. In this situation, the only useful parameters determined by the Coulter Counter Model S Plus are the white blood cell count, hemoglobin, and platelet count.

21. Any time the instrument has not been cycled for any period of time, the sweep flow lines must be checked for the presence of air bubbles.

COULTER COUNTER MODELS S PLUS II, III, IV, AND V

Coulter Electronics, Inc. has modified the basic Coulter Counter Model S Plus and improved the instrument's capabilities. Because the basic operating unit shows only minor changes, only a brief description of the changes will be given here. The major addition, the data terminal, however, will be described in more detail.

The Coulter Counter Model S Plus II uses a reagent system that has been modified slightly from the one used in the Model S Plus. This has resulted in the reporting of lymph number and %, and the RDW is calculated as a true C.V. (coefficient of variation). This model also is capable of determining and reporting the number of lymphocytes per μl of blood and the % of lymphocytes present. A data terminal may also be used with this instrument that essentially provides many quality control capabilities (including $\overline{X}_B$ analysis), the ability to flag abnormal results, and white blood cell, red blood cell, and platelet histograms. A matrix printer plotter replaces the previously used X-Y recorder and is capable of printing all information displayed by the data terminal.

The Coulter Counter Model S Plus III adds an automated sampler handler. This permits up to 32 patient samples to be loaded onto a tray. The instrument will then automatically obtain the sample from the original sealed collection tube. Throughput on this instrument is over 115 samples per hour.

The Coulter Counter Model S Plus IV, in addition to the modifications made in the S Plus II, uses a 100 μl patient sample in place of the 1.0 ml of blood that was previously required. This instrument also uses approximately 25% less reagents.

The Coulter Counter Model S Plus V has

been improved over the Model S Plus IV by its ability to pierce the cap of the test tube, making it unnecessary to remove the top from the test tube to obtain the blood sample.

A brief description of the newer aspects of these various Coulter Counters follows.

Red Blood Cell Histogram and Red Cell Distribution Width

On all Coulter Counter Models S Plus, the red blood cell dilution contains red blood cells, white blood cells, and platelets. Those particles between 2 and 20 fl in size are categorized as platelets. Particles greater than 36 fl are counted as red blood cells. (White blood cells are counted along with the red blood cells, but because of their low numbers in relationship to the red blood cells, they are felt to be insignificant.) As the red blood cells are counted, their size (MCV) is also determined. This information is used to create the red blood cell histogram, where the number of red blood cells are plotted on the vertical axis of the graph and the size of the red blood cell is plotted on the horizontal axis. Normally, the red blood cell histogram will be almost symmetric with a single peak (Fig. 197a). The tail seen to the left of the curve may represent large or clumped platelets, electrical interference, or red blood cell fragments. The larger tail on the right of the curve is termed the *foot* and may represent red

blood cells that may have been stuck together when going through the aperture.

The red cell distribution width (RDW) represents the coefficient of variation of the red blood cell size and is determined by the following formula for the Coulter Counter S Plus Models II, III, IV, and V:

$$\text{RDW (CV\%)} = \frac{\text{S.D. (of RBC sizes)} \times 100}{\text{MCV}}$$

Before the RDW is calculated, the lower portion of the histogram, containing the two tails, is excluded from the calculations. If a relatively large secondary population of red blood cells is present (Fig. 197b), this will be detected by the instrument because the two populations are well separated. In these instances, the RDW will be flagged by the instrument. If, however, the second population of red blood cells present is not that distinctly different from the other red blood cells present (Fig. 197c), the RDW will not be flagged, but the result should be markedly increased. The normal range for the RDW determined in this manner is 11.5 to 14.5%.

White Blood Cell Histogram, Lymph Number, and Lymph Percentage

The Coulter Counter S Plus Models consider all particles larger than 45 fl to be white blood cells. In addition to counting the white blood cells, the instrument determines the size of the cells. This information is then used to plot the histogram

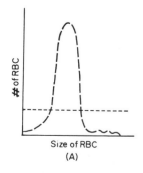

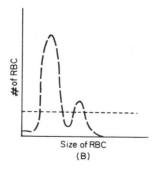

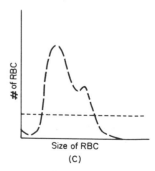

Fig. 197. RBC histograms. **A.** Normal distribution of red blood cells. **B** and **C.** Abnormal distribution of red blood cells.

as previously described for red blood cells. Using the specific Coulter reagent system, the nucleated cells in the size range of 45 to 99 fl have been found to be normal lymphocytes. Those cells between 99 and 450 fl are normally considered to be the non-lymphocytic cells. The percentage of white blood cells that are lymphocytes is calculated by the instrument. The number of lymphocytes is then calculated by the instrument by multiplying the percentage of lymph cells by the white blood cell count. A normal white blood cell histogram (Fig. 198) will show two distinct populations of white blood cells that are separated at approximately 45 fl, 99 fl, and 450 fl. If nucleated red blood cells are present, these are characteristically indicated by the lack of a valley at 45 fl or a peak in the curve at 45 to 50 fl. A significant number of abnormal white blood cell types may be indicated by a curve showing little to no valley at 99 fl. If certain abnormal white blood cell histograms are obtained, the white blood cell count as projected on the data terminal will be backlit.

$\overline{x}_B$ and Quality Control

The $\overline{x}_B$ (pronounced x bar B) is used as a quality control check for hematology instruments. Essentially, it is a weighted moving average of the patient's red blood indices (MCV, MCH, and MCHC) and is calculated by the Coulter Counter data terminal using a relatively complex mathematical formula. Studies have shown that the population of patients in medium to large hospitals show relatively stable val-

ues for the red blood cell indices. Also, in the calculations used here by the instrument, less weight is given to the extremely high or low patient result.

Basically, each successive group of 20 patient results are grouped into a batch. As each patient blood is tested, the mean ($\overline{x}_B$) value from the previous batch (of 20 patient samples) is subtracted from the respective current red blood cell index (MCV, MCH, or MCHC). The square root of the resultant number is then determined. After 20 patient blood specimens have been analyzed, the sum of the square roots for each of the three indices is added up and divided by the number of patient samples (usually 20). This number is then squared and added to or subtracted from the respective previous $\overline{x}_B$ value obtained to derive the $\overline{x}_B$ value for this current batch of patient samples. This new mean value is then used to help determine the $\overline{x}_B$ value for the next batch of 20 blood specimens. Each laboratory should have its own set of target values for each of the indices. Once set, the $\overline{x}_B$ value for each index in each batch should fall within ±3% of the target value. If, however, an instrument or reagent problem exists, this will be indicated by one or more of the red blood cell indices moving consistently in one direction (up or down) or in the $\overline{x}_B$ value falling outside of the allowable laboratory preset range. The recommended target values are ±3% of (1) 89.5 (MCV), (2) 30.5 (MCH), and (3) 34.0 (MCHC).

The hemoglobin bias, RBC % difference, and hematocrit percentage difference are further calculations made by the instrument to be used in detecting where specific instrument problems lie. The *hemoglobin bias* is defined as the difference between what the hemoglobin value should be (assay value) and the hemoglobin value the instrument actually reads (average of last five control values in file No. 1).

Data Terminal

The data terminal receives information from the analyzer unit and sends it to the

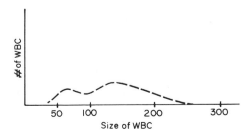

Fig. 198. WBC histogram (normal).

printer and the matrix printer plotter. It determines the lymph percentage, calculates the lymph number, and provides a very complete quality control program. The following is a brief summary of the data terminal available for use with the Coulter Counter Model S Plus IV (Fig. 199).

The program used in the data terminal is made up of six parts, each of which is termed a *menu*. The main menu of the data terminal lists these six menus as:

1. Specimen analysis menu.
2. Data entry menu.
3. Start-up menu.
4. Control data menu.
5. Special tests menu.
6. Prime menu.

Each of these menus may be displayed alone and is further broken down into submenus. The primary functions that may be carried out in each menu are outlined below.

In the *specimen analysis* menu, the patient samples are run; the operator may delete the last sample run from the $\bar{x}_B$ analysis; the $\bar{x}_B$ may be turned off or on; and there is a submenu for $\bar{x}_B$ review. In $\bar{x}_B$ review, the last batch of $\bar{x}_B$ values may be reviewed; the entire last batch of $\bar{x}_B$ values may be deleted; $\bar{x}_B$ values for the last 20 batches are listed; the red and white blood cell values in the current $\bar{x}_B$ batch of blood specimens are listed; $\bar{x}_B$ graphs (MCV, MCH, MCHC, hemoglobin bias, red blood cell percentage difference, and hematocrit percentage difference) for the previous 20 batches may be displayed; and the hemoglobin may be set for the hemoglobin bias. During sample analysis, the patient results are displayed following completion of the instrument cycle: white blood cell, red blood cell, and platelet histograms, white blood cell count, all red blood cell parameters, platelet count, MPV (mean platelet volume), lymph percentage, and lymph number. Information about the $\bar{x}_B$ is also given: $\bar{x}_B$ on or off and whether the pre-

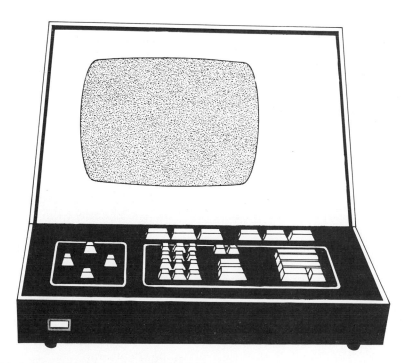

Fig. 199. Data terminal, Coulter Counter Model S Plus IV.

vious batch of patient samples was within or outside of the acceptable range.

The *data entry* menu allows the operator to enter information into the data terminal: operator number; hospital I.D. number; critical value ranges for each parameter so that the abnormal results may be flaggged by the data terminal; acceptable ranges for the $\overline{x}_B$ values, ramp and precision voltages, reagent lot numbers, assay values, and limits for up to nine different quality control types; set the print size for the matrix printer plotter; and set automatic printing of histograms if desired.

The *start-up menu* is used primarily in setting up the instrument each morning and displays: the previously run result, limits and histograms for the background count; the previously run ramp and precision results, limits, and histograms; a start-up log (background, precision and ramp result, and reagent lot numbers); the previously run reproducibility check (result, limits, and histograms) and a method for deleting this information; and the previously run carry-over result (result, limits, and histograms) and a method for deleting these results from the data terminal.

In the *control data* menu, the operator may select the control file; enter the control values as they are run; review the previously run control values, assay, and limits for each of the nine control files; delete the results of the last control sample; review all of the previous control results (up to 40 sets for each control); review control graphs for each parameter of each control; and delete all information from any control file.

The *special tests* menu allows the operator to perform checks on memory, data terminal screen, graphics, ticket printer, recorder, matrix printer plotter, keyboard, and the battery.

The *prime* menu allows the operator to run patient samples through the instrument without their being included in the $\overline{x}_B$ analysis.

As stated previously, all information displayed on the data terminal may be printed on the matrix printer plotter by depressing the plot key on the data terminal.

ORTHO ELT-8/ds HEMATOLOGY ANALYZER

The Ortho ELT-8/ds hematology analyzer is a fully automated eight-parameter (test) cell counter that utilizes a laser beam in counting and sizing cells and smaller particles (platelets). The instrument performs white and red blood cell counts, platelet counts, hemoglobin, and hematocrit, and calculates the red blood cell indices (MCV, MCH, and MCHC).

The Ortho ELT-8/ds is made up of two main components: the *sample handler* and the *data handler*. A third module, the *page printer*, is optional and may be hooked into the data handler to obtain a printed copy of information displayed on the data handler (Fig. 200).

COMPONENTS OF THE SAMPLE HANDLER

The control or patient sample is aspirated, diluted, mixed, and analyzed by the sample handler (Fig. 201).

1. The *power button* turns the instrument on and off.
2. The *printer assembly* provides printed results of the eight parameters, test number, and date.
3. The *sampler* has three components: a *sip tube*, through which the sample is aspirated, a retractable *waste bucket* to collect the reagent during the wash period, and the *wash block*, which provides an external wash of the sip tube.
4. The *optical bench*, where the actual counting and sizing of cells and platelets occurs, consists of the laser, focusing lens, flow channel, blocker bar, objective lens, aperture, and photodetector.
5. The *colorimeter assembly* is where

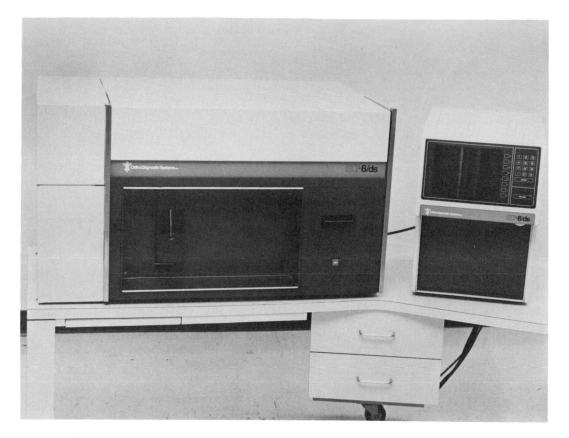

Fig. 200. Ortho ELT-8/ds Hematology Analyzer.

the hemoglobin is read at a wavelength of 540 nm.

6. The *air compressor* supplies 22 to 30 psi of air pressure to the accumulator.

7. The *pressure gauges* monitor the air reservoir pressure. A *regulator* reduces pressure from 22 to 30 psi to 9 psi in the reagent containers.

8. *Reagent bottles:* Two Isolac (saline diluent), one Cyanac (cyanmethemoglobin reagent), and one Lysac (lysing reagent).

9. The *air dump system* reduces the air pressure in the reagent bottles when the instrument is in standby.

10. The *waste bucket control* consists of solenoid switches V14 and V15 that control the air cylinder to place the wash bucket in the in or out position.

11. The *programmer switches,* S1 through S10, regulate the timing of the instrument during sample testing.

12. The *accumulator* pressurizes Isolac to 22 to 30 psi for refilling the pumps on the 3-RPM cam assembly.

13. The *cam assemblies* (2) are blocks that have a rotating shaft at the base. The 1-RPM cam is located behind the 3-RPM cam.

14. The *pumps* (12) move the reagents and blood through the system. Pumps 2 though 5 are located on the 1-RPM cam assembly, are filled with Isolac pressurized to 9 psi, and function in the count portion of sample testing. Pumps 6 through 13 are on the 3-RPM cam assembly. Pump 6 is filled with Cyanac at a pressure of 9 psi. Pump 7 contains Lysac at a pres-

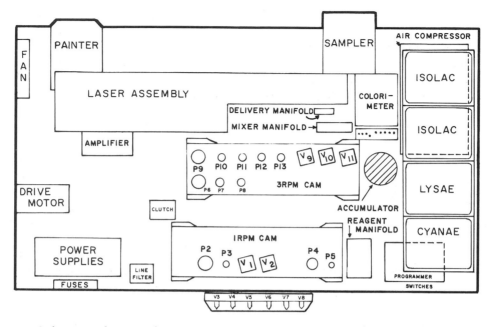

Fig. 201. Ortho ELT-8/ds Hematology Analyzer. View from the top of the sampler handler (the cover has been removed).

sure of 9 psi. Pumps 8 through 13 are filled with Isolac, are pressurized to 22 to 30 psi, and function in sample aspiration and dilution. On all pumps, the side opening is the input port and the top opening is the output port. (Pump 9 has an additional side opening, which is an output port.)

A. Pump 2 supplies the RBC sheath.

B. Pump 3 supplies the drive for the RBC count.

C. Pump 4 supplies the boost for the WBC count.

D. Pump 5 supplies the drive for the WBC count.

E. Pump 6 supplies Cyanac for the hemoglobin dilution and for the hemoglobin blank.

F. Pump 7 supplies Lysac for the WBC dilution.

G. Pump 8 supplies the drive for the 1:19 WBC dilution.

H. Pump 9 supplies the Isolac for the 1:63 and 1:600 dilutions.

I. Pumps 10 and 11 aspirate the blood sample.

J. Pumps 12 and 13 supply the drive for the 1:63 and 1:600 dilutions, respectively.

15. The *slide valves* (5) (V1, V2, V9, V10, and V11) direct the flow of reagents and the blood sample. These valves are comprised of three sections. The two outside sections remain stationary, whereas the middle section will move up and down during the cycle to open or close fluid pathways.

16. The *poppet valves* (6) (V3 through V8) will direct the flow of fluids or air through the system. In these valves, the bottom opening is the input port, and the top opening is the output port.

17. The *manifolds* (3) function as a meeting and mixing place for the blood sample and reagents. The *reagent manifold* supplies 9 psi from the reagent reservoirs to other parts of the system. The *mixer manifold* houses and mixes the sample dilutions. The

delivery manifold delivers the WBC dilution to the flow channel and splits the Isolac sheath into two portions.

18. The *power supply* regulates and supplies the necessary electrical power to the instrument components.

19. The *fuses* (8) prevent electrical overload.

OPERATION OF THE SAMPLE HANDLER DURING CYCLE

1. Prior to use, the tip of the sip tube contains a 5-μl air bubble to separate the blood sample from the diluent already in the lines. When the back plate switch is pressed, pumps 10 and 11 stroke down, causing 100 μl of the blood sample to be drawn up into the sip tube (behind the air bubble). The blood sample travels through valve 11, where it is split into two segments, one for the RBC, hematocrit, platelet count, and hemoglobin dilution, and the other portion for the WBC. The sample then enters the mixer manifold. (This occurs during the first 6 seconds of the 60-second cycle.)

2. Pumps 9 and 12 are activated and dilute the blood sample 1:63 with Isolac for the RBC dilution (7 to 13 seconds).

3. Pump 6 adds Cyanac to the front portion of the RBC dilution, making a 1:126 dilution for the hemoglobin. This solution is then mixed (8 to 13 seconds).

4. Pumps 9 and 13 dilute and drive the second segment of the 1:63 dilution to give a 1:600 dilution. The solution is then mixed (14 to 20 seconds).

5. Pump 2 creates the sheath flow through the flow channel, whereas pump 3 forces the RBC dilution through the flow channel for the determination of the red blood cell count, hematocrit, and platelet count. (Begins at approximately 21 seconds into the cycle.)

6. A hemoglobin blank reading is taken 4 to 5 seconds into the cycle. Approximately 10 seconds after the cycle has begun, the diluted blood sample arrives in the hemoglobin cuvette, where it is stored and is read (by measuring the amount of light passing through the solution) between 30 and 40 seconds into the cycle.

7. During steps 3, 4, and 5 above, the second segment of the blood sample (WBC) is drawn into the mixing manifold and is diluted with Lysac, and a 1:19 dilution is made by the action of pumps 7 and 8. The dilution is mixed and then moved by pump 8 into the WBC storage coil, where it remains for a short period to ensure complete lysis of the red blood cells (8.5 to 33 seconds).

8. The diluted WBC sample is forced out of the storage coil and into the delivery manifold. Valve 4 opens up to allow the Isolac to pass through and into the flow channel to create the sheath. The WBC dilution is forced out of the delivery manifold and through the flow channel (33 to 40 seconds).

9. Counting of cells, platelets, and hematocrit determination in the flow cell. The flow cell contains a very narrow fluid channel. Prior to and during the sample entry into the flow cell, two streams of Isolac are forced through the channel, creating a laminar flow. When empty, the opening through the flow channel has a diameter of 250 μm. When the Isolac is flowing through the channel, it completely covers all inner surfaces of the channel. The stream of Isolac flowing adjacent to the sides of the channel travels at the slowest rate of speed, whereas the stream of Isolac near the center of the chamber flows

at the fastest rate of speed. The diluted blood sample is forced through the center of this flow and is carried along with the fastest moving Isolac. The diameter of the sample stream is about 18 μm and it travels at a speed of about 55 mph. Therefore, the cells travel through the flow channel in single file and are counted and sized using the laser beam (See Figure 202). This laser beam is situated on one side of the flow cell and directs its beam through the flow cell and onto a sensor. When there are no cells passing through the flow cell, the laser beam is completely focused onto a blocker bar (on the collecting lens), which blocks the laser beam from hitting the sensor or photodetector. When cells or platelets pass through the flow chamber, each individual particle passing through the laser beam will cause a scattering of this beam. This scattered light then falls on the collecting lens and passes through to the photodetector, where it is changed to a voltage pulse corresponding in magnitude to the size of the particle. Red blood cells are differentiated from platelets in three ways. (1) A voltage threshold has been preset in the instrument and, when counting the 1:600 RBC dilution, all voltage values lower than the threshold are considered to be plate-

lets and all voltage values higher than the threshold are classified as red blood cells. (2) The instrument also takes into consideration the refractive index of the particle, which is different for red blood cells and platelets. (3) The time of flight through the counting zone is determined by noting the point at which the forward tip of the particle first enters the counting area and the time at which the tail end of the particle leaves the counting zone. The hematocrit is determined by the sum of the integrated voltages for the red blood cells.

A. The 1:600 RBC dilution enters the flow chamber 20 seconds into the counting cycle, and the platelets and red blood cells are counted for the next 10 seconds. The platelet and red blood cell counts are then corrected for coincidence. At 30 seconds into the cycle, the hematocrit is determined.

B. At the conclusion of the counting cycle for the 1:600 dilution, the 1:19 WBC dilution is introduced into the flow chamber and counted as described above. The white blood cell count is not corrected for coincidence.

10. Beginning at 6 seconds into the sample cycle, a complete system wash is begun and each pump is refilled.

A. Valve 5 opens, allowing the outside of the sip tube to be washed with Isolac (6 to 13 seconds).

B. Valve 2 shifts to the up position to refill pump 6 with Cyanac, pump 7 with Lysac, and pumps 8 through 13 with Isolac. The mixer manifold, RBC and WBC whole blood storage lines, and the inner portion of the sip tube are washed with Isolac from pumps 9, 10, and 11 (17 to 20 seconds).

C. Valve 2 again shifts to the up position, and reagent is supplied to

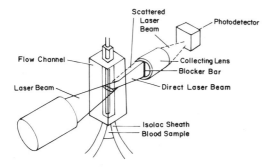

Fig. 202. Optical subsystem of the Ortho ELT-8/ds Hematology Analyzer.

pumps 6 through 13. The mixer manifold, RBC and WBC whole blood storage lines, and the inner portion of the sip tube are washed for a second time with reagent, which passes through pumps 9, 10, and 11. Valve 11 will also be washed during this process (cycle begins at 36 seconds).

D. The 3-RPM cam is reactivated, and pumps 10 and 11 aspirate, drawing in Isolac from valve 2 (40 seconds into the cycle).

E. Isolac is driven through the RBC lines (46 seconds).

F. Cyanac is forced into the mixer manifold and then rinses and fills the hemoglobin cuvette (for the hemoglobin blank reading, which will be taken at the beginning of the next instrument cycle). All samples lines and parts (including the flow channel) are rinsed (47 seconds).

G. The outside of the sample tube is washed with Isolac again, and pumps 10 and 11 draw back very slightly to aspirate the 5 μl of air that will precede the next blood sample aspirated into the instrument (58 to 60 seconds).

11. When all tests have been performed in the sample handler, this information is forwarded to the data handler, where the MCV, MCH, and MCHC are calculated. This information is then forwarded to the printer in the sample handler and is displayed on the data handler CRT.

DATA HANDLER

The data handler has two primary functions: (1) It accepts information from the operator concerning numeric identification and operating instructions, and (2) it processes information from the sample handler, calculates red blood cell indices, and transmits this information to the printer in the sample handler and the page printer module and CRT screen.

The data handler contains a *CRT screen*, which serves as a means of communication between the operator and the instrument and between the sample handler and the data handler. Associated with the CRT, along the right front side of the data handler, are a series of keypad *select switches* that are used to select various functions of the instrument. The select switches each have a LED (light emitting diode), that indicates the functions available. Further to the right is the *keyboard*, which is utilized by the operator to enter numeric information.

Through the software program in the data handler, the operator gains access to the operational functions. The table of contents of the software is termed the *base page*, and, when displayed, it lists the six operational modes (main pages) available to the operator. A keypad select switch is used to select the specific operational mode desired. The CRT will then display this mode, termed a *main page*, listing all possible options available (these functions are termed *subpage functions*).

Following is an outline of the six main pages and their subpage functions.

1. *Date* is the operational mode in which the operator may enter the date in any one of three different ways: month, day, year; day, month, year; or Julian.

2. The *calibration* mode is used to verify the ELT-8/ds calibration and is also used in recalibrating the instrument. In this mode, the samples for verifying the calibration of all eight parameters are run; the background for the platelet count is verified; the calibrating samples are processed; and the samples run in the calibration or in any operating mode may be viewed (results, histograms, and hemoglobin reaction display) and printed out.

3. The *control runs* mode is primarily

used for processing quality control samples. There are eight quality control *libraries* in the data handler, each one capable of storing a different control level, which is determined by the operator. In this mode, the operator selects the control library into which a control sample is to be entered; the assay value for the control may be entered; the previous three control values (which have just been entered) may be deleted; and the samples run in any operating mode may be viewed (results, histograms, and hemoglobin reaction display) and printed out. In addition, the *Q.C. library* subpage mode (within the control runs mode) allows the operator to view the control data in all libraries; to remove or restore the numeric data from the statistics (but not from the CRT display); to print out the results from any library; to view and print out Levey-Jenning charts of the control data; and to enter or erase all quality control information (to reuse the library).

4. The *run sequence* mode is used for the processing of patient samples. In this mode, the operator may enter up to 66 patient I.D. numbers in the order in which the patient samples will be run; or an accession number may be used, where the number will be increased by one digit each time a sample is run through this mode. All samples run in this mode that are within the operating range of the instrument will enter the moving average program. The numeric data from the last 20 samples processed will be stored, and a printout may be obtained on any one of these samples. During sample processing, the results and histograms may be displayed on the CRT if desired. There is a moving average library in which numerical results of Levey-Jenning

information may be viewed, deleted, edited, entered, or printed out.

5. The *test-options* mode enables the user to perform electronic checks of the data handler and is also used by field service.

6. The *standby* mode is utilized to maintain the instrument in a hold position. It keeps the electronics on but depressurizes the sample handler.

OPERATION OF THE ELT-8/ds

1. *Start-up*

   A. Perform a visual inspection of the instrument: (1) Empty the waste container. (2) Check the reagent levels and fill if necessary. Clean the sample station.

   B. Press return on the data handler to access the base page. Enter the date.

   C. Access the calibration mode and perform a fluid subsystem wash: (1) Aspirate an air sample two times. Gently tap pumps 10 and 11 to remove any bubbles that may be present. (2) Run five samples of Ortho flushing solution. (3) Aspirate an air sample three times. It is suggested that the subsystem wash be performed at start-up, midday, and at shutdown.

   D. Access start cal background (in the calibration mode) and determine that the duplicate background counts check within ± 100 of previous background counts and are below 500.

   E. Press return to access the calibration mode (main page) and prime the instrument with two whole blood samples.

   F. Access start cal (calibration mode) 7/8 and run 4 to 10 samples of the calibrator material. Check the precision of the instrument by ensuring that all C.V.s are within range. If they are not, trouble shoot system. Make certain the averaged results for each parameter are within ± 1 S.D. of posted calibration values. If they are not, recalibrate.

G. Repeat step F above in the start cal plt mode if platelets were not included in that step.

H. Access the control runs page and select the appropriate quality control library. Run the quality control samples and ensure that they are within the acceptable ranges.

2. *Processing of patient samples*

A. Access the run sequence mode. Follow your particular laboratory's procedure for the identification of the patient sample.

B. Wipe the outside of the sip tube with a piece of clean gauze. Place the tube of blood under the sip tube and insert the sip tube at least ½ inch into the blood. Press the back plate switch. After the system beep sounds, remove the tube of blood.

C. Place a report form in the printer, located in the right side of the sample handler.

D. Review the results of the CRT when they appear. Remove the ticket from the printer when printing is complete.

E. At the completion of the sample run, place the instrument in standby by accessing the standby mode on the data handler.

F. Just prior to shutting the instrument down each day, access the calibration mode and perform a subsystem wash as previously described. Place the instrument in the standby mode.

3. *Weekly maintenance procedures*

A. Remove all of the covering panels from the instrument and check the valves, pumps, and connectors and tubing for crystalline deposits. Wipe away any deposits with a damp cloth. Ensure that the valves move freely and are aligned. The pumps and the connectors and tubing should be checked for leaks and replaced as needed. Clean the area around the cams and cam shafts.

B. Perform the sip tube back and forward flushes and the flow channel flush as outlined in the instrument's maintenance manual.

C. Clean the sip tube wash station funnel with warm water.

D. Replace the covers and clean the exterior of the instrument.

4. *Monthly maintenance procedures*

A. Remove the instrument covers as necessary.

B. Rinse all reagent containers at least two times with fresh reagent.

C. Clean the wash block slide with gauze and lubricate both the wash block slide and jackshaft with 3-in-1 oil.

D. Clean the cams as outlined in the instrument's maintenance manual.

E. Remove the filter in the data handler, clean in warm water and detergent, dry, and replace. (See the instrument's maintenance manual for the procedure.)

DISCUSSION

1. *Deadtime alarm.* On the ELT-8/ds, deadtime has been defined as the duration of time that each cell is being seen and counted by the instrument while in the flow cell. More specifically, the deadtime is that amount of time from the moment the instrument sees the forward tip of the cell as it enters the counting area until it sees the tail end of the cell as it leaves the counting area. This deadtime calculation serves two purposes: (1) The cumulative deadtime is used to correct the red blood cell and platelet

counts for coincidence. (2) It detects problems (instrument malfunction, patient abnormalities, or operator errors). If the deadtime value for a particular count is significantly larger than normal, an audible beep will be given by the instrument and the CRT will display RBC (PLATELET) DEADTIME IS XX%, UPPER LIMIT IS 12% (30%). Patient abnormalities causing this alarm may be agglutinated red blood cells, rouleaux of the red blood cells, extremely high red blood cell or platelet count, or platelet aggregates.

2. *Red and white blood cell histograms.* The red and white blood cell histograms are real-time graphic illustrations of the number and relative sizes of the cells. The number of cells is plotted on the vertical axis of the graph, and the size of the cell is plotted on the horizontal axis. On the red blood cell histogram, the tail on the right side of the graph probably represents red blood cells stuck together when they were counted. This is used to correct the red blood cell count.

3. *Platelet channel interference and platelet histogram.* The platelet histogram is a graphic illustration of the number and size of the platelets counted by the instrument. As described for the red and white blood cell histograms, the Y, or vertical, axis represents the number of platelets, and the X, or horizontal, axis represents the magnitude of the pulses (size). In the ELT-8/ds, the X axis is divided into 80 channels, which are numbered 1 through 80. The majority of platelets fall into channels 7 through 10 on the histogram. Channels 56 through 59 are monitored for interference. If the ratio between the number of particles counted in channels 56 to 59 to the number of particles detected in chan-

nels 7 to 10 exceeds a preset limit, the instrument will beep, and the CRT will display PLATELET INTERFERENCE IS XX%, UPPER LIMIT IS 10.0%. This alarm indicates that particles significantly larger than platelets have been detected and have been counted as platelets. Generally, these particles are extremely small red blood cells, red blood cell fragments, or giant platelets. Under these circumstances, a manual platelet count should be performed.

4. *Hemoglobin reaction display.* The hemoglobin reaction may be displayed on the CRT. This graphic illustration plots the amount of light passing through the hemoglobin cuvette (on the Y axis) just prior to, during, and immediately following the sample reading by the instrument. The X axis represents the time elapsed.

5. *Moving averages.* The moving average is essentially a weighted moving average of a group (batch) of patients' red blood cell indices (MCV, MCH, and MCHC). This mathematical formula was published in 1974 by Brian Bull. It is based on the fact that groups of patients will show relatively stable values for the red blood cell indices. In the ELT-8/ds, the operator may choose the batch size from 1 to 99. The recommended number of patients in a batch, however, is 20. The batch average for each red blood cell index is then compared to a previously set target value and, under normal circumstances, should not vary from this target value by more than 3%. A larger variation is generally due to an instrument malfunction, but may also be seen if the group of patients in the batch are abnormal to like degrees (e.g., many microcytic patients). In cases where there is instrument malfunction, it should be noted which red blood cell indices

fall out of the range, as an aid in troubleshooting the problem. In the ELT-8/ds, all eight parameters are included in the moving averages program. For the RBC, WBC, hemoglobin, hematocrit, and platelet count, a ±20% difference from the target value is recommended. A difference of ±3% from the target value is obtainable on the MCV, MCH, and MCHC.

Bibliography

1. Ackerman, G.A.: Substituted naphthol AS phosphate derivatives for the localization of leukocyte alkaline phosphatase activity, Lab. Invest., *11*, 563, 1962.
2. American Optical Corporation: *Reference Manual Series 10 Microstar Advanced Laboratory Microscopes*, Scientific Instrument Division, Buffalo, New York, 1974.
3. Ames Division, Miles Laboratories, Inc.: *Operating Manual Hema-Tek Slide Stainer*, Elkhart, Indiana, 1974.
4. Ames Division, Miles Laboratories, Inc.: *Operating Manual Hema-Tek II Automated Slide Stainer*, Elkhart, Indiana, 1978.
5. Bainton D., and Farquhar, M.: Differences in enzyme content of azurophil and specific granules of polymorphonuclear leukocytes, J. Cell Biol., *39*, 299, 1968.
6. Baltimore Biological Laboratory: *Instruction and Technical Data Manual, Fibrometer Precision Coagulation Timer*, Baltimore Biological Laboratory, Baltimore, Maryland, 1962.
7. Becton, Dickinson and Company: *Laboratory Procedures Using the Unopette Brand System*, Becton, Dickinson and Company, Rutherford, New Jersey, 1977.
8. Becton, Dickinson and Company: *Platelet Retention Column*, Becton, Dickinson and Company, Rutherford, New Jersey, 1978.
9. Betke, K., Marti, H.R., and Schlicht, I.: Estimation of small percentages of foetal haemoglobin, Nature, *184*, 1877, 1959.
10. Beutler, E.: A series of new screening procedures for pyruvate kinase deficiency, glucose-6-phosphate dehydrogenase deficiency, and glutathione reductase deficiency, Blood, *28*, 553, 1966.
11. Biggs, R., and Douglas, A.S.: The thromboplastin generation test, J. Clin. Pathol., *6*, 23, 1953.
12. Biggs, R., and MacFarlane, R.G.: *Human Blood Coagulation and Its Disorders*, Blackwell Scientific Publications, Oxford, 1962.
13. Bio/Data Corporation: *Operating Instructions and Methods Manual, Platelet Aggregation Profiler Model PAP-4*, Hatboro, Pennsylvania, 1982.
14. Blackburn, E.K.: The clinical management of hemophilia and allied disorders. *Recent Advances in Blood Coagulation*, Poller, L., ed., J. & A. Churchill Ltd., London, 1969.
15. Boggs, D.R.: The kinetics of neutrophilic leukocytes in health and in disease. Semin. Hematol., *4*, 359, 1967.
16. Boggs, D.R., and Winkelstein, A.: *White Cell Manual*, 3rd ed., F.A. Davis, Philadelphia, 1975.
17. Bowie, E.J.W., et al.: *Mayo Clinic Laboratory Manual of Hemostasis*, W.B. Saunders Company, Philadelphia, 1971.
18. Brecker, G., and Cronkite, E.P.: Morphology and enumeration of human blood platelets. J. Appl. Physiol., *3*, 365, 1950.
19. Breen, F.A., Jr., and Tullis, J.L.: Ethanol gelation: A rapid screening test for intravascular coagulation, Ann. Intern. Med., *69*, 1197, 1968.
20. Breen, F.A., Jr., and Tullis, J.L.: Ethanol gelation test improved, Ann. Intern. Med., *71*, 433, 1969.
21. Briere, R.O., Golias, T., and Batsakis, J.G.: Rapid qualitative and quantitative hemoglobin fractionation. Cellulose acetate electrophoresis, Am. J. Clin. Pathol., *44*, 695, 1965.
22. Buckell, M.: The effect of citrate on euglobulin methods of estimating fibrinolytic activity, J. Clin. Pathol., *11*, 403, 1958.
23. Bull, B.S., and Brailsford, D.: The Zeta sedimentation ratio, Blood, October 1972.
24. Bull, B.S., Schneiderman, M.A., and Brecker, G.: Platelet counts with the Coulter Counter, Am. J. Clin. Pathol., *44*, 678, 1965.
25. Canalco: Hemoglobin analysis, Disc Electrophoresis Newsletter, *3*, 2, 1963.
26. Carrell, R.W., and Kay, R.: A simple method for the detection of unstable haemoglobins, Br. J. Haematol., *23*, 615, 1972.
27. Cartwright, G.E.: *Diagnostic Laboratory Hematology*, Grune & Stratton, Inc., New York, 1963.
28. Cline, M.J.: *Leukocyte Function*, Churchill Livingstone, New York, 1981.
29. Cocchi, P., Mori, S., and Becattini, A.: N.B.T. tests in premature infants. Lancet, *2*, 1426, 1969.
30. Cohen, Z.A.: The metabolism and physiology of the mononuclear phagocytes. In *The Inflammatory Process*, Zweifach, B.W., Grant, L., and McCluskey, R.T., eds., Academic Press, New York, 1965.
31. Colfs, B., and Verheyden, J.: A rapid method for the determination of serum haptoglobin, Clin. Chim. Acta, *12*, 470, 1965.
32. Copeland, B.E.: Statistical tools in clinical pathology, In *Todd-Sanford Clinical Diagnosis by Laboratory Methods*, 15th ed., Davidsohn, I., and Henry, J.B., eds., W.B. Saunders Company, Philadelphia, 1974 (15th ed. only).
33. Coulter Electronics, Inc.: *Coulter Counter*

Model S-Plus Operator's Manual, Coulter Electronics, Inc., Hialeah, Florida, 1977.

34. Coulter Electronics, Inc.: *Instruction and Service Manual for the Model S Coulter Counter*, Coulter Electronics, Inc., Hialeah, Florida, 1970.

35. Coulter Electronics, Inc.: *Coulter Counter Model S-Plus IV with Data Terminal Product Reference Manual*, Hialeah, Florida, 1983.

36. Coulter Electronics, Inc.: *Instructional and Service Manual for the Coulter Counter Model Fn*, Hialeah, Florida, 1970.

37. Coulter Electronics, Inc.: *Instruction Manual for Coulter Thrombo-fuge*, Coulter Electronics, Inc., Hialeah, Florida, 1974.

38. Coulter Electronics, Inc.: *Instruction Manual for Coulter Zetafuge*, Coulter Electronics, Inc., Hialeah, Florida, 1973.

39. Dacie, J.V., and Lewis, S.M.: *Practical Haematology*, 5th ed., Churchill Livingstone, New York, 1975.

40. Dade Diagnostics, Inc., American Hospital Supply Corporation: *Data-Fi Fibrinogen Determination Reagents*, Dade Division, American Hospital Supply Corporation, Miami, Florida, 1982.

41. Daland, G.A., and Castle, W.B.: A simple and rapid method for demonstrating sickling of the red blood cells: The use of reducing agents, J. Lab. Clin. Med., *33*, 1082, 1948.

42. Davidsohn, I., and Nelson, D.A.: The blood, In *Todd-Sanford Clinical Diagnosis by Laboratory Methods*, 15th ed., Davidsohn, I., and Henry, J.B., eds., W.B. Saunders Company, Philadelphia, 1974 (15th ed. only).

43. Diggs, L.W.: Laboratory tests in the diagnosis of sickle cell disease: part III, *Hematology*, produced by National Committee for Careers in the Medical Laboratory of the American Society of Clinical Pathologists and the College of American Pathologists, 1973.

44. Diggs, L.W., Sturm, D., and Bell, A.: *The Morphology of Human Blood Cells*, Abbott Laboratories, North Chicago, Illinois, 1975.

45. Dougherty, W.M.: *Introduction to Hematology*, 2nd ed., C.V. Mosby Company, St. Louis, 1976.

46. Dutcher, T.: Normal cells in the peripheral blood. *Hematology*, produced by National Committee for Careers in the Medical Laboratory of the American Society of Clinical Pathologists and the College of American Pathologists, 1973.

47. Duke, W.W.: The pathogenesis of purpura haemorrhagica with especial reference to the part played by the blood platelets. Arch. Intern. Med., *10*, 445, 1912.

48. Eli Lilly and Company: ART coagulation test advocated in pre-surgery cases, Clinical Laboratory Forum, 5, 4, 1970.

49. Evelyn, K.A., and Malloy, H.T.: Microdetermination of oxyhemoglobin, methemoglobin, and sulfhemoglobin in a single sample of blood, J. Biol. Chem., *126*, 655, 1938.

50. Fahey, J.L., Barth, W.F., and Solomon, A.: Serum hyperviscosity syndrome, JAMA, *192*, 464, 1965.

51. Fareed, J., Messmore, H.L., and Bermes, E.W.: New perspectives in coagulation testing, Clin. Chem., *26*, no. 10, 1380, 1980.

52. Fertman, M.H., and Fertman, M.B.: Toxic anemias and Heinz bodies, Medicine, *34*, 131, 1955.

53. Finch, C.A.: *Red Cell Manual*, University of Washington, Seattle, Washington, 1969.

54. Freeman, J.A.: The microscope. In *Todd-Sanford Clinical Diagnosis by Laboratory Methods*, 15th ed., Davidsohn, I., and Henry, J.B., eds., W.B. Saunders Company, Philadelphia, 1974 (15th ed. only).

55. Gambino, S.R., et al.: The Westergren sedimentation rate, using K_3EDTA, Techn. Bull. Regist. Med. Techn., *35*, 1, 1965.

56. Garnham, P.C.C.: *Malaria Parasites and Other Haemosporidia*, Blackwell Scientific Publications, Oxford, 1966.

57. General Diagnostics: *Coag-A-Mate 2001 Operator's Manual*, Morris Plains, New Jersey, 1979.

58. General Diagnostics, *Coag-A-Mate Dual Channel Operator's Manual*, General Diagnostics, Morris Plains, New Jersey, 1974.

59. General Diagnostics: *Coag-A-Mate • X2 Operations Manual*, Warner-Chilcott, Morris Plains, New Jersey, 1981.

60. General Diagnostics: *Simplate, Bleeding Time Device*, General Diagnostics, Morris Plains, New Jersey, 1977.

61. Geometric Data Corporation: *The Hemaprep Automatic Blood Smearing Instrument Instruction Manual*, Geometric Data Corporation, Wayne, Pennsylvania, 1974.

62. Gerarde, H.W., and Anderson, E.: *Hematology Laboratory Procedures Using the Unopette Disposable Diluting Pipette*, Becton, Dickinson and Company, Rutherford, New Jersey, 1968.

63. Graham, R.C., Lundholm, U., and Karnovsky, M.J.: Cytochemical demonstration of peroxidase activity with 3-amino-9-ethylcarbazole, J. Histochem. Cytochem., *13*, 150, 1965.

64. Griffin, D., and Greeban, L.: *Practical Charting Technics in Quality Assurance Programs*, Dade Division, American Hospital Supply Corporation, Miami, Florida, 1971.

65. Haight, V.: *White Blood Cell Morphology*, New London, Connecticut, 1978.

66. Ham, T.H.: Studies on destruction of red blood cells. Chronic hemolytic anemia with paroxysmal nocturnal hemoglobinuria, Arch. Intern. Med., *64*, 1271, 1939.

67. Hardisty, R.M., and Ingram, C.I.C.: *Bleeding Disorders; Investigation and Management*, Blackwell Scientific Publications, Oxford, 1965.

68. Hardisty, R.M., and Macpherson, J.C.: A one-stage factor VIII assay and its use on venous and capillary plasma, Thromb. Diath. Haemorrh., *7*, 215, 1962.

69. Harker, L.A.: *Hemostasis Manual*, 4th ed., F.A. Davis, Philadelphia, 1974.

70. Harris, J.W.: *The Red Cell, Production, Metab-*

olism, Destruction: Normal and Abnormal, Harvard University Press, Cambridge, Massachusetts, 1965.

71. Hartmann, R.C., and Jenkins, D.E.: The "sugar-water" test for paroxysmal nocturnal hemoglobinuria, N. Engl. J. Med., *275,* 155, 1966.

72. Hartsock, R.: Fundamental teachings in hematology, *Hematology,* produced by National Committee for Careers in the Medical Laboratory of the American Society of Clinical Pathologists and the College of American Pathologists, 1973.

73. Hattersley, P.G., and Hayse, D.: The effect of increased contact activation time on the activated partial thromboplastin time, Am. J. Clin. Path., *66,* 479, 1976.

74. Hayhoe, F.G.J., and Flemans, R.J.: *An Atlas of Haematological Cytology,* Wiley-Interscience, John Wiley & Sons, Inc., New York, 1970.

75. Helena Laboratories: *Sickle Cell Hemoglobinopathies,* Helena Laboratories, Beaumont, Texas, 1979.

76. Helena Laboratories: *Titan III Citrate Hemoglobin Procedure,* Helena Laboratories, Beaumont, Texas, 1972.

77. Hellman, R.S.: *Hematology Laboratory Manual,* University of Washington Medical School, Seattle, Washington, 1969.

78. Hicks, N.D., and Pitney, W.R.: A rapid screening test for disorders of thromboplastin generation, Br. J. Haematol., *3,* 227, 1957.

79. Hillman, R.S., and Finch, C.A.: *Red Cell Manual,* 2nd ed., F.A. Davis, Philadelphia, 1974.

80. Hutchison, H.E.: *An Introduction to the Haemoglobinopathies and the Methods Used for their Recognition,* Edward Arnold, Ltd., London, 1967.

81. Ivy, A.C., Nelson, D., and Beecher, G.: The standardization of certain factors in the cutaneous "venostasis" bleeding time technique, J. Lab. Clin. Med., *26,* 1812, 1940.

82. Jacob, H.S., and Jandl, J.H.: A simple visual screening test for glucose-6-phosphate dehydrogenase deficiency employing ascorbate and cyanide, N. Engl. J. Med., *274,* 1162, 1966.

83. Johnson, S.A., and Greenwalt, T.J.: More sensitive tests and tests of platelet function, *Coagulation and Transfusion in Clinical Medicine,* Little, Brown, and Company, Boston, 1965.

84. Kaplow, L.S.: Substitute for benzidine in myeloperoxidase stains, Am. J. Clin. Pathol., *63,* 451, 1975.

85. Katayama, I., and Yang, J.P.S.: Reassessment of a cytochemical test for differential diagnosis of leukemic reticuloendotheliosis, Am. J. Clin. Pathol., *68,* 268, 1977.

86. Koepke, J.A., Rodgers, J.L., and Ollivier, M.J.: Pre-instrumental variables in coagulation testing, Am. J. Clin. Pathol., *64,* 591, 1975.

87. Koepke, J.A., ed.: *Differential Leukocyte Counting CAP Conference/Aspen 1977,* College of American Pathologists, 1977.

88. Lampasso, J.A.: Error in hematocrit values produced by excessive ethylenediaminetetrace-tate, Techn. Bull. Regist. Med. Techn., *35,* 109, 1965.

89. Lampasso, J.A.: Changes in hematologic values induced by storage of ethylenediaminetetrace-tate human blood for varying periods of time, Techn. Bull. Regist. Med. Techn., *38,* 37, 1968.

90. Langdell, R.D.: Coagulation and hemostasis, In *Todd-Sanford Clinical Diagnosis by Laboratory Methods,* 15th ed., Davidsohn I., and Henry, J.B., eds., W.B. Saunders Company, Philadelphia, 1974 (15th ed. only).

91. Lathem, W., and Worley, W.E.: The distribution of extracorpuscular hemoglobin in circulating plasma, J. Clin. Invest., *38,* 474, 1959.

92. Lee, R.I., and White, P.D.: A clinical study of the coagulation time of blood, Am. J. Med. Sci., *145,* 495, 1913.

93. Lenahan, J.G., and Smith, K.: *Hemostasis,* General Diagnositics, Morris Plains, New Jersey, 1979.

94. Lewis, A.E.: *Principles of Hematology,* Appleton-Century-Crofts, New York, 1970.

95. Lillie, R.D., and Fullmer, H.M.: *Histopathologic Technic and Practical Histochemistry,* McGraw-Hill, New York, 1976.

96. Linman, J.W.: *Principles of Hematology,* The Macmillan Company, New York, 1966.

97. Loh, W.P.: A new solubility test for a rapid detection of hemoglobin S, J. Indiana State Med. Assoc., *61,* 1651, 1968.

98. Losowsky, M.S., Hall, R., and Goldie, W.: Congenital deficiency of fibrin-stabilizing factor, Lancet, *2,* 156, 1965.

99. Lynch, M., et al.: Cell organization and functions, In *Medical Laboratory Technology and Clinical Pathology,* W.B. Saunders Company, Philadelphia, 1969.

100. Magath, T.B., and Winkle, V.: Technic for demonstrating "L.E." (lupus erythematosus) cells in blood, Am. J. Clin. Pathol., *22,* 586, 1952.

101. Marchand, A.: Circulating anticoagulants: Chasing the diagnosis, Diag. Med., *13,* June, 1983.

102. Marder, V.J., and Conley, C.L.: Electrophoresis of hemoglobin on agar gels: Frequency of hemoglobin D in a Negro population, Bull. Johns Hopkins Hospital, *105,* 77, 1959.

103. Maronde, G.R., et al.: A quality control system utilizing duplicate patient specimens, Am. J. Med. Technol., *40–4,* 165, 1974.

104. McDonald, G.A., Dodds, T.C., and Cruickschank, B.: *Atlas of Haematology,* 4th ed., Churchill Livingstone, New York, 1978.

105. McManus, J.F.A.: Histological demonstration of mucin after periodic acid, Nature, *158,* 202, 1946.

106. Medical Laboratory Automation, Inc.: *Operator Instruction Manual for the Electra 600 Automatic Clotting Time Recorder,* Medical Laboratory Automation, Inc., Mount Vernon, N.Y., 20, 1973.

107. Medical Laboratory Automation, Inc.: *Operator's Manual, MLA Electra 700,* Mount Vernon, New York, 1981.

108. Miale, J.B.: *Laboratory Medicine, Hematology,*

396 BIBLIOGRAPHY

6th ed., The C.V. Mosby Company, St. Louis, 1982.

109. Mielke, C.H., et al.: The standardized normal Ivy bleeding time and its prolongation by aspirin, Blood, *34*, 204, 1969.

110. Milstone, H.: A factor in normal human blood which participates in streptococcal fibrinolysis, J. Immunol., *42*, 109, 1941.

111. Murano, G., and Bick, R.L., eds.: *Basic Concepts of Hemostasis and Thrombosis: Clinical and Laboratory Evaluation of Thrombohemorrhagic Phenomena*, CRC Press, Inc., Boca Raton, Florida, 1980.

112. Nalbandian, R.M., et al.: Dithionite tube test—a rapid, inexpensive technique for the detection of hemoglobin S and non-S sickling hemoglobin, Clin. Chem., *17*, 1028, 1971.

113. Nalbandian, R.M., et al.: Automated dithionite test for rapid, inexpensive detection of hemoglobin S and non-sickling hemoglobinopathies, Clin. Chem., *17*, 1033, 1971.

114. National Committee for Clinical Laboratory Standards: *Standardized Method for the Human Erythrocyte Sedimentation Rate (E.S.R.) Test*, National Committee for Clinical Laboratory Standards, Villanova, Pennsylvania, 1977.

115. Nelson, D.A., and Davey, F.R.: Hematology and coagulation, In *Todd-Sanford Clinical Diagnosis and Management by Laboratory Methods*, 15th ed., Davidsohn, I., and Henry, J.B., eds., W.B. Saunders Company, Philadelphia, 1974 (15th ed. only).

116. Nevalainen, D.E., Herbst, G.H., and Sage, B.H.: *Hematology: Laboratory Evaluation of Blood Cells,* Abbott Laboratories, Dallas, 1977.

117. Ortho Diagnostic Systems: *ELT-8/ds Laser Hematology Analyzer Training Manual*, Westwood, Massachusetts, 1982.

118. Ortho Diagnostic Systems, Inc.: *Ortho ELT-8/ds Hematology Analyzer Operator Reference Manual*, Westwood, Massachusetts, 1982.

119. Owen, C.A., et al.: *The Diagnosis of Bleeding Disorders*, 2nd ed., Little, Brown, and Company, Boston, 1975.

120. Patrick, C.W., Haight, V., and Evans, V.S.: *The Erythrocytes Volume 1*, ASMT Education & Research Fund, Inc., Bellaire, Texas, 1974.

121. Palmer, I.: Basic spectrophotometry for the medical technologist, Am. J. Med. Technol., *25*, 341, 1959.

122. Park, B.H., Fikring, S.M., and Smithwick, E.M.: Infection and nitroblue-tetrazolium reduction by neutrophils, Lancet, *2*, 532, 1968.

123. Parpart, A.K., et al.: The osmotic resistance (fragility) of human red cells, J. Clin. Invest., *26*, 636, 1947.

124. Perkins, H.A., et al.: Neutralization of heparin in-vivo with protamine: a simple method of estimating the required dose, J. Lab. Clin. Med., *48*, 223, 1956.

125. Platt, W.R.: *Color Atlas and Textbook of Hematology,* J.B. Lippincott, Philadelphia, 1969.

126. Porter, I.A., and Turk, C.C.: Microscopy and the morphology of micro-organisms, *A Short Textbook of Microbiology*, W.B. Saunders Company, Philadelphia, 1965.

127. Proctor, R.R., and Rapaport, S.I.: The partial thromboplastin time with kaolin, Am. J. Clin. Pathol., *36*, 212, 1961.

128. Quick, A.J.: *Bleeding Problems in Clinical Medicine*, W.B. Saunders Company, Philadelphia, 1970.

129. Randolph, T.G.: Differentiation and enumeration of eosinophils in the counting chamber with a glycol stain, J. Lab. Clin. Med., *34*, 1696, 1949.

130. Rapaport, S.I., and Ames, S.B.: Clotting factor assays on plasma from patients receiving intramuscular or subcutaneous heparin, Am. J. Med. Sci., *234*, 678, 1957.

131. Richards, O.W.: Phase microscopy, Wallerstein Laboratories, *15*, 155, 1952.

132. Richards, O.W.: *The Effective Use and Proper Care of the Microscope*, American Optical Corporation, Scientific Instrument Division, Buffalo, New York, 1958.

133. Salzman, E.W.: Measurement of platelet adhesiveness. A simple in-vitro technique demonstrating an abnormality in von Willebrand's disease, J. Lab. Clin. Med., *62*, 724, 1963.

134. Schmidt, R.M., and Brosius, E.M.: *Basic Laboratory Methods of Hemoglobinopathy Detection*, HEW Pub. No. (CDC) 74-3266, U.S. Dept. of Health, Education, and Welfare, Public Health Service, Center for Disease Control, Atlanta, 1974.

135. Schneider, C.L.: Rapid estimation of plasma fibrinogen concentration and its use as a guide to therapy of intravascular defibrination, Am. J. Obstet. Gynecol., *64*, 141, 1962.

136. Seaman, A.J.: The recognition of intravascular clotting, Arch. Intern. Med., *125*, 1016, 1970.

137. Shaffer, J.G., and McQuay, R.M.: Medical protozoology, In *Todd-Sanford Clinical Diagnosis by Laboratory Methods*, 15th ed., Davidsohn, I., and Henry, J.B., eds., W.B. Saunders Company, Philadelphia, 1974 (15th ed. only).

138. Sheehan, H.L., and Storey, G.W.: An improved method of staining leukocyte granules with sudan black B, J. Path. Bact., *59*, 336, 1947.

139. Shepard, M.K., Weatherall, D.J., and Conley, C.L.: Semiquantitative estimation of the distribution of fetal hemoglobin in red cell populations, Bull. J. Hopkins Hosp., *110*, 293, 1962.

140. Sherwood Medical, Lancer Division: *Operator's Manual, Lancer Coagulyzer II*, St. Louis, Missouri, 1981.

141. Sherwood Medical, Lancer Division: *Operator's Manual, Lancer Coagulyzer Jr. III*, St. Louis, Missouri, 1981.

142. Sigma Chemical Company: *Glucose-6-phosphate Dehydrogenase Deficiency in Blood,* Sigma Technical Bulletin no. 202. Sigma Chemical Company, Saint Louis, Missouri, 1979.

143. Sigma Chemical Company: *Glutathione Reductase Deficiency in Blood*, Sigma Tentative Technical Bulletin no. 190, Sigma Chemical Company, Saint Louis, Missouri, 1981.

144. Sigma Chemical Company: *Pyruvate Kinase*

Deficiency in Red Blood Cells, Sigma Technical Bulletin no. 205, Sigma Chemical Company, Saint Louis, Missouri, 1981.

145. Silverman, E.M., and Ryden, S.E.: The nitroblue tetrazolium (NBT) test: A simple reliable method and a review of its significance, Am. J. Med. Tech., 40–4, 151, 1974.

146. Singer, K., Chernoff, A.I., and Singer, L.: Studies on abnormal hemoglobins. 1. Their demonstration in sickle cell anemia and other hematologic disorders by means of alkali denaturation, Blood, 6, 413, 1951.

147. Spinco Division, Beckman Instruments Incorporated: *Preliminary Instruction Manual for Model R-101 Microzone Electrophoresis Cell*, Spinco Division, Beckman Instruments Incorporated, Palo Alto, California, 1963.

148. Sundberg, R.D.: Lymphocytogenesis in human lymph nodes, J. Lab. Clin. Med., 32, 777, 1947.

149. Sundberg, R.D., and Broman, H.: The application of the Prussian blue stain to previously stained films of blood and bone marrow, Blood, 10, 160, 1955.

150. Thompson, R.B., and Holloway, C.H.: Observations on the sickling phenomenon, Am. J. Med. Technol., 29, 379, 1963.

151. Thomson, J.M., ed.: *Blood Coagulation and Hemostasis, a Practical Guide*, Churchill Livingstone, New York, 1980.

152. Tocantins, L.M., and Kazal, L.A.: *Blood Coagulation Hemorrhage and Thrombosis; Methods of Study*, Grune & Stratton, Inc., New York, 1964.

153. Triplett, D.A.: *Laboratory Evaluation of Coagulation*, American Society of Clinical Pathologists Press, Chicago, Illinois, 1982.

154. Triplett, D.A., Harms, C.S., Newhouse, P., and Clark, C.: *Platelet Function*, Educational Products Division, Am. Soc. Clin. Path., Chicago, Illinois, 1978.

155. Turner, R.C., and Holman, R.R.: Automatic lancet for capillary blood sampling, Lancet, 2, 712, 1978.

156. Walton, J.R.: Uniform grading of hematologic abnormalities, Am. J. Med. Technol., 39, 517, 1973.

157. Ware, A.G., and Seegers, W.H.: Two-stage procedure for the quantitative determination of prothrombin concentration, Am. J. Clin. Path., 19, 471, 1949.

158. Warner, E.D., Brinkhous, K.M., and Smith, H.P.: The titration of prothrombin in certain plasmas, Arch. Path., 18, 587, 1934.

159. Weatherall, D.J., and Clegg, J.B.: *The Thalassemia Syndromes*, 2nd ed., Blackwell Scientific Publications, Oxford, 1972.

160. Wellcome Reagents Limited: *Thrombo-Wellcotest. Rapid Latex Test for Detection of Fibrinogen Degradation Products*, Wellcome Research Laboratories, Beckenham, Kent, England, 1981.

161. Willard, H.H., Merritt, L.L., and Dean, J.A.: Visual colorimetry. Photoelectric colorimetry. In *Instrumental Methods of Analysis*, D. van Nostrand Company, Inc., Princeton, New Jersey, 1958.

162. Williams, W.J., et al.: *Hematology*, McGraw-Hill Book Company, New York, 1977.

163. Winkelstein, A., and Craddock, G.C.: Lymphoid physiology, Am. J. Med. Technol., 36, 361, 1970.

164. Wintrobe, M.M., et al.: *Clinical Hematology*, 8th ed., Lea & Febiger, Philadelphia, 1981.

165. Wolf, P.L., et al.: *Practical Clinical Hematology*, John Wiley & Sons, New York, 1973.

166. Yam, L.T., Li, C.Y., and Crosby, W.H.: Cytochemical identification of monocytes and granulocytes, Am. J. Clin. Path., 55, 283, 1971.

167. Zuck, T.F., Bergin, J.J., Raymond, J.M., and Dwyre, W.R.: Implications of depressed antithrombin-III activity asssociated with oral contraceptives, Surg. Gynecol. Obstet., 133, 609, 1971.

Index